Kiss My Asparagus

An essential guide to nutrition's role in health and disease

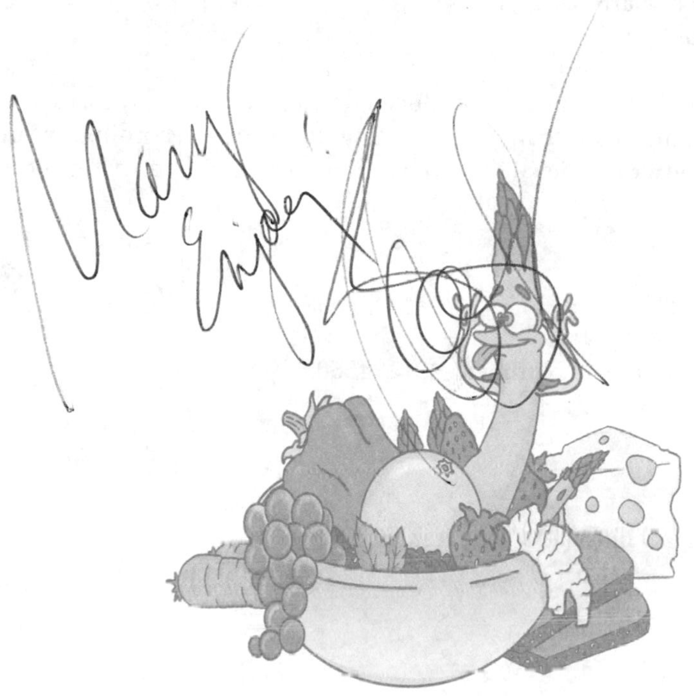

BARB BANCROFT

WELLWORTH PUBLISHING

ISBN 13: 978-0-9723541-8-9

Library of Congress Control Number: 2012945607

Cover art and original illustrations by Ashley J. Long

Wellworth Publishing
Oregon USA
www.wellworthpublishing.com

Printed in the United States of America

Dedication

J. K. and Connie.
You left the table way too soon.
My thoughts and love will be with you both, always.

Thank you. Thank you. Thank you.

Mom and Dad. Thank you for continuing to support all of my hare-brained ideas. I still have one more big idea…I need to run it by you. You're the best.

Ashley Long. It's been ten years and you're still making magic with your cartoons. Many, many thanks for your professionalism and your patience.

Emily Hermann, RN, BSN. Thank you for your meticulous research and being my fact-finder and fact-checker.

Rae Stith. You are a genius with words. Your input is always trusted and invaluable—as is your friendship.

Jeannine Dal Pra. The next Masterchef and a phenom in the kitchen.

Joey, Jack and Spencer. All my sweet furry "kids"—Joey and Spencer for taking me for needed walks between chapter revisions, revisions, and more revisions. And Jack, for functioning as my little hairball paper weight.

Jean Sheldon. Thank you. Nothing would ever get done without your gentle push.

Before you begin!

You will notice that I have used the generic term "average" American throughout the text. Just exactly what is an "average" American? The term is used rather loosely as you can imagine—an "average" American living in Duluth may be quite different from the "average" American living in Daytona Beach. Suffice it to say, the "average" American is red, yellow, black and white; male gender, female gender, transgender, heterosexual, bisexual, homosexual, and asexual; blonde-haired and blue-eyed, black-hair and brown-eyed, gray-haired with cataracts, and blue-haired and cross-eyed. We're different in many ways but we're all "average" Americans. Hey, and what about our fabulous Canadian friends? They're just as interestingly "average" as we are in the United States. But the one thing we ALL have in common is our love of food—we ALL love to eat. When appropriate, I have added gender-based, ethnic-based, and geographically-based findings.

There are also many numbers scattered throughout the book. These numbers describe amounts (tablespoons, teaspoons, ounces, kilograms, milliliters and liters) and doses (milligrams and micrograms). I have checked, rechecked, and checked again for the accuracy of these numbers. However, as much as I hate to admit it, there may be an error somewhere. So please always recheck numbers. Read the label before tossing back a vitamin or mineral.

And, last but not least—I would enjoy hearing comments from any and all of you about the book. Please send comments to me via my website, www.barbbancroft.com, or either of my personal email addresses, bbancr9271@aol.com or barbbanc@gmail.com.

Buon Appetito! Bon Appétit! Buen Apetito!
APetyt Buena! Guten Appetit!

Eat well, eat healthy, eat slowly!

I know a man who gave up smoking, drinking, sex and rich food. He was healthy right up until the time he killed himself.
—Johnny Carson

Addicted to love, addicted to alcohol, addicted to *junk-food?* To your brain, sugar, salt, and fat are akin to cocaine, nicotine, and heroin. Whoa, did I say cocaine, nicotine, and heroin? Yes. There is now compelling evidence that the above trio of junk-food indulgences (sugar, salt, and fat) can alter your brain chemistry in the same way as the above trio of highly addictive drugs.

Let's first start with the rat studies. Researchers offered rats sugar syrup, similar to the concentration of sugar in a typical non-diet soda beverage consumed by humans, alongside regular rat feed and water. After only 30 days on the sugar syrup, the rats developed behavior and brain changes that were chemically identical to morphine-addicted rats. They binged on the sugar syrup and showed agitated behavior when deprived of the solution—typical signs of withdrawal.

Some of the biggest brain changes were in the area of the nucleus accumbens. This is the area of the brain, in both rats and humans, associated with reward. When something is rewarding, the nucleus accumbens releases dopamine—the neurotransmitter of pleasure. In other words, the experience was so fabulous, let's do it over and over and over again! Dopamine is vital for learning, memory, decision-making and sculpting the reward circuitry. The rats' brains released dopamine each time they binged on the sugar solution. Repeated use "dulls" the brain's reward system, resulting in heavier use to get the same feeling. In other words, this can lead to compulsive eating.

The rat studies in the early 2000s paved the way for human studies. Researchers found that addiction changes in the brain of obese individuals mimicked those found in rats. One of the studies showed a dopamine deficiency in the brains of obese individuals that was virtually identical to that seen in drug addicts. Other studies showed that even when individuals are shown their favorite foods, an area of the brain involved in decision-making called the orbital frontal experiences a surge of dopamine. The same area is activated when cocaine addicts are shown a bag of white powder. (Trivedi B. Junkie food. *New Scientist.* September 2010;38–41)

Albedo. This is the white stuff that sticks to the orange segments. In other words, it's the underside of the orange peel. Is it worth eating? Absolutely. It contains carbohydrates and vitamin C, but it's especially rich in pectin, a soluble fiber that helps to lower cholesterol. Albedo also contains numerous molecules that are currently being studied for their nutritional benefits—including nobiletin, tangeretin, and sinestetin—obviously anything that ends with "etin" must be good for "eatin." What do these "etins" do for the orange? They actually comprise the immune system of the orange and help protect it from fungi, pests, and predators. They also help protect the orange from human consumption because this particular layer isn't that tasty, and is generally described as being bitter. But let's get back to the other functions of nobiletin, tangeretin, and sinestetin. These molecules may have anti-inflammatory effects, cholesterol- lowering effects, cancer-prevention effects, and anti-fungal effects. One of the major problems is that you might have to eat quite a large dose of albedo to benefit from all its healthful properties. (Dr. Renee Goodrich, Associate Professor of Food Science and Human Nutrition, University of Florida, 2009; Dr. Sheldon S. Hendler, co-editor of The Physician's Desk Reference for Nutritional Supplements, 2009)

Albumin. Serum albumin is the most abundant plasma protein. It is produced in the liver and forms a large proportion of all plasma proteins. Human serum albumin normally constitutes about 60% of the total plasma proteins. Its main function is to regulate the colloidal osmotic pressure of blood, which is a fancy way of saying it "holds water in the vascular space." Its second major function is to "bind" various components of blood, including electrolytes such as calcium, sodium, and potassium. Its third major function is to bind drugs. Once drugs are absorbed they become either "protein-bound," which actually means "albumin-bound" or the drug is "free." The portion of the drug that is "free" is the functioning portion of the drug, whereas the "bound" form of the drug is unable to function. (Think of "bound" as having your arms and legs tied—try to get up and walk and you will realize that you are not "free" to do so.) Some drugs are highly protein bound, meaning that almost all of the drug is bound to albumin, and other drugs are "loosely" protein bound, meaning that the drug is hanging on for dear life and any other drug with stronger binding capacities can knock the drug off its binding sites. Once the drug is "knocked off" or displaced from albumin, the drug becomes free. This can result in drug toxicity. Another cause of drug toxicity is low albumin levels—not enough albumin to bind all of the drugs someone is taking. Low albumin is clinically referred to as hypoalbuminemia and it may be caused by liver disease, kidney disease, significant burns, protein-losing enteropathy (entero=small intestine, patho=disease), malabsorption (in the small intestine), *malnutrition*, and malignancy (cancer). High serum albumin (hyperalbuminemia) is almost always caused by dehydration.

ALCOHOL

Alcohol. Can alcohol really contribute to health benefits? It appears that the answer is yes. The good news is that moderate alcohol intake can fit into a healthy lifestyle and can even offer benefits for the estimated 100 million Americans who choose to imbibe responsibly. One of the first research publications to extol the healthy attributes of alcohol was published in 1979. Did you hear the uproar? It's been over thirty years since that momentous publication and studies continue to demonstrate the many health benefits of alcoholic beverages—in moderation, of course.

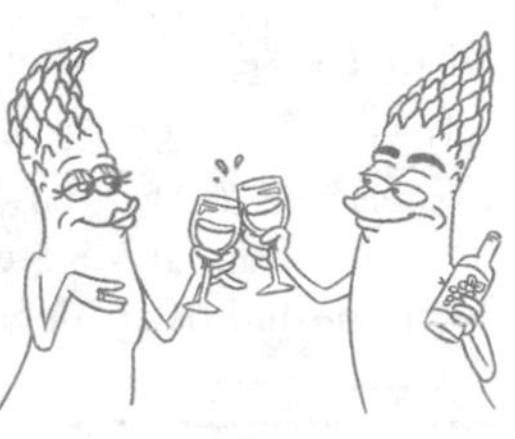

But first, what constitutes a drink? Apparently the average American has not been made aware of a "healthy serving" of alcohol. In fact, 54% couldn't identify a standard serving of alcohol for distilled spirits, wine and beer. Here are the sobering facts:

One standard "healthy" alcohol serving is equal to:

- One 12-ounce beer, 150 calories
- 5 ounces of wine, any color, 100 calories
- 1.5 ounces of 80-proof distilled spirits, 100 calories

Remember, moderation is the key. Disease and death rates in the U.S. each year are highest in those who indulge in excessive drinking. There are 79,000 deaths annually due to excessive alcohol intake, according to the 2010 Dietary Guidelines for Americans. So, zip it after two cocktails and always have a designated driver.

Alcohol and Alzheimer's disease. A 2009 report from the Alzheimer's Association suggests that a regular, moderate intake of alcohol, especially wine, is associated with a reduced risk of dementia in middle-aged adults with no established dementia at baseline. What does "moderate intake" mean to those of us who like to partake of the grape? In this particular report, a moderate intake of one to two drinks per day was associated with a 37% reduction in dementia in patients with normal cognition at the start of the study. Excellent news for us oenophiles.

How about the good old American way of thinking? *Well, if one to two glasses of wine is protective, won't a bottle mean better protection?* Noooooooo, not exactly...heavy drinking (more than 14 drinks per week) doubles the risk of developing dementia.

Why is it that along with the good news there's always the bad news? For older adults with mild cognitive impairment (MCI) at the beginning of the study, moderate alcohol consumption was associated with a more rapid rate of decline. So, if you're already having significant memory impairment problems, it would behoove you to nix the booze.

You might be saying to yourself, well, I don't drink at all, so I must be protecting my brain from the ravages of alcohol. Whoa, not so fast. The 2009 report also showed that participants who consumed 1 to 6 drinks per week had 54% lower odds of developing dementia than did abstainers. The best results were those who had 1 to 2 drinks per day. So, a little dab will do ya' when it comes to booze and protecting the brain. Pop that cork! (Alzheimer's Association: ICAD (2009). Sink KM, et al. Moderate alcohol intake is associated with lower dementia risk. GEMS Study; Mukamal KJ, et al. (2003) Prospective study of alcohol consumption and risk of dementia in older adults. *JAMA* 289:1405–1413)

They tell you that you will lose your mind as you grow older. What they don't tell you is that you won't miss it. —Malcolm Crowley (1898–1989)

Alcohol and cancer. Excessive alcohol intake is associated with an increased risk of a wide variety of cancers—from the oral cavity to the prostate with a few stops along the way. Alcohol is on the list as a "convincing cause" of cancers of the mouth, pharynx (throat), larynx (voice box), esophagus, and liver.

The combination of tobacco and alcohol is a deadly duo for the above cancers. This may be because alcohol acts as a solvent, promoting the breakdown products of cigarette smoke to enter the cells lining the digestive tract. Alcohol may also slow down the cell's ability to repair DNA damage caused by chemicals in tobacco.

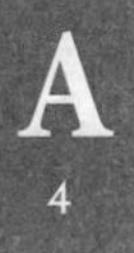

Alcohol is on the list of "probable causes" for cancers of the colon, rectum and breast. Why breast? It's certainly not a part of the gastrointestinal tract. (American Cancer Society, 2010)

Moderate alcohol intake is considered a double-edged sword for women. The good news is that moderate drinking, one to two drinks per day, appears to protect against Alzheimer's disease and stroke; to reduce the risk of heart disease; and does not contribute to an enlarged heart (cardiomyopathy) or cirrhosis of the liver. The bad news is that one to two drinks per day ***may*** increase the risk of breast cancer due to the metabolism of alcohol into estrogen-like substances by the liver. This may provide more "fuel" for estrogen-related cancers in the body—many researchers believe that excess estrogen may be a contributor to the development of breast cancer. Estrogen is a growth hormone, therefore providing more of the hormone may trigger an excessive, uncontrolled growth.

A February 1998 study in the *Journal of the American Medical Association* found that among women who averaged one or fewer drinks per day, the breast cancer risk was 9% higher than it was among nondrinkers. This means that one more woman per 10,000 develops breast cancer per year due to alcohol intake. To put it another way—the risk without alcohol consumption is 11 of every 10,000 women; the risk with one or fewer drinks per day is 12 of every 10,000 women. Among women reporting two to five drinks per day, breast cancer rates rose by 41%. A study of more than 30,000 Italian women, published in the March 4, 1998 *Journal of the National Cancer Institute,* also found a connection between increasing amounts of alcohol and breast cancer. Researchers calculated that slightly more than one drink a day combined with little physical activity accounted for 20% of breast cancers in postmenopausal women, and more than 40% among premenopausal women.

Ok, so those are 25-year-old studies...anything new? Yes, studies continue to link breast cancer with alcohol consumption; the greater the amount of alcohol consumed, the greater the risk. The risk is considered a "modest" risk and the risk is associated with a type of breast cancer that has the best prognosis—the estrogen receptor (ER) and progesterone receptor (PR) positive breast cancers. (Zhang SM, et al. Alcohol consumption and breast cancer risk in the Women's Health Study. *American J of Epidemiology* 2009;170:308–317; Deandrea S, et al. Alcohol and breast cancer risk defined by estrogen and progesterone receptor status: A case-controlled study. Cancer Epidemiology, Biomarkers and Prevention. August 2008;2025)

Is there any good news? A study of 90,000 women demonstrated that for women who drink one to two drinks a day and also take more than 300 µg (.3 mg) of folate (folic acid) per day, breast cancer risk reverts to that of a nondrinker. Folate is essential for DNA synthesis, and unfortunately, alcohol blocks the absorption of *folate. So, the solution of taking more than 300 µg overrides the absorption problem,* enabling women to maintain its cancer-protective properties. Check your multivitamin and make sure it contains at least 300 µg of folate—most multivitamins contain 400 µg of folate. However, before you get all excited about this finding, many other studies have pointed out a relationship between epithelial cancers, such as breast cancer and a *high* intake of folate...so, at the moment, be prudent with your consumption of alcohol *and* folate. Don't assume that popping a multivitamin with every Maker's Mark will protect your breasts. (*Journal of the American Medical Association,* May 5, 1999)

A

5

Alcohol and type 2 diabetes. Alcohol consumption in moderation has been shown to improve insulin sensitivity, which not only helps to control blood glucose but may also help to stave off type 2 diabetes. Research in the *Journal of the American Medical Association* published in 2002 found that after eight weeks, the group that drank 30 grams of alcohol daily (about two drinks) had lower fasting insulin levels and improved insulin sensitivity compared to those who didn't drink at all.

Alcohol and drug interactions. Interactions between alcohol and numerous drugs have been reported. The two mechanisms proposed for this interaction include an alteration of albumin binding sites and the inhibition or induction of CYP 2C9. What's CYP 2C9? CYP is the acronym for cytochrome P, the name for the group of enzymes located in the liver and small intestine that is responsible for the metabolism of drugs. The 2C9 is one of those enzymes.

An increase in blood alcohol levels competes for albumin binding sites, making highly protein-bound drugs more active as they are displaced from their binding sites. Once displaced, the drug becomes "free" or more active, which in turn can result in drug toxicity. A couple of drugs to be aware of with this reaction are digoxin and warfarin (Coumadin). (American Heart Association, 2010;Alcohol, Wine, and Cardiovascular Disease. http://www.heart.org/HEARTORG/GettingHealthy/NutritionCenter/Alcohol-Wine-and-Cardiovascular-Disease)

Alcohol and gastric bypass surgery. Gastric bypass surgery leaves the patient with a stomach the size of a shot glass. As a result, alcohol is absorbed into the bloodstream much faster than usual, resulting in blood alcohol levels that spike faster after ingestion. Blood alcohol levels also take longer to decline in gastric bypass patients, resulting in an increased risk of alcohol abuse. Studies have shown that a 5-ounce glass of red wine increases the blood alcohol level to close to 0.09%, slightly above the legal limit of 0.08%. (Seppa N. Bypass's Big Boon. *Science News* (September 10, 2011).

Alcohol and hangovers. The liver and stomach metabolize alcohol into acetyl aldehyde via an enzyme known as alcohol dehydrogenase. Acetyl aldehyde is metabolized into acetyl coenzyme A and either eliminated from the body or used in the synthesis of cholesterol and fatty acids. The average American can metabolize the alcohol in 13 ounces (400 ml) of wine (3.2 drinks) in approximately five to six hours. If more alcohol is consumed than that amount, the body will have an excess amount of wine with an insufficient amount of alcohol dehydrogenase to metabolize the excess. The excess alcohol accumulates in the blood and not only interferes with the metabolic functions of the liver it also interferes with the ability of the kidney to reabsorb water.

The "over-served" individual will urinate excessively and lose copious amounts of electrolytes and minerals, including magnesium, sodium, calcium, and zinc. Lactic acid levels increase and contribute to the feeling of lassitude and malaise. Blood vessels in the dura covering the brain dilate and throb, and the stomach lining is irritated, resulting in gastric upset and abdominal pain. The end result is the familiar "hangover." The hangover symptoms will finally resolve once the body has produced enough additional alcohol dehydrogenase to metabolize the alcohol "overload" in the bloodstream.

I feel sorry for people who don't drink, because when they get up in the morning, they're not going to feel any better all day. —Phil Harris

---

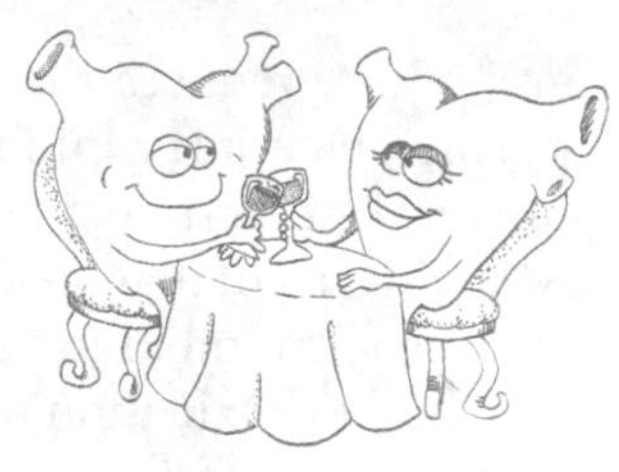

Alcohol and heart disease. A 2010 report in the American Heart Association continues to associate moderate alcohol consumption with a decreased risk in cardiovascular disease. This is good news for those who enjoy a cocktail in the evening. Moderate alcohol consumption increases the "good" HDL (high density lipoprotein) fraction of total cholesterol. HDLs provide anti-inflammatory effects, lipid-clearing effects, and anti-oxidant effects—all of which have been shown to reduce the risk of heart attacks, strokes, and peripheral arterial disease.

Previous studies have linked alcohol consumption with an increase in tissue plasminogen activator (tPA), the enzyme associated with dissolving fibrin clots in the blood vessels. This study found that the highest tPA levels were in study participants who consumed two or more alcoholic drinks per day.

In addition, components of red wine, including the flavonoids and resveratrol, have been shown to reduce heart disease risk. Resveratrol has anticoagulant and anti-platelet properties, both of which reduce the risk of clotting.

How much alcohol is considered to be cardioprotective? We're back to the "usual" healthy amount discussed in the first section on alcohol with a twist on gender differences. Moderate alcohol intake is defined as one 12-ounce beer or one 5-ounce glass of wine or 1.5 ounces of 80-proof spirits such as bourbon, vodka, gin, or scotch for women. Men can consume twice that amount for cardioprotection—in other words, two 12-ounce beers, two 5-ounce glasses of wine, or two 1.5 ounces of 80-proof spirits. Does that mean that everyone should immediately throw this book down and kick back a shot or two of Jack Daniels? No, not exactly.

The health benefits of an alcoholic drink a day are substantially smaller than those offered by 30 minutes of exercise a day and eating a proper diet. Jeez, nothing like buzz kill. My suggestion? Thirty minutes of exercise followed by an ice-cold brewski.

Of course, there are a few caveats when it comes to the decision to imbibe. If you don't drink you certainly don't have to start drinking to protect your heart. There are many ways to protect the cardiovascular system that don't involve alcohol. Two major reasons to abstain from alcohol include pregnancy and established liver disease, such as chronic hepatitis. Any amount of alcohol can damage a developing fetal brain and any amount of alcohol can contribute to the progression of chronic hepatitis. Just say NO with either of these two conditions. (American Heart Association 2010. Alcohol, Wine, and Cardiovascular Disease. http://www.heart.org/HEARTORG/GettingHealthy/NutritionCenter/Alcohol-Wine-and-Cardiovascular-Disease)

Alcohol benefits without the alcohol. What's up with that statement? How can that happen? According to studies by Corder and Dohadwala, 10–12 ounces of purple grape juice per day can also protect the heart. Purple grape juice reduces the stickiness of platelets within 14 days. In addition, purple grape juice inhibits oxidation of the bad LDL-cholesterol and improves the function of endothelial cells that line the blood vessels. Now, just what does all of that mean? Reducing platelet stickiness reduces the ability of clots to form in blood vessels, an obvious benefit for reducing heart attacks and strokes. Oxidation of LDL-cholesterol prevents this "bad" fat/lipid from packing the arteries that supply the heart and the brain. And, if endothelial cells that line the blood vessels have improved function, cholesterol cannot enter the cells to form the fat "plaques." Grape juice has also been shown to improve arterial vasodilation which in turn lowers blood pressure. Interestingly, the findings only apply to red grapes, not white or green grapes. Why? It has to do with a chemical in red grapes called resveratrol, a potent antioxidant found in the skin of red grapes. See chapter R for more on resveratrol.

Previous studies touting the benefits of grape juice were all supported by Welch's Grape Juice Company. Studies supported by any company that makes the product may tend to be a bit biased; however, the current studies did not receive their funding from Welch's. (Corder R. Red wine, chocolate, and vascular health: developing the evidence base. *British Medical Journal.* 2008;94:821-823; Dohadwala MM, Vita JA. Grapes and cardiovascular disease. *J of Nutrition* 2009;149:1788; Park YK et al. Concord grape juice supplementation reduces blood pressure in Korean hypertensive men: double-blind, placebo-controlled intervention trial. *Biofactors.* 2004;22:145–147. Castilla P, et al. Concentrated red grape juice exerts antioxidant, hypolipidemic, and antiinflammatory effects in both hemodialysis patients and healthy subjects. *Am J Clin Nutr* 2006;84:252–256)

Alcohol and herbal extracts. Many consumers have no idea that alcohol is a common ingredient in many herbal extracts. In fact, some herbal preparations have as much as 55% alcohol. Most herbal preparations sold in health food stores have the alcohol content listed on the label. Read it! This is especially important if you are considering using the herbal product for a child, a diabetic, a pregnant woman, a patient with liver disease, or a recovering alcoholic. Some of the ginseng products sold in convenience, health food and video stores can contain up to 34% alcohol. Of 55 ginseng-containing vials tested by the government, only seven were alcohol free. (*Environmental Nutrition,* March 1998)

Alcohol and liver disease. How much alcohol does it take to kill a liver? Clinically evident alcoholic liver disease is unlikely until the individual has imbibed excessively for at least six to ten years. A conservative threshold amount for this level of disease in men is 70–80 grams per day (about 6 ounces of 86-proof liquor, a six-pack of beer, or a 750 ml bottle of wine). A conservative threshold amount for women for this level of disease is 35–40 grams daily.

Alcohol and longevity. In a literature review published in 2008 in the *Journal of the American Dietetic Association,* moderate drinking was found to consistently reduce mortality rates and disease risk among middle aged

(45–65 years) and older (>65 years) adults. Moderation is, once again, the mantra, as you'll see in the next section.

Alcohol and murder. Despite national differences, alcohol use clearly contributes to homicide, especially among those who heavily binge drink. Overall, 57% of U.S. homicides are attributed to alcohol. (Landberg J. and Norström T. Alcohol and homicide in Russia and the United States: A comparative analysis. *J Stud Alcohol Drugs* 2011 Sept;721–723)

Alcohol and nosebleeds. Since alcohol is known to have numerous effects on the clotting system, it could be assumed that individuals who imbibe with gusto might have an increase in bleeding problems. A study in the September 10, 1994 *British Medical Journal* confirms this association. Investigators compared 140 patients arriving at the ER with epistaxis (the medical term for a nosebleed) to 113 age- and sex-matched controls arriving at the ER with other conditions of the ear, nose, and throat. All patients were admitted to the hospital. Alcohol consumption was quantified by questionnaires within a day after admission. Both the nosebleed group and the control group had approximately 35% nondrinkers; however, the nosebleed group had 45% stating that they were regular drinkers vs. the control group with only 30% regular drinkers. Patients in the nosebleed group also had a higher mean alcohol intake of 33 drinks per week vs. seven per week for the control group. A mean of 33 drinks per week? I'm getting a nosebleed thinking about drinking an average of 5 alcoholic beverages a day…no surprise with the nosebleeds in this group.

ASPARAGUS TIP

Before you attribute *all* of your nosebleeds to platelet dysfunction or alcohol consumption, remember that the *number one* cause of nosebleeds in the average American is *nose-picking,* or "digital manipulation of the nasal septum." Some people are chronic obsessive nose-pickers. The medical term for this somewhat annoying and ghastly habit is "rhinotellexomania."

Spontaneous superficial mucous membrane bleeds such as nosebleeds are usually the result of platelet abnormalities. Alcohol has been shown not only to interfere with the ability of platelets to function, but to also suppress the bone marrow's ability to produce platelets. Most likely the platelet count is low as well. Patients with significant nosebleeds and/or low platelet counts should be asked about alcohol consumption—and not just, "Do you drink alcohol?" The question should be, "Do you drink alcohol and how much do you drink on a daily basis? Tell the whole truth and nothing but the truth!"

Alcohol and pancreatitis. People who drink as little as 1.35 ounces of the hard 80-proof spirits (vodka, bourbon, gin, and scotch) have a 10% high-

The Yuck Factor

I'm sure many of you have wondered, at some point in time, whether or not snot has any nutritive value or physiologic value. Dr. Friedrich Bischinger, a leading Austrian pediatrician, extols the virtues of nose-picking. He states: "With the finger you can get to places you just can't reach with a handkerchief, keeping your nose far cleaner." He goes on to say, "And eating the dry remains of what you pull out is a great way of strengthening the body's immune system." Ingesting the bacteria from your nose helps inoculate the body against illness, which may be why this instinctual behavior evolved. Dr. Bischinger also recommends that parents encourage children to pick their nose; somewhat of a new approach to the habit, wouldn't you agree? (*The Week*, April 9, 2004)

er risk for an acute attack of pancreatitis. Drinking 6.7 ounces on any one occasion increases the risk to 52%. Acute pancreatitis is considered a life-threatening emergency. Interestingly, beer and wine don't increase the risk for acute pancreatitis. (Omid Sadr-Azodi, MD, PhD, Department of Gastroenterology, Karolinska University Hospital, Stockholm, Sweden)

Alcohol: prenatal exposure and adolescent alcoholism. A 14-year follow-up of single-born children examined the role of prenatal alcohol exposure and the subsequent development of alcohol problems in adolescence. In a multivariate analysis, prenatal alcohol exposure was more predictive of adolescent alcohol use than a family history of alcohol problems. The implications of this study are numerous. At the very least it implicates maternal alcohol use as an important risk factor in the development of alcohol use in the offspring. In addition, prenatal exposure should be examined when studying the potential heredity of alcoholism. Finally, this study also adds to the growing literature on the delayed effects of both stress and teratogens (an agent that can disturb the development of an embryo or fetus), such as prenatal alcohol exposure, on behavior that may not be apparent until adolescence or adult life. (Baer JS, et al. Prenatal alcohol exposure and family history of alcoholism in the etiology of adolescent alcohol problems. *J Stud Alcohol* 1998 Sept;59:533–43)

A more recent study followed children with prenatal maternal alcohol exposure and the onset of subsequent alcohol disorders. Follow-ups occurred at 6 months, 5 years, 14 years, and 21 years. Mothers who had 3 or more drinks per day during pregnancy, especially during the early stages of pregnancy, were 2.47 and 2.04 times more likely to have children with early and late onset of alcohol disorders, with the effect stronger for early onset alcohol disorders. (Alati R, et al. In utero alcohol exposure and prediction of alcohol disorders in early adulthood. *Arch Gen Psych* 2006;63:1009–16)

Alcohol and rheumatoid arthritis. Researchers from the U.K. questioned 873 people with rheumatoid arthritis and 1004 people without rheumatoid arthritis. They found that non-drinkers were four times more likely to have rheumatoid arthritis than people who drank at least 10 days per month. This study also showed that alcohol consumption was also linked with fewer and milder rheumatoid arthritis symptoms. (Källberg H. Alcohol consumption is associated with a decreased risk of rheumatoid arthritis: Results from two Scandinavian case-control studies. *Ann Rheum Dis* 01 Feb 2009;68(2):222-7)

Alcohol and stroke. Since many of the same risk factors associated with ischemic heart disease (decreased blood flow and lack of oxygen to the heart muscle) are the same as for ischemic stroke (decreased blood flow and lack of oxygen to the brain), it stands to reason that a little toddy might actually protect against cholesterol buildup in the major vessels supplying the brain. A little booze goes a long way, as evidenced by the 1999 study published by researchers at New York Presbyterian Hospital-Columbia University. They found that moderate alcohol consumption does indeed reduce the risk of ischemic stroke due to fatty plaque accumulation in the main arteries supplying the brain. Moderate consumption raises the good HDL-cholesterol which helps prevent fat plaque formation in the major arteries supplying the brain. Don't overdo it! The same study showed that drinking copious amounts of alcohol (more than seven drinks per day) did not protect against stroke. In fact, heavy drinkers, those who consumed more than seven drinks per day, had an increased risk of different type of stroke known as a hemorrhagic stroke (a bleed inside the brain).

The current research continues to support moderate alcohol consumption (1 to 2 drinks per day) with a reduction in ischemic strokes. More than 2 drinks per day have been shown to increase the risk of stroke, so moderation continues to be the operative word when hearts and brains need protection. (National Stroke Association, 2010)

A
11

Alcohol and *Helicobacter pyloric* **infection of the stomach.** Alcohol may damage the stomach lining and facilitate the adherence of *Helicobacter pylori (H. pylori)* to the stomach lining. A recent study confirmed that *H. pylori* is more likely to be present when alcohol, especially wine and spirits, were consumed. The greater the consumption, the greater the association with *H. pylori* infection. (Zhang L, et al. Relationship between alcohol consumption and active *Helicobacter pylori* infection. Alcohol and Alcoholism: International Journal of the Medical Council on Alcoholism 2010;45(1):89–94)

Alcoholism and women. The former 3:1 male-to-female ratio for developing alcoholism is narrowing as more women, especially young women, are experiencing more serious problems with alcohol. A survey conducted by the Gallup Organization (2009) reports there are 4.5 million women in the U.S. with a drinking problem, and 2.5 million who consume at least 60 drinks per month. The alcoholic beverage most frequently consumed by women is wine (50%), and the average age at which women start drinking

Terms used for alcohol use, abuse, and abstinence...

Dipsomania (dip-suh-MAY-nee-uh)—an insatiable, periodic craving for alcohol. Etymology: from the Greek dipsa (thirst) + mania (excessive enthusiasm or craze (wordsmith.org)

Teetotalism refers to either the practice of or the promotion of complete abstinence from any form of alcohol. A person who practices (and possibly advocates) teetotalism is called a **teetotaler** or **teetotaller.** The teetotalism movement was first started in Preston, England in the early 19th century. Where did the name come from? One of the stories gives credit to a member of the Preston Temperance Society, Dicky Turner. He had a tendency to stutter, and in a speech he said that nothing would be accepted as far as drinking except a "tee-tee total abstinence." If you are a teetotaler you can also be "on the wagon," as in "on the water wagon," or you can be "straight" and/ or "sober."

The phrase, **"Three sheets to the wind,"** which today means a completely inebriated individual, is derived from sailing lingo. However, it has nothing to do with the actual sails, but everything to do with the chains that were used to regulate the angle of the sails, referred to as sheets. When the sheets were loose, the boat would become unstable and tipsy, resembling an individual who has been over served.

is 13. Liquor is the second choice for women (24%) and beer comes in last (21%).

Alcoholism is a greater problem physiologically for women than it is for men. Women are twice as likely to die of alcoholism-related illnesses including cirrhosis of the liver and cardiomyopathy (an enlarged heart) as are male drinkers of the same age. In fact, the incidence of cirrhosis and cardiomyopathy occurs a full 10 years earlier in women compared to men.

Women become intoxicated more easily than men. Women have 30% less gastric alcohol dehydrogenase (GAD), the enzyme located in the stomach lining begins the metabolism of alcohol. Since less of this enzyme is present in women, alcohol is absorbed directly through the stomach lining without being metabolized into a more *inactive* form. Therefore, alcohol is absorbed as a more *active* metabolite and is directly toxic to the female heart, liver and brain. And, since alcohol "hits" her brain sooner and in a more concentrated form, she gets a bit tipsier a bit quicker—hence the "cheaper drunk" moniker.

Alcoholism as a by-product of our ancestral nutritional physiology. What's that all about? Sounds like a fancy, convoluted way of making excuses for our overindulgent nature when it comes to imbibing. Genes for alcohol addiction may have persisted in the human lineage for the same reason as those for fat accumulation. Modest amounts of alcohol are known to reduce the risk for heart disease and, in turn, improve survival. Humans predisposed to a little snort had the survival advantage, and would more likely pass that survival advantage on to their ancestors. This particular genetic trait, useful hundreds of thousands of years ago, is no longer advantageous. Humans no longer have to forage through the underbrush for food and fermenting fruit (sugar/alcohol) to survive. All we have to do today is walk to the corner tavern for that "winning" combination of a hamburger, fries, and cold beer. (*New England Journal of Medicine,* May 5, 1999)

"Alcohol on the breath" is a misnomer used by just about everyone, including medical personnel. Pure alcohol (ethanol) has absolutely no odor and therefore it is not possible to smell it on someone's breath. What one actually smells is juniper berry in gin, fusel oil in whiskey, fermented grape in wine, hops in beer, or the acetaldehyde metabolite of alcohol (the morning after breath—whew!)

Alcoholism…Are you ready to clean up your act? Head straight to Minnesota, the "Land of 10,000 Treatment Centers," the "Halfway State," or "Minnesober." Located within the state boundaries are 236 outpatient treatment programs, 56 inpatient programs, 46 halfway houses, 35 detoxification centers, and 29 extended care facilities—give or take a few. One chemical dependency service estimates that half of the 500 patients who enter that facility each year from out-of-state decide to stay in Minnesober permanently.

Alcohol and fruit? Adding alcohol to purees of blended fruit increases the level of healthy antioxidants. Now that's a bonus. So all of you out there who love the froofroo drinks with the strawberries and pineapple chunks, rejoice! You have just raised your antioxidant levels to a new high, along with your glass and your mood! (U.S. Department of Agriculture, 2007)

Alcohol and proof. The PROOF is in the numbers. A proof is the number that expresses the alcoholic strength of liquor. To figure out the proof, take the liquor's percentage of alcohol by volume, and simply multiply that number by two. Here are some notable numbers:

1 Proof — the maximum proof allowable for "non-alcoholic" beer
2.8 Proof — Maximum strength Robitussin
53.8 Proof — Listerine antiseptic
10 Proof — Most American beer
48 Proof — World's strongest beer (Sam Adams' Utopias MMII)
80 Proof — Most distilled spirits (Scotch, Gin, Bourbon)
196 Proof — Strongest commercially available drink on record, distilled from potatoes in the early 20th century Estonia. For the record, it's impossible to make a 200 Proof alcohol. At that level, it begins to pull moisture from the air, diluting itself back down to less than 98 percent alcohol.

Allergies to food—the numbers. The presence of food allergy has been increasing over the past two decades. For example, the prevalence of peanut allergy doubled over a 5-year time span in the late 1990s through the early 2000s.

An estimated 2.2 million school-aged kids have food allergies. Although the public perception of prevalence is higher (around 25–33%), oral challenge testing puts the figures between 6% and 8% for infants and young children and 2.0–3.5% for adults. Is there a rosy outlook for food allergies? NO. Unfortunately the incidence of food allergies continues to rise as evidenced by the yearly increase in emergency room visits. (*Journal Allergy Clin Immunol.* 2001;107:191–193)

Emergency room visits for food allergy symptoms topped 1,000,000 between 2001 and 2005, according to a study in the December 2010, *Journal of Allergy and Clinical Immunology.* That's about 200,000 visits for each of those five years. About 90,000 of those visits each year were for anaphylaxis, a potentially fatal reaction to food. A study from the 1990s hypothesized that only 30,000 emergency room visits were for anaphylaxis each year.

Allergies to food—who's at risk? Children with latex allergy, atopic dermatitis, allergies to pollen, asthma, and allergic rhinitis will experience higher rates of food allergies. The risk of food allergies is four times greater with a positive family history of asthma. Actually a positive personal or family history of any food allergy is also considered to be a risk for subsequent food allergies.

Allergies—foods that trigger. The eight foods that trigger 90% of the traditional food allergies are milk, eggs, peanuts, tree nuts (e.g. walnuts, almonds and pecans), fish, shellfish, soybean, and wheat. Sesame seed are also an important emerging food allergen in the U.S. The first 3 foods listed above—milk, egg, and peanuts—cause the most reactions with population prevalence rates of 2.5%, 1.3%, and 0.8% respectively. (The Food Allergy and Anaphylaxis Network, 2010)

Kids tend to grow out of their allergies to cow's milk, eggs, and soy; however, allergies to peanuts and tree nuts, seafood, and seeds tend to persist throughout adulthood. Only 20% of infants with peanut allergy will outgrow the allergy. (Sampson H. Update on food allergy. *J Allerg Clin Immuno*l 2004;113:805-19; Sicherer S, Munoz-Furlong A, Sampson H. Prevalence of peanut and tree nut allergy in the U.S. determined by means of a random digit dial telephone survey: A 5-year follow-up study. *J Allerg Clin Immunol* 2003;112(5):1203–1207)

Allergic reactions to food. The length of time between ingestion and symptoms can help to distinguish between the two main types of allergic reactions to food protein: IgE*-mediated reactions (also known as immune-mediated reactions) and non-IgE mediated reactions. IgE-mediated reactions can produce signs and symptoms within 20 minutes of ingestion of the food vs. 2 hours to several days for the non-IgE reactions. Symptoms of non-IgE allergic food reactions—protracted vomiting and/or diarrhea, and dehydration—can resolve within 72 hours of food avoidance.

IgE-mediated reactions can be more serious, even life-threatening, because of the possibility of anaphylactic shock. An estimated 150 people die each year of fatal food anaphylaxis. Factors that increase the risk of fatal anaphylaxis to food include a history of severe reactions to the offending food, underlying asthma, delayed use of epinephrine, and symptom denial among adolescents and young adults. The most common food allergy that causes fatal and/or nearly-fatal allergic reactions is a peanut allergy. The incidence is rising in the U.S. with at least one to two percent of the U.S. population having a peanut allergy. As mentioned earlier, it is also the one food allergy that the majority of children most often do NOT outgrow.

Anaphylaxis—foods that trigger anaphylaxis. Many foods have been implicated in triggering anaphylaxis in addition to the traditional foods that cause food allergies. The following list is in addition to the "usual suspects": berries (blackberries, blueberries, raspberries, and strawberries), chocolate, corn, fish, legumes (green peas, lima beans), peaches, pork, and tomatoes.

Food-dependent, exercise-induced anaphylaxis is rare, but may occur after eating a food that usually produces an allergic reaction three to four hours prior to exercising. As an individual exercises and the body temperature rises, symptoms may occur that include itching, tightness in the chest, and light-headedness. Women are especially vulnerable to this response, so it is advisable not to eat the foods that trigger any reaction within three to four hours of exercising.

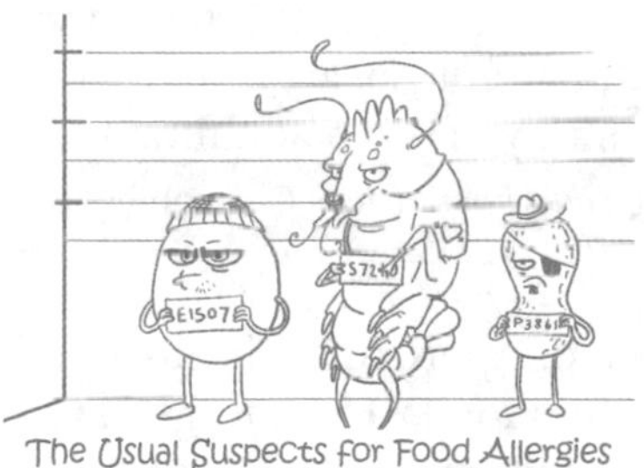
The Usual Suspects for Food Allergies

The last potential risk for food allergies exists with genetically modified (GM) foods. The problem for people with allergies is that GM foods may contain allergenic proteins from a different species of food. Fortunately this is not a huge risk; however, it could be potentially dangerous for super-allergic individuals.

Allergies to cow's milk. The most common food allergy in children is to cow's milk. The bad news is approximately 6–8% of infants are allergic to milk as are 2–3% of toddlers. The good news is that 80–90% of those milk-allergic toddlers will be able to tolerate milk by the age of five. Only 0.1 to 0.5% of adults are allergic to milk. Let's talk specifics. As mentioned earlier, it is possible to "outgrow" milk allergies.

*What is IgE? IgE stands for Immunoglobulin E, a protein produced by the immune system in response to an allergen (a substance that can induce allergies). There are many allergens, including foods, as mentioned above, as well as pollen, dust mites, ragweed, and animal dander. When IgE is produced by the immune system in response to an allergen, it attaches to "mast cells" and drills a hole in the mast cell membrane. Mast cells release histamine. Histamine must be the "bad guy" because every other shelf in Wal-Mart, Kmart and Target contains hundreds of boxes and bottles containing "antihistamines."

When histamine is released, blood vessels vasodilate: fluid is released into the tissues, resulting in drippy eyes and runny noses; histamine causes the eyes, nose and throat to itch; histamine causes the bronchioles of the respiratory tract to swell and breathing becomes difficult; histamine causes fluid to move into the gastrointestinal tract and "sh#!t happens"...in other words, copious amounts of explosive diarrhea. If all of this occurs at once, it's called "anaphylactic shock"—the throat starts to itch, lips swell, the skin turns bright red (due to the vasodilation), the blood pressure falls to zero (this is known as hypotension and is due to the systemic vasodilation), and breathing is labored with wheezing. This condition is a medical emergency and needs to be treated immediately.

It appears as if the old central dogma that kids with cow's milk allergy need to avoid ALL products with cow's milk, including baked products, might just be thrown out the proverbial window. A specific protein in cow's milk appears to be the culprit, and interestingly this culprit is inactivated by heat. Researchers gave baked products with milk, including waffles and muffins, to milk-allergic children and found that 75% of children were able to eat the baked products without an allergic reaction. The 25% of the kids that had reactions, even to the heated foods, also had the largest reactions when allergy skin testing was performed. So the stronger the reaction, the more likely that baked products will not be in your future until you are at least five years old, and perhaps you might have to wait until you reach adulthood to consume a waffle or muffin. (*The Journal of Allergy and Immunology Online* July 14, 2008;*Journal of the American College of Nutrition* (24:582S, 2005)

Allergies to foods that cross-react with pollen. Approximately 25–33% of Americans believe that they are allergic to certain foods. Don't forget that the actual number is 6–8% for infants and young kids and only 2.0–3.5% of adults. So, how about all of the folks who think they are allergic to foods? Every time they eat a certain food they have the classic reaction of itchy or swollen lips, scratchy throat, and gastrointestinal upset with cramping and diarrhea.

What's going on then? It appears as if people who are highly sensitive to pollen (a factor outside the food chain) can also experience an allergic response when they eat certain foods that cross-react *with* pollen. Specific foods such as celery, tomatoes, potatoes, seeds, nuts, and fruits, can trigger this syndrome, known as oral allergy syndrome (OAS). Heat usually destroys the protein in foods that cross-react with pollen. In contrast, cooking food has ***no*** effect on the majority of foods that cause traditional food allergies.

The specific proteins (allergens) in the major foods associated with allergies have been identified. Milk allergens are the alpha, beta, and kappa caseins or the "curd" portion of milk, as well as beta-lactoglobulin in whey. The allergenic proteins of egg include ovomucoid, ovalbumin, ovotransferrin, and lysozyme. Peanut (Ara h 2 and Ara h-6 and other Ara h family members), shrimp (tropomyosin), soy (Gly m BD 28K), and fish (parvalbumin) allergens are the culprits.

Here's a question for you: If you are allergic to walnuts as a tree nut, can you also be allergic to pecans, another tree nut? Yes, and this is referred to as cross-reactivity. Among patients allergic to one tree nut, 15–40% will have allergy to at least one other tree nut. Thirty to 100 percent of patients allergic to fish are allergic to more than one species of fish. Twenty-five percent of patients with one grain allergy will react to at least one other grain. So, should we restrict all members of a food family because of an allergic reaction to one member of the family? No, not necessarily. The current recommendation is to *not* automatically restrict all members of a food family because of an allergic reaction to one member of the family. But, included in the current recommendation—be aware of this reaction.

Allergies to latex have made a meteoric rise in the past 20 years due to the increased use of latex gloves and other products containing latex (condoms, anyone?). High-risk groups include health care workers, beauticians, food handlers and couples smart enough to practice safe sex with latex condoms. Latex, which comes from a certain species of the rubber tree, has proteins that cross-react with avocados, bananas, kiwi-fruit, passion fruits (especially for those wearing latex condoms), water chestnuts, Brazil nuts, and tomatoes. Eating foods that cross-react with latex won't always cause an allergic reaction in latex-sensitive individuals; however, it is important to make high-risk groups aware of the problem.

ASPARAGUS TIP

Anyone with a history of food allergies or history of anaphylaxis to anything (food, bee stings, drugs) should carry an EPI PEN (a prefilled syringe with epinephrine in it) with them at all times. Epinephrine is a potent vasoconstrictor and prevents the blood pressure from dropping to zero. It also gives the heart a boost, which in turn keeps the blood pressure elevated. Epinephrine opens up the airways (bronchodilation) and helps the patient breathe. The EPI PEN should be used within 10 minutes of the initial symptoms of anaphylactic shock. One of the reasons that the EPI PEN fails is that a person having symptoms waits too long to use it. (*Annals of Allergy, Asthma and Immunology* 100:570, 2008)

Allergies to peanuts. Peanut allergy causes an estimated 15,000 emergency room visits each year and nearly 100 deaths. Although peanuts are a ground nut and a peanut allergy is different from a tree nut allergy (walnuts, pecans, almonds), there are similarities. Even trace amounts of peanut can cause a reaction in extremely sensitive individuals. One peanut allergy patient used a knife to spread mayonnaise on his sandwich a few days *after* the knife had been used to spread peanut butter. He immediately developed anaphylactic shock from the exposure to the peanut butter.

Of course, everyone has proposed their own theory of why the immune system has gone nuts over peanuts. The "hygiene hypothesis" gets a lot of credit for the increase in nut allergies. This hypothesis basically says that infants and toddlers are not getting dirty enough. In other words, germophobic moms are loathe to allow their precious pumpkins to dig in the dirt, to crawl through the crunchy fall leaves, to swap mud pies with their fellow playmates, and to just enjoy the outdoors. Critters in dirt (especially little helminths, or parasitic worms) help to prime the immune system into a pathway that prevents allergies. If the child is not exposed to dirt early in life the immune system takes an entirely different pathway, the pathway that increases the risk not only of allergies, but of autoimmune diseases (which, by the way, are also on the rise).

Another theory blames the food processing system that alters the natural proteins found in foods and adds nonfood substances that have never before been consumed in large amounts. Other theories put the onus on the lack of certain vitamins (such as vitamin D) and still other theories throw in the obesity card. In other words, our kids are not getting enough sunlight and our kids are too fat. All theories; nothing proven at this point.

You might be surprised to know that peanut sources are rather ubiquitous. For example they are contained in diaper rash ointment used on baby's bottoms. How about breast milk, or other milk formulas? Yes, indeed. The maternal ingestion of peanuts can result in peanut proteins passing to the infant via breast milk. Peanut oil, by the way, also crosses through breast milk. Fortunately, the grade of peanut oil sold in the United States and Europe contains no detectable proteins and is thus not allergenic. Unfortunately, in other countries peanut oil may contain enough of the protein to cause an allergic reaction.

Other hidden sources include baby massage oil, airplane cabin dust and skin creams. Peanuts are the base ingredient for many vitamin D supplements. Small amounts of peanuts may be present in veggie burgers, packaged gravy powder, prepared sauces, and even baked goods. Even multivitamins have been shown to list peanut oil as one of the ingredients. Some food manufacturers are "de-flavoring" peanuts and disguising them to taste like other nuts. Many of those same companies refuse to guarantee that their products are peanut-free for this very reason. Peanut sensitivity increases the risk of cross-sensitization to other types of nuts and may increase the risk of allergies to milk and eggs.

Families with multiple allergies should be especially aware of the risk of peanuts. Peanuts or food containing peanuts should not be given to children under the age of two. Some experts suggest increasing the age to seven in families with allergic histories.

Approximately one in three individuals who has had a near-fatal anaphylactic reaction to peanuts, and who has been rescued with epinephrine, will have a recurrence of anaphylaxis within four hours, and will need a second injection. (*Cutis* 2000 (65): 285)

See Chapter P for more on Peanut and Peanut Butter allergies.

Allergies to peanuts and genetic engineering. Most allergic reactions to peanuts are triggered by the same eleven proteins. Scientists have identified two proteins (Ara h 2 and Ara h 6) that are the worst offenders and cause the most intense allergic reactions. Researchers are using the process of genetic engineering to deactivate these genes and make a non-allergic plant. That's good news for all of the peanut allergy sufferers in the world. (Chu Y et al. Reduction of IgE binding and nonpromotion of *Aspergillus flavus* fungal growth by simultaneously silencing Ara h 2 and Ara h 6 in Peanut. *J Agric Food Chem* 2008;56(23):11225-233)

Almonds. Almonds are considered to be one of the top choices for cardiovascular health. The tree *(Prunusdulcis)* that produces almonds is native to southwestern Asia. Most almond trees today are found in California. The tree bears large, hard, green fruit with an oval seed that is covered with a tough shell. Its nuts come in two types: sweet and bitter. The nutmeat is used to make marzipan and nougat. One ounce of almonds provides 6 grams of protein.

Almonds also contain a significant amount of calcium, but there's one big drawback. The amount of calcium in a whole cup of almonds is 378 milligrams, 78 more milligrams than a cup of milk that contains 300 milligrams. And that's good, *riiiight?* Perhaps… if all you're looking at is the calcium content of the almonds. Unfortunately, if you toss down an entire cup of almonds you would be consuming **eight** times more calories than drinking a single glass of milk, so is the trade-off in pounds gained worth the extra amount of calcium? Nope. (Christina Stark, nutritionist, Cornell University, 2009)

Almonds are also a rich source of vitamin E, an antioxidant necessary for maintaining the integrity of cell membranes, and protecting cells from the process of "oxidation"—which can be harmful in many ways. Almonds are a great source of monounsaturated fatty acids that help to reduce LDL-cholesterol (one of the "bad" cholesterols) and help to increase HDL-cholesterol (the "good" cholesterol). Almonds contain many of the vitamins found in the "B" family—riboflavin (B2), niacin (B3), thiamine (B1), pantothenic acid (B5), folate (B9), and pyridoxine (B6). Almonds are gluten-free, hence, the darling of the celiac food producers. Almonds can be used in the preparation of gluten free foods and used as alternatives to foods that contain wheat. Almond butter can be used by individuals that have peanut allergies. Almonds are also a great source of various minerals including potassium, manganese, iron, magnesium, zinc, and selenium. WOW, what's *not* to love about almonds? Nuttin'.

What is considered to be the healthy "dose" of almonds? Usually a healthy "dose" of any form of a nut is considered to be an ounce. So, it takes approximately 23 almonds (¼ cup) to make one "dose" for a mid-afternoon snack.

Alpha linolenic acid. Alpha linolenic acid is an omega-3 fatty acid found in soybean (tofu, edamame), canola oil, flaxseeds, flaxseed oil, chia seeds, and walnuts. Women who eat foods containing high amounts of alpha linolenic acid, particularly oil-based salad dressings and mayonnaise, five to six times per week, have a significantly reduced risk of developing fatal ischemic heart disease.

Lest one forget—oil-based salad dressings and mayonnaise are also calorie dense (a fancy way of saying "very high in calories"), so don't drench the salad in salad dressing. Too many calories, even the good omega-3 fatty acid calories, can lead to weight gain. Weight gain, in and of itself, is a risk factor for heart disease.

The World Health Organization recommends that adults consume 0.8 to 1.1 grams of alpha-linolenic acid daily. So, gulp down a handful of walnuts followed by a tablespoon of flaxseed, and a small bowl of edamame. What the heck is edamame? Flip over to Chapter E and you'll get the scoop.

Aluminum and Alzheimer's disease. Let's finally put this one to rest, shall we? The first connection between aluminum as a causative factor in Alzheimer's disease was made in the 1970s when Canadian researchers reported that the brains of Alzheimer's patients contained 10 times more aluminum compared to the brains of healthy control patients. No studies have duplicated these findings. Cooking with aluminum pots and pans adds up to 2.5 mg of aluminum to the daily American diet. However, tomato sauce cooked in an aluminum pot for two hours and then stored overnight in that same pot was found to contain only .0024 mg of aluminum per cup. By comparison, food additives, like certain leavening or emulsifying agents, add about 10 times that much or 26–50 milligrams of aluminum. Buffered aspirin contains 125–725 mg, and antacids, 850–5,000 mg. Even with those amounts, no study has proven that aluminum is a cause of Alzheimer's disease. So, that's the aluminum story. End of story. (Alzheimer's Organization, Alz.org; accessed 12-21-2010; *Cook's Illustrated*, January/February 2012)

Android obesity. It may come as a surprise to many average Americans that your waist size ***should*** be smaller than your hip size. Android obesity occurs when the waist is larger than the hips and you are shaped like an "apple." Androgens (the adrenal gland form of the male hormone testosterone) tend to move fat around the waist. Adrenal glands produce androgens in both men and women. Estrogen, from the ovaries, counteracts the androgens from the adrenal glands and helps maintain a smaller waistline. The bad news…once women reach menopause and the ovaries bite the dust, the adrenal androgens take the opportunity to move fat around the waistline. Can this dreaded complication of menopause be prevented? Yes, by watching what you eat, walking, walking, walking, and by taking estrogen replacement therapy. Did I mention walking?

A waist/hip ratio can give you an idea if you are creeping toward the apple shape—so can a quick look in a full-length mirror. In a study of over 40,000 middle-aged female nurses, women with a waist-to-hip ratio of greater than 0.88 (apple-shaped) were three times more likely to have a heart attack or die of heart disease over an eight-year period than women with a waist-hip ratio below 0.72 (pear-shaped). (*Journal of the American Medical Association*, December 2, 1998)

Stop what you are doing *right now*. Pour yourself two shots of Jack Daniels. Drink one shot. Yank a tape measure out of that all-purpose drawer in the kitchen and measure your waist size and hip size. Divide the hip number into the waist number. For women the result should be less than 0.85 and for men the result should be less than 0.95. Drink the second shot if your hip-to-waist ratio exceeds the above measurements. Anything greater than the above measurements and you have an increased risk of coronary artery disease, stroke, and diabetes.

"I'm in shape. Round is a shape." —Anonymous

Angiotensin Converting Enzyme Inhibitors (ACE Inhibitors) and potassium-containing foods. What drugs are known as the ACE inhibitors and what do they do? The bottom line is they inhibit the production of angiotensin II.

Angiotensin II is a very potent chemical that causes the muscles surrounding blood vessels to contract, thereby narrowing the blood vessels. The narrowing of vessels increases the pressure within the vessels and leads to hypertension. Angiotensin II also triggers the release of a hormone, aldosterone, from the adrenal gland. When aldosterone is released, it zips over to the kidneys and instructs them to save sodium and water and to excrete potassium.

So how do we make angiotensin II? Angiotensin II is converted from angiotensin I in the blood vessels by an enzyme called angiotensin converting enzyme, or ACE. ACE inhibitors are medications that inhibit the activity of the enzyme ACE. When angiotensin II is inhibited, the blood vessels dilate, and blood pressure is reduced. Don't forget that if you can't make "angie" you can't make "al" (aldosterone). If aldosterone cannot be produced, sodium and water will be excreted into the toilet and potassium will be conserved.

This inhibition of angiotensin II and aldosterone results in lower blood pressure. A lower blood pressure also makes it easier for the heart to pump blood and improves the function of a failing heart. In addition, the progression of kidney disease due to high blood pressure or diabetes is slowed. Sounds great, right? Yep, but there's always a downside or two.

As far as diet is concerned, potassium-containing foods can be a problem when a patient is on an ACE inhibitor. Since aldosterone is inhibited by the drug, potassium is retained by the kidney. If a patient is also consuming too many foods that contain too much potassium, a potentially life-threatening condition called hyperkalemia can result. See Chapter P for the most common foods that contain potassium, but here's a quick list to get you started: potatoes, oranges, bananas, prunes, cantaloupe, apricots…just to name a few. Hyperkalemia is the medical term for excess potassium in the blood. Too much potassium can contribute to a cardiac arrhythmia that is potentially fatal. SOOO…a couple of precautions are necessary. One of those precautions is to reduce potassium-containing foods and the other precaution is to carefully monitor the potassium level in patients taking ACE inhibitors.

How do you know if you are on an ACE inhibitor? Take out all your pill bottles and look for any drug that has the last name "pril." There are lots of ACE inhibitors on the market so look for benazepril (Lotensin) captopril (Capoten), lisinopril (Zestril, Prinivil) enalapril (Vasotec), perindopril (Aceon), quinapril (Accupril), and my very favorite, ramipril ("Ram a pril right down your throat," also known as Altace).

Some other drugs to be aware of that also have potassium-retaining properties include spironolactone (Aldactone), eplerenone (Inspra), trimethoprim-sulfamethoxazole (Bactrim, Septra), triamterene (Dyrenium), amiloride (Midamor), and the birth control pill, Yaz.

ANOREXIA

Anorexia. Anorexia is the Greek word for loss of appetite. Anorexia is a clinical symptom in some patients with depression and/or alcoholism. It may be seen at the beginning of fevers and numerous illnesses (such as liver infections or hepatitis), disorders of the GI tract (especially the stomach) and addiction (especially cocaine and methamphetamine). Many prescription medications, including chemotherapy for cancer and digoxin for heart failure, have the undesired side effect of causing anorexia and weight loss.

Patient had waffles for breakfast and anorexia for lunch.
—Note from a patient's hospital chart

Anorexia nervosa. Anorexia nervosa is an eating disorder marked by excessive fasting. It occurs more often in females between the ages of 12 and 21; however, it can also occur in males and in older females. The individual with anorexia nervosa has an intense fear of gaining weight, even when they are underweight. This fear does not diminish as weight loss progresses. The patient claims to feel fat even when emaciated. A loss of 25% or more of the original weight may occur. No known physical illness accounts for the weight loss. There is a refusal to maintain body weight over a minimal normal weight for body and size. Persons with anorexia nervosa may develop ritualistic eating habits such as cutting their food into tiny pieces. They may eat one M&M per day by cutting it into four pieces and having each piece as a treat four times a day. This is an eating disorder that is life-threatening. According to a study done by Crow, crude mortality rates are 4% for anorexia nervosa, the highest for any specified eating disorder. (Crow SJ et al. Increased mortality in bulimia nervosa and other eating disorders. *Am J Psych.* 2009;166:1342–1346)

Anorexia nervosa in males. Four weight loss goals that are more commonly held by males with anorexia nervosa than by females:

1) To avoid teasing brought on by being overweight
2) To improve athletic performance (wrestlers, jockeys)
3) To avoid a medical illness their father had
4) To improve a homosexual relationship

(Anderson A, Cohn L, Holbrook T. Eating disorders. In: Making Weight: men's conflicts with food, weight, shape, and appearance. Carlsbad, Calif: Gürze, 2000:32–37)

Anorexic pigs. The incessant focus on lean meat and selective breeding has led to a problem that sounds vaguely like an oxymoron—anorexic pigs. A researcher at the University of Wales has identified pigs, typically young females, that don't eat enough to maintain their pig-appropriate figure. Studies using these pigs may shed some light on possible genetic causes of anorexia and eventually lead to better therapies. (*Nutrition,* July/August 1999.)

Anticoagulants and food. Foods that are high in vitamin K may interfere with the effectiveness of anticoagulants such as heparin and warfarin (Coumadin, Dicumarol, Panwarfin). Rich sources of vitamin K include most dark green leafy greens (kale, collards, lettuce, spinach, turnip greens, dandelion greens, Swiss chard), asparagus, broccoli, Brussels sprouts, cabbage, cauliflower, and some oils like canola and soybean. Herbal supplements that are known to interact with warfarin include dong quai, ginseng, gingko, glucosamine, feverfew, and garlic. Green tea also has a large amount of vitamin K.

Antioxidants. This is a term thrown around all the time in clinical nutrition journals, cardiology journals, oncology journals, neurology journals and even Prevention magazine and the Ladies Home Journal. Antioxidants are powerful vitamins and chemicals that sop up "oxidants" or "free radicals." In large amounts, the process of oxidation can damage tissues and trigger a chain reaction that deposits cholesterol into the walls of the major arteries in the body—the coronary arteries, cerebral arteries, aorta, renal arteries, and femoral arteries, resulting in decreased blood flow to all of the major organs and the extremities. Oxidation can also trigger mutations of certain oncogenes predisposing an individual to cancer. So, it only makes sense that "antioxidants" can either prevent these processes or slow them down.

The most potent antioxidant vitamins include vitamin C and vitamin E. Extra virgin olive oil contains powerful antioxidants. However, if it loses its "virginity" so to speak, and it is processed to create a milder, "light" olive oil, it also loses its powerful antioxidant property. Carotenoids, the pigments that give many fruits and vegetables their yellow and orange colors, also act as antioxidants. Lycopene, a specific carotenoid found in tomatoes, is a powerful antioxidant that is "unleashed" when the tomato is cooked. Flavonoids are potent antioxidants found in berries—blueberries, raspberries, cranberries, strawberries, and blackberries. Blueberries are number one in this category. Resveratrol, found in the skins of red and purple grapes is also a potent antioxidant.

Should you go out and buy those expensive antioxidant formulas that you see on late-night TV? No. Period. Every nutrition expert in the world, and there are a lot of them, concurs that antioxidants are best ingested from food sources—red wine, or grape juice, extra version olive oil, fruits and vegetables. The only antioxidant not available in the quantities needed from food sources is vitamin E, and as you will read in the vitamin chapter (V), vitamin E in large doses causes more harm than benefit.

APPLES

Apple facts. There are nearly 10,000 varieties of apples, but approximately twenty varieties make up 90% of the apples produced in the United States. The Golden Delicious apples are the most popular yellow apples in the U.S. Granny Smith apples are tart and ideal for baking in pies. McIntosh apples are eaten fresh or made into applesauce. McIntosh apples are the parent apple to the newer Cortland variety. Cortland apples are used in salads due to the fact that they don't turn brown as quickly as other apples do when cut, sliced, and diced. One pound of apples is equal to three to four medium apples and to three cups of sliced apples.

Apples are filled with vitamin C, protein, pectin, natural sugars, copper, and iron. The apple's major vitamin contribution to the world of nutrition is vitamin C. Its major mineral contribution is potassium. The pectin in the apple is a natural anti-diarrheal agent that helps to solidify stool. Shaved raw apple has been used as an herbal remedy for diarrhea, and purified pectin has been used as an ingredient in over-the-counter anti-diarrheal products. The pectin pushers of the world also claim that pectin lowers cholesterol by interfering with cholesterol absorption in the bowel. Apples are also a great source of water—raw apples are 84% water.

"An apple a day keeps the doctor away." This proverb comes from the ancient Romans, who believed the apple had magical powers to cure illness.

"An apple a day keeps claustrophobia away." Researchers at the Smell and Taste Treatment Center Foundation in Chicago tested various odors to determine if the odor had any influence on the perception of space. Test subjects found that the smell of green apples made a room appear to be larger than it actually was. The researchers were unable to explain this phenomenon; however, they mentioned that the smell of green apples might be helpful to individuals with claustrophobia.

Apple of one's eye. The apple of one's eye is the pupil, which in the ninth century was likened to an apple. At that time the eye was believed to be a solid round mass.

Apple, as in Adam's apple. This eponym refers to the anterior protuberance of the thyroid cartilage, usually seen in men due to the growth of this cartilage at puberty secondary to testosterone. According to *Brewer's Dictionary of Phrase and Fable* the name comes from the superstition that a piece of the forbidden fruit which Adam ate stuck in his throat and caused the swelling. However, there is no mention in the Bible that the so-called forbidden fruit was actually an apple. Another interpretation was offered by Professor Alexander Gode in the *Journal of the American Medical Association* (1968;(206):1058). Professor Gode proposed that the Latin term *pomum Adami* ("Adam's apple") is really an early error in translation of the Hebrew *tappuach ha adam,* which means "male bump." The mistake could have easily been made because a single Hebrew word means both "bump" and "apple," and the Hebrew word for "man" eventually became the proper name "Adam."

The apple and William Tell (c. 1250). William Tell, a Swiss patriot, was a legendary crossbow marksman who defended Bürglen against Austrian oppression. Legend has it that William Tell refused to bow in homage to an

Austrian governor's hat placed in the Town Square. His punishment was to take a bow and arrow and shoot an apple off of his son's head at a distance of 80 paces. He performed the feat without a problem and later took his revenge by killing the same Austrian governor whose hat was placed in the Town Square.

The apple and Isaac Newton. Newton's formulation of the laws of gravity was supposedly triggered by observing the fall of an apple.

The apple and Apple computers—how did Apple computer get it's name? Perhaps Steve Jobs wanted to honor Sir Issac Newton. One of the earliest Apple Computer logos featured Sir Isaac Newton under an apple tree. Another account gives credit to Rob Janoff of Regis McKenna Advertising in 1977. He designed the Apple logo with the apple representing "the acquisition of knowledge." Steve Jobs subsequently added the rainbow colors to the logo to emphasize Apple II's superior color output. This leads us to the third, and most unlikely theory which incorporates the rainbow (gay flag colors) and naming the Apple computer as a tribute to an early genius in the world of mathematics and computers, Alan M. Turing. What does his name have to do with an apple? Apparently he was exposed as a gay man in the early 1950s. He was arrested for his homosexuality, which at the time was a felony offense under British law. He avoided prison by agreeing to chemical castration via female hormone injections. His reputation was ruined and his security clearance was revoked. Two years later he committed suicide by eating a single bite of an apple laced with cyanide. (Gore G. Understanding the Enigma of the Apple Computer Logo. www.GregGore.com)

Apple juice. Ninety-eight percent of all apple juices sold in the U.S. are pasteurized in order to prevent the natural enzyme action that would otherwise turn sugars into alcohol, eventually producing an alcoholic beverage known as apple cider. Pasteurization also protects apple juice from molds and bacteria including a potentially deadly strain of bacteria, *E. Coli O157:H7*, found in the bowels of cows. How in the world could this bacteria contaminate apple juice?

Here's the scenario. Cow manure is used as fertilizer. Apples drop off the tree into the cow manure. There is no "five-second rule" here. As soon as that apple hits a bed of cow manure it becomes contaminated with millions of pathogens. If *E. Coli O157:H7* just happens to be in that particular pile of cow manure then the apple is coated with the deadly bacteria. It only takes 10 to 100 pathogens to make you sick or even to kill you.

Several deaths have been attributed to unpasteurized apple juice contaminated with *E. Coli O157:H7*. The contaminated apples are used to make apple juice. If the apple juice has not been pasteurized and is sold at roadside stands, yard sales, bake sales, farmer's markets and fund-raisers, the consumer can acquire the deadly *E. Coli O157:H7* infection. Buyer beware. The

FDA has mandated that a warning be placed on any and all juices that have not been pasteurized. In fact, to be on the safe side, all juices sold in stores now must be pasteurized.

Can kids get too much apple/fruit juice? Yes. The American Academy of Pediatrics (AAP) has updated its guidelines for juice consumption in kids and now recommends the following:

1) no fruit juice for infants under 6 months as it offers no nutritional benefit for this age group

2) limit juice to 4–6 ounces a day for kids between 1–6 years

3) limit juice to 8–12 ounces a day for kids between ages 7–18.

(http://aappolicy.aapublications.org/cgi/content/full/pediatrics;107/5/1210)

Note to parents: A typical small juice glass holds 4–6 ounces. On average, an 8-ounce serving has 120 calories. Juices that are 100% juice have 11–16 grams of sugar for every 3 ounces, a relatively high amount of sugar. Beverages labeled "fruit drink" are usually almost entirely made of sugar. Consuming large amounts of sugar increases the risk of dental cavities. To protect teeth, the AAP advises parents not to put babies to bed with a bottle of juice. Allowing young children to carry "sippy cups" or boxes of juice around all day also promotes cavities. A second concern is diarrhea and stomach cramps. Much of the sorbitol, the key sugar in juices, is not absorbed in the small intestine, causing abdominal pain and diarrhea if juice is consumed in copious amounts. And, not only is excess juice contributing to malnutrition in our children, especially when it takes the place of milk in the daily diet, it is also contributing to the major epidemic of childhood obesity due to its large sugar and calorie load.

Appleseed, Johnny. John Chapman (1774–1845), was born in Leominster, Massachusetts. On what should have been his wedding day (his fiancée died prior to the wedding) in 1797, he left Massachusetts and traveled westward through Ohio, Indiana, Michigan, Iowa, and Minnesota to plant apple trees. Contrary to popular belief, Johnny did not just "scatter" the seeds as depicted in many stories about his life. Johnny actually was a dedicated nurseryman and helped establish homesteads for settlers and plant the apple trees. The law required that each settler plant 50 apple trees during their first year on the homestead. Because of the poor transportation systems that existed in the late 1700s and early 1800s, apples were an essential component of the early settlers' diets. Johnny Appleseed died on March 18, 1845 in Fort Wayne, Indiana after close to fifty years of travel and planting apple orchards.

Apple seeds. Apple seeds may be hazardous to your health if swallowed in large quantities. Parents should be especially aware of the apple seed's potential to poison since swallowing only a few seeds can be fatal in small children. Educating the young and the old about the dangers of apple seeds is imperative. Yikes! Why is that? Apple seeds contain amygdalin, a naturally occurring cyanide/sugar compound that degrades into hydrogen cyanide in the stomach. Don't panic if a teenager or adult accidentally swallows one apple seed. One seed is not enough cause cyanide poisoning. However, as mentioned, swallowing a few seeds can have potentially lethal consequences to a small child.

Apricots. Ounce for ounce, dried apricots are richer in nutrients and fiber than fresh apricots. It takes five pounds of fresh apricots to make one pound of dried apricots. Drying only removes the water, not the nutrients. In fact, dried apricots have twelve times the iron, seven times the fiber, and five times the vitamin A of the fresh fruit. In some studies with laboratory animals, dried apricots have been as effective as liver, kidneys, and eggs in treating iron-deficiency anemia.

The bark, leaves, and inner stony pit of the apricot all contain amygdalin (the same compound found in apple seeds), the naturally-occurring compound that degrades to release hydrogen cyanide in your stomach. Cases of fatal poisoning from apricot pits have been reported, especially in kids mistaking the pits for candy. The extract of apricot pits, known as the drug Laetrile, has been used in the past by alternative practitioners to treat various types of cancer. The presumed mechanism of action is that cyanide destroys the tumor enzyme beta-glucuronidase, an enzyme necessary for cell division. Numerous studies have yet to confirm this mechanism of action, and Laetrile has been banned for use in the United States; however, you can go South of the Border into Mexico to purchase Laetrile for use in treating certain forms of cancer. Does it work? *No,* Laetrile has *not* been shown to be effective against established cancers.

Eating an apricot *without* the pit provides a rich source of beta-carotene. According to the American Cancer Society, beta carotene may help to lower the risk of certain cancers of the head and neck, including cancers of the esophagus and larynx. (American Cancer Society, 2010)

Artichokes, globe. Vitamin C, iron, fiber, and potassium are the major contributions to the world of nutrition made by this prickly plant. Artichokes are low in calories and low in fat, not to mention delicious. Some folks are sensitive to the essential oils contained in artichokes and can develop a contact dermatitis from skin contact with those oils. Globe artichokes also con-

THE YUCK FACTOR

Each apricot pit releases about 1.5 milligrams of cyanide. The lethal dose for an adult is approximately 100 milligrams.

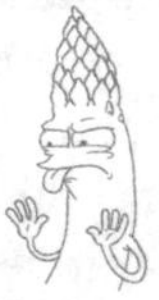

tain cynarin, a sweet-tasting chemical that dissolves in water and saliva to sweeten the flavor of anything you eat right after eating the artichoke.

Artificial food dyes and attention deficit disorder. Attention deficit hyperactivity disorder (ADHD) is one of the most common behavioral disorders in children affecting 3–7% of school-aged children. The essential features of ADHD include a pervasive pattern of hyperactivity-impulsivity and/or inattention, which is observed before the age of 7 years and occurs for a minimum of 6 months. In the early 1970s, research conducted by Dr. Benjamin Feingold found that when hyperactive children were given a diet free of artificial food additives and dyes, symptoms of hyperactivity were reduced. Oh, that it should be so easy!! Parents would rejoice world over if it was just a matter of eliminating artificial food dyes. Three decades after Dr. Feingold's declaration in 1975, hundreds of studies have supported his findings. Unfortunately, the more rigorous studies didn't completely support his findings. Many of the findings have been inconsistent and confusing. Now, that being said, let's look at some of the nutrients involved and the findings of the most recent clinical studies.

Hyperactivity and inattention are common symptoms associated with marginal zinc, iron, and magnesium deficiencies. Significant negative correlations have been seen between both serum ferritin (a measure of iron stores) and zinc levels and parental reports of hyperactive behavior. In addition, some kids with ADHD who are taking supplements containing zinc, iron, and magnesium have shown improvement in behavior. The same theory holds true with omega-3 fatty acids. Studies have shown that diets low in omega-3 fatty acids can predispose children to ADHD, and that the supplements containing omega-3s have been shown to decrease the symptoms in children with ADHD.

So what about artificial food dyes? Adding natural pigments to foods has been around for thousands of years. It's estimated that there are somewhere between 2,500 and 3,000 food additives used today, many of which help to maintain the consistency, freshness and safety of foods. However, not all additives have beneficial effects—some are just tossed in for cosmetic purposes. For example, margarine would be white without the addition of a yellow food dye. In the 1890s the dairy industry pushed for regulations that would ban the margarine makers from adding yellow to make their margarine look like butter. Anti-coloring laws were enacted in 30 states, and some legislatures mandated that margarine be dyed pink. To get around the legislation, some margarine manufacturers sold yellow dye packets with their products so that consumers could color their margarines at home. In the mid-1800s bread manufacturers added chalk to bread to make it whiter than white.

Many of the additives just "tossed in" are artificial or synthetic. Nine synthetic food dyes have been approved by the United States Department of Agriculture (USDA). Companies prefer the ease of using synthetic dyes over natural dyes such as colors derived from grapes, saffron, paprika, carrots, beet roots, and algae. Our intake of food dyes has increased by five-fold over the past 60 years—in parallel with our intake of processed foods, including breakfast cereals, snack foods, soft drinks, and baked foods.

The most used food dye is Allura red, or Red Dye No. 40. It's found in strawberry-flavored drinks, ice creams, and cream cheeses; some Nutri-Grain bars; licorice; and most other red sweets. It was approved by the FDA in 1971 and, in terms of consumption, is currently the most-used food dye.

After 40 years of research into food additives and ADHD, what's the bottom line? The first finding is that it's a tough subject to test. Some studies showed that food additives *did* lead to an increase in hyperactivity in a small portion of children, whereas other studies did not show that same result in all children. One of the problems with the studies was that different age groups were tested. Once the studies were all thrown into a blender and evaluated, findings showed that preschoolers appeared to be more sensitive to food additives than older children and adolescents. Individual variations are common, so let's just throw in another variable—genetics. And, the findings have to do with a histamine degradation gene. Interesting. A few studies have shown that 1) there are histamine receptors in the brain, and 2) food additives can trigger histamine release, and 3) genetic differences in the histamine degradation gene impair histamine clearance. Toss all of those findings in with the fact that drugs used in the treatment of ADHD also affect the histamine system. The drugs are methylphenidate (Ritalin, Concerta, Metadate) and atomoxetine (Strattera).

So, what should a practitioner advise parents? If parents are concerned about the artificial food additives, have them make careful food selections, choosing as many natural foods as possible. They should attempt to limit foods with synthetic food dyes, such as Captain Crunch cereals and the neon-hued Fruit Loops—especially in the younger, preschool-aged children. Stress that only a portion of the children with ADHD will respond positively to the removal of synthetic food dyes, but it's worth a try. (Cornier E. Attention deficit/hyperactivity disorder: a review and update. *J Pediatr Nurs.* 2008;23:345–357; Stevenson J et al. The role of histamine degradation gene polymorphisms in moderating the effects of food additives on children's ADHD symptoms. *Am J Psychiatry.* 2010;167:1108–1115; Kanarek RB. Artificial food dyes and attention deficit hyperactivity disorder. *Nutrition Reviews.* 2011;69(7):385–391; Bell L. The color of controversy. *Science News.* August 27, 2011:22–25)

Asparagus. Asparagus is a member of the lily family, for all of you lily lovers. Under ideal temperature conditions, an asparagus spear can grow 10 inches in a 24-hour period. A well cared for asparagus field will generally produce for about 15 years without being replanted. When you are picking asparagus at the grocery store, remember that the larger the diameter, the better the quality!

Asparagus is a nutrient-dense food. The major contribution to the world of nutrition by the asparagus is its high folate level of 135μg or 66% of the recommended daily intake for a man (current recommended daily intake, or RDI, is 200 μg) and 73% of the RDI for a woman (current recommendation is 180 μg for a woman). If a woman is in the mode or the mood to get pregnant the FDA recommends 400 μg of folate per day to prevent neural tube defects. Asparagus is also a great source of potassium, fiber, pyridoxine (vitamin B6), vitamin A,vitamin C, and thiamine (vitamin B1). Asparagus has no fat, contains no cholesterol, and is low in sodium. Indeed, you should KISS your asparagus.

So what's not to love? Well…

Asparagus cause a filthy and disagreeable smell in the urine, as everybody knows. (Treatise of All Sorts of Foods Louis Lemery, 1702)

So, why does eating asparagus make your urine smell funky—kind of like, well, asparagus? The culprits are various sulfur compounds identified as:

- methanethiol
- dimethyl sulfide
- dimethyl disulfide
- bis (methylthio)methane
- dimethyl sulfoxide
- dimethyl sulfone

The first two are the most pungent of the six compounds, while the last two provide a sweet aroma. A mixture of these compounds form what is referred to as the reconstituted asparagus urine odor. The onset of the asparagus urine smell is remarkably rapid. It has been estimated to start within 15 to 30 minutes after ingestion.

In the past, scientists believed that only people who inherited a certain gene formed the sulfur compounds found in asparagus. Now they know that everyone forms this pungent by-product, but only 22% of the population inherits the autosomal dominant gene that enables them to actually smell it. FYI: I'm one of the 22%. (Waring RH, et al. (1987). The chemical nature of the urinary odour produced by man after asparagus ingestion. *Xenobiotica* 17(11):1363–1371; Mitchell, S.C. (2001). Food idiosyncrasies: beetroot and asparagus. *Drug Metabolism and Disposition.* 29(4):539–543.Somer, E. (August 14, 2000). *Eau D'Asparagus.* WebMD. http://www.webmd.com/content/article/43/1671_51089. Retrieved 2006-08-31.)

Tastes like asparagus.

"When cicadas come out of their skin," says biologist Gene Kritsky, "they taste like cold, canned asparagus." We can try it out every 13 to 17 years when cicadas appear during the months of May and June.

Aspartame (NutraSweet, Equal). Aspartame is a no-calorie sugar substitute found in over 1,500 products. It was FDA approved for human consumption in 1974. Since that time over 90 countries have also approved aspartame as a safe sugar substitute. Aspartame is 200 times sweeter than table sugar. As a comparison, saccharin is 500 times sweeter than table sugar.

Controversy concerning the safety of aspartame has continued to proliferate thanks to the Internet; however, most experts agree that it is safe. Here are the current findings from the American Dietetic Association (ADA)—as of April 2009.

The ADA project looked at several questions raised by the media and others over recent years. The final analysis, posted on the ADA Evidence Analysis Library (EAL) web site, puts these questions to rest. For example, there have been claims that low calorie sweeteners like aspartame could have a rebound effect that stimulates the appetite and encourages people to consume more food. The ADA analysis found: There is good evidence that aspartame does not affect appetite or food intake. This consensus statement was given a grade 1, the highest grade in the EAL scale.

As a corollary to the above statement, naysayers have implied that low calorie sweeteners actually "make" people gain weight. The ADA committee looked at studies in adults and concluded that using aspartame in the context of a reduced calorie diet either does not affect weight nor is associated with increased weight loss. This body of research was also given a grade 1.

Myths about aspartame's supposed "negative effects" have proliferated on the Internet for years. The committee evaluated peer-reviewed research from the scientific literature on this topic and concluded that: ***"Aspartame consumption is not associated with adverse effects in the general population."*** Once again, the committee found that the support for this statement is grade 1.

The one exception as far as aspartame safety is concerned is for individuals diagnosed with phenylketonuria (PKU), a rare genetic disease in which the body cannot metabolize the amino acid phenylalanine (a component of aspartame.)

A few adverse reactions to aspartame tend to crop up in a small group of individuals. These reactions include headaches, allergic reactions, behavioral changes, and seizures. However, scientific studies have not been able to prove a clear connection between the aforementioned symptoms to the sweetener. And, as to the speculation that aspartame causes brain tumors, there is absolutely no scientific basis for an increased risk. Does this mean that you can drink 27 diet drinks a day containing aspartame? Absolutely

The Yuck Factor

The accumulation of phenylalanine is neurotoxic and can cause significant brain damage in developing babies and children. Hence, a big MR. YUCK sticker for aspartame in infants and kids with PKU.

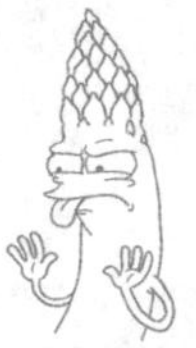

not. Even though aspartame is safe, foods that contain the sweetener are usually low in nutrients and should be limited in a healthy diet.

Aspirin from food. Salicylates (aspirin) are naturally present in fresh fruit and vegetables. Manufacturers also add salicylates (as antioxidants) to processed foods. Salicylates are also used as antioxidants in cosmetics and are absorbed through the skin. The total amount an average person obtains from these several sources is approximately 125 mg per day, an amount that inhibits platelet aggregation and reduces the risk of myocardial infarction. (By comparison, a "baby" aspirin, or one-fourth of a full aspirin, is 81 mg.) Could this exposure to salicylates via food and cosmetics explain the declining rate of heart disease mortality since the 1960s? Fresh fruit and vegetables did not become available for year-round consumption until the mid-1950s. This was also the same time the manufacturers began adding salicylates to processed foods and long before the average American became diet-conscious.

A rule of thumb in the matter of medical advice is to take everything any doctor says with a grain of aspirin. —Goodman Ace (1899–1982)

ATKINS DIET

Atkins diet. *Dr. Atkins New Diet Revolution* claims that carbohydrates (carbs) are the culprits of weight gain. The Atkins diet sets strict limits on the amount of carbohydrates one can consume in a 24-hour period. The claim is that if you limit carbs, you will burn fat stores. His diet is heavy on meat, poultry, seafood, eggs, cheese, butter, cream, oil, nuts, some (non-starchy) vegetables, and artificial sweeteners. Nutritionally there are some problems with his diet. For starters, the saturated fat content is off the chart. It is also low in fruit, whole grains and fiber, resulting in a major complaint of Atkins' devotees: constipation. Low carbs can also result in a whopping case of halitosis, especially during the induction phase when you can hardly look at a carbohydrate without gaining weight.

One of the reasons weight loss occurs with the Atkins diet is that fewer calories are consumed. Interestingly, when one has fewer choices to make, one chooses fewer foods. On average, the high-protein eaters consume about 450 calories less than high-carbohydrate eaters. High-protein foods also have a much higher "satiety value" than high carbohydrate foods. In other words, eating lots of protein is more likely to make you feel full and stop eating.

One of the interesting benefits of the Atkins diet concerns cholesterol, of all things. Naysayers were screaming that since the diet was high in saturated fats the cholesterol level would skyrocket and the risk of heart disease would skyrocket right along with it. Interestingly this didn't happen. What did happen was the healthy HDL-cholesterol started inching its way up as the carbohydrate intake inched its way down. And, HDL is an independent variable in reducing the risk of cardiovascular disease, so any small increase in HDL helps to decrease the risk of heart disease.

Atkins diet and drugs. The Atkins diet and the South Beach diet are two well-known high protein diets that espouse the loss of copious amounts of weight while gorging oneself with as much protein as one can possibly eat in any given day and reducing carbohydrate intake to virtually nothing during the induction phase of the diet. And, while these diets were receiving a bit of flak about their trans and saturated fats and subsequent possible effects on cholesterol, no one appeared to be too interested in how a high protein/low carbohydrate diet might affect drugs that were highly protein bound in the plasma—until anticoagulation clinicians began to report more INR fluctuations in patients on high-protein, low carbohydrate diets. (Thomas JA. Drug-nutrient interactions. *Nutr Rev* 1995;53(10):271–82)

OK, before we go on, let me explain the acronym, INR. INR stands for International Normalized Ratio, a fancy way of saying how well the anticoagulant warfarin, also known by its brand name, Coumadin, is working. When a patient is taking warfarin, the INR should be maintained between 2 and 3 to prevent clotting. There are exceptions to this rule, but this number is generally accepted as the "norm" in patients taking warfarin. Now, let's move on to the rest of the story.

Once a dose of a highly protein-bound drug such as warfarin is taken, a certain proportion of it binds to albumin in the plasma. As a "bound" drug, warfarin has no anticoagulant effect. The amount of drug that remains "free," or the nonprotein bound drug, is the amount of drug that is considered to be therapeutic.

High protein diets increase the amount of plasma proteins, including albumin, which, in turn, *increase* the amount of drug binding, causing a *decrease* in the amount of "free" drug, which, of course, is the functioning form of the drug. The effect becomes most pronounced within 10 days of the induction phase of the diet, resulting in a decrease in warfarin available to prevent clots (a reduction in the INR); therefore, the dose of warfarin may need to be increased. If the dose isn't increased, patients are at high risk of developing blood clots within two weeks of starting the diet. Instruct patients to advise their health care professional prior to initiating a high-protein, low-carbohydrate diet.

Other highly protein-bound drugs that may be affected by high-protein, low-carbohydrate diets include diazepam (Valium), fluoxetine (Prozac), simvastatin (Zocor), and valproic acid (Depakene, Depakote).

A single high protein meal can also reduce the effect of levodopa/carbidopa (Sinemet) in the treatment of Parkinson's disease. Advise the patient that it would be best to take most of the daily recommended proteins with the evening meal in order to receive the full effects of levodopa/carbidopa during the day. (Jefferson JW. Drug and diet interactions: Avoiding therapeutic paralysis. *J Clin Psychiatry* 1998;59 (suppl 16):31–39)

I've been on a diet for two weeks and all I've lost is two weeks.
—Totie Fields (1931–1978)

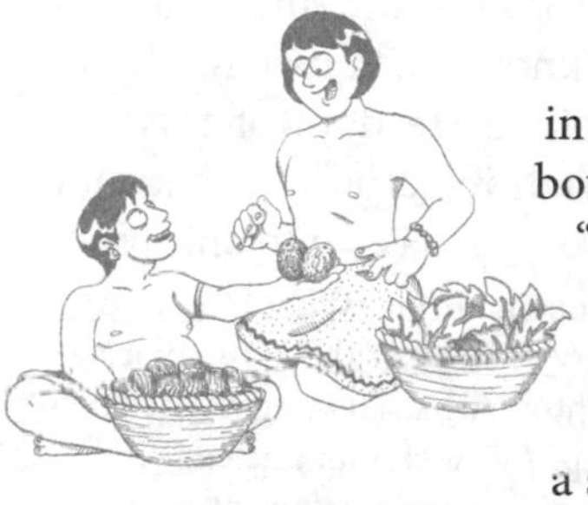

Avocado. This fruit was introduced to Europe in the early nineteenth century by an Argentinian botanist, Jorge Avocado (1798–1868). The word "avocado" comes from the Aztec word "ahuacatl," meaning testicle, a reference to the shape of the fruit. One can only guess at this reasoning, but since the avocado is shaped somewhat like a scrotal sac and it hangs off of an avocado tree in pairs, the assumption can be made that this is what the Aztecs had in mind when "ahuacatl" rolled off their tongues. The fruit is sometimes called an avocado pear or alligator pear (due to its shape and the rough green skin). The word ahuacatl can be compounded with other words, as in ahuacamolli, meaning "avocado soup or sauce," from which the Mexican Spanish word guacamole is derived.

The avocado is an unusual fruit in that 16% of its total body weight is fat, primarily monounsaturated fat. Approximately 75% of the calories from an avocado come from the monounsaturated fats. The major contribution of the avocado to the world of nutrition is high soluble and insoluble fiber, vitamins A, C, E and K, folate, and the mineral potassium. Avocados have 60% more potassium than bananas. Because potassium is excreted in the urine, potassium-rich foods are recommended for patients taking potassium-wasting diuretics including furosemide (Lasix), and hydrochlorothiazide (HCTZ). One avocado contains 1,000 mg of potassium. Another benefit of the potassium-rich avocado is the reduction in the risk of stroke. A 1998 Harvard School of Public Health analysis of data from the long-running Health Professionals Study shows 38% fewer strokes among men who ate nine servings of high potassium foods a day vs. those who ate less than four servings. Among men with high blood pressure, taking a daily 1,000 mg potassium supplement reduced the incidence of stroke by 60%. Of course, the preference is to eat foods high in potassium. Flip again to chapter P for all of the foods that are high in potassium.

Avocados and toxicity to animals. There is documented evidence that cats, dogs, cattle, goats, rabbits, rats, birds, fish, and horses can be severely harmed or even killed when they consume avocado leaves, bark, skin and pits. Avocado leaves contain a toxic fatty acid derivative known as persin, which in sufficient quantity can cause symptoms that include gastrointestinal irritation, vomiting, diarrhea, respiratory distress, congestion, pericardial effusions (fluid accumulation around the tissues of the heart), and even death. Birds also seem to be particularly sensitive to this toxic compound. Feeding avocados or guacamole to any non-human animal should be avoided completely. Negative effects in humans seem to be primarily in allergic individuals.

Avocados also contain large amounts of serotonin and may interact with serum tests for a type of endocrine tumor known as a carcinoid that also secretes serotonin. Eating an avocado within three days of this test may give a false positive reading. Other foods high in serotonin that may also cause a false positive reading on this test are bananas, eggplant, pineapples, plums, tomatoes, and walnuts. (University of California, What kind of fruit is the avocado?; Stradley, Linda (2004). All About Avocados: History of the Hass Avocado. What'sCookingAmerica.net. Newberg, OR: self-published. http://whatscookingamerica.net/avacado.htm. Retrieved 2008-05-13.Etymonline.com. http://www.etymonline.com/index.php?search=avocado. "Avocado Fun Facts." California Avocado Commission. http://www.avocado.org/about/fun_facts. Retrieved 2008-06-03. Clipsham, R. "Avocado Toxicity". http://kgkat.tripod.com/avocado.html. Retrieved 2007-12-29)

Avocado swap for butter. Replace butter with an avocado spread. Butter is loaded with saturated fats, whereas avocados contain the good heart health monounsaturated fat, the major antioxidant vitamin E, and the blood pressure controlling nutrient potassium. Per tablespoon, you'll save over 75 calories per swap and you'll still delight in that creamy satisfaction you enjoy from butter.

ASPARAGUS TIP

Avocados are high in potassium and great for lowering blood pressure as long as you're not on blood pressure drugs known as ACE inhibitors. ACE inhibitors conserve potassium and this could lead to dangerous levels of serum potassium.

High avocado intake has also been shown to have a beneficial effect on serum cholesterol levels. Specifically, after a seven-day diet rich in avocados, hypercholesterolemia patients showed a 17% decrease in total serum cholesterol levels. These subjects also showed a 22% decrease in both LDL-cholesterol (harmful cholesterol known as Low Density Lipoprotein) and triglyceride levels and 11% increase in good HDL-cholesterol.

Avocado is also known to promote healthy skin and hair. Although many people use it as a facial mask, it is most beneficial when eaten.

Bread that is sliced with an axe is bread that is too nourishing.
— Fran Leibowitz

BACON

Bacon. If you're going to eat bacon, at least cook it in the healthiest way possible. Instead of frying bacon in the skillet, cook it in the microwave oven. Microwaving bacon diminishes the formation of harmful nitrosamine chemicals produced when cooking cured meats such as bacon and ham. (Miller BJ et al. Formation of N-nitrosamines in microwaved vs. skillet-fried bacon containing nitrate. *Food and Chem Toxicol* 1989;27(5):295–99)

Bacon as a processed food. Would it be a surprise to anyone that 68% of bacon's calories come from fat, almost half of which is saturated? One strip of bacon contributes 30 milligrams of cholesterol to the daily intake. Add three strips to those three scrambled eggs, with 200 milligrams of cholesterol per egg and your breakfast contains 690 milligrams of cholesterol, more than twice the recommended daily amount.

Eating foods rich in saturated fat can increase cholesterol levels, increasing the risk of cardiovascular disease. Cardiovascular disease is not the only health risk of eating bacon.

Bacon is considered a type of red meat and is a member of the dreaded "processed meat" group. Processed meat is preserved via smoking, curing, or salting. The American Institute for Cancer Research (AICR) has made the statement that no amount of processed meat is considered safe to eat. Who else belongs to the processed meat group? Ham, sausage, hot dogs, bologna, salami, pepperoni, and pastrami all belong to this group.

Many researchers have concluded that regular consumption of processed meats may lead to higher risk for prostate cancer, colon cancer and several other cancers. It's not clear exactly how processed meat raises cancer risks, but it most likely has to do with the nitrates which are often used as preservatives in processed meat. The nitrates change into N-nitroso (nitrosamine) compounds that promote DNA mutations. Polycyclic aromatic hydrocarbons have also been implicated as carcinogens and are produced during processing.

ASPARAGUS TIP

It's Saturday morning and you're sitting at a restaurant and your Grand Slam Double By-pass breakfast comes with a choice of 3 pieces of bacon or two pork sausage links. Hmmmm...what to choose? Is one better than the other? Or should I say, is one the lesser of two evils? Actually, the answer is yes and the answer is bacon. Here's a handy comparison:

Two pork sausage breakfast links (45 g) have 140 calories, 12 grams fat, 4 grams saturated fat, 30 mg cholesterol, 7 grams protein, and 310 mg sodium.

Three hickory smoked bacon strips, pan-fried (26 g) have 120 calories, 9 grams fat, 3.8 grams saturated fat, 30 mg cholesterol, 7.5 grams protein, and 435 mg sodium.

HISTORICAL HIGHLIGHT

Where did the phrase "bringin' home the bacon" come from? There are quite a few theories for the origin of this phrase. In the eighteenth century the term *bacon* was a slang term for the rewards brought home by thieves. In the twelfth century, a noblewoman from Dunmon, England, stated that any person who would kneel at the front door of the church and swear that, "For 12 months and a day he has never had a household brawl or wished himself unmarried," could claim a side of bacon. Needless to say, she didn't part with too many sides of bacon—rumor has it that only eight men won the prize of "bringing home the bacon." One last possibility is that the phrase refers to greased pig contests held at county fairs, where the contestant who captured the greased pig won the prize and therefore *brought home the bacon.*

BANANAS

Bananas. The banana is the number one selling fruit in the world. The average American consumes 28 pounds of bananas per year. Bananas are shaped like a smile, have no bones or seeds, contain no cholesterol, don't leak, come in their own wrappers, ripen off the plant, are fun to play with, are picked off a giant herb plant, are 99.8% fat free, contain fiber, vitamins and potassium, and are a natural diet food. What's not to love? And, if you're looking for a major dose of potassium, one large banana contains 1,000 mg.

When the skin of the banana is yellow-green, 40% of its carbohydrates are starch; when the skin is fully yellow and the banana is ripe, only 8% of the carbohydrates are still starch. Ninety-one percent of the starches have been broken down into sugars—glucose, fructose, and sucrose. The high sugar content of the banana makes it a perfect source for a high-energy snack.

A single banana is called a finger, whereas a bunch of bananas is called a hand.

The International Banana Association has a helpful hint for the use of banana peels—the inside of a banana peel makes an excellent shoe polish.

A typical banana travels 4000 miles before being eaten.

A foodless world would have the disastrous effect of robbing one's initiative. Ambition has no place in a society that refuses its members the opportunity to become top banana. —Fran Leibowitz

Bananas and latex allergies. Certain foods such as bananas, Brazil nuts, chestnuts, kiwi fruit, avocado, and tomato demonstrate cross-reactivity with latex, most likely because of a resemblance to a latex protein component. These foods have been responsible for anaphylactic reactions in latex-sensitive persons, while many other foods, including figs, apples, celery, melons, potatoes, papayas, and pitted fruits such as cherries and peaches have caused progressive symptoms beginning with oral itching.

In 1944, to let the public know that bananas should be allowed to ripen at room temperature, not in the refrigerator, United Fruit commissioned a song and a character named Chiquita Banana. The song was so popular that it was once played on the radio 376 times in one day. And, here it is…

I'm Chiquita banana and I've come to say
Bananas have to ripen in a certain way
When they are fleck'd with brown and have a golden hue
Bananas taste the best and are best for you
You can put them in a salad
You can put them in a pie-aye
Any way you want to eat them
It's impossible to beat them
But, bananas like the climate of the very, very tropical equator
So you should never put bananas in the refrigerator.

The banana the first fruit you eat when you come into this world, and the last fruit you eat on your way out. Bananas appeal to the very young and the very old, especially when a lack of teeth is a concern. Ken Bannister, proprietor of The International Banana Club and Museum, 2524 El Molino Avenue, Altadena, CA

Bananas, Rice, Applesauce, and Toast diet. The BRAT diet. The BRAT diet was historically advocated by physicians, nurses, and nutritionists as a bland, "refeeding" diet after a child was rehydrated from a gastrointestinal (GI) bout of diarrhea and vomiting. This low-fiber diet was believed to decrease GI distress. But, this diet is NO longer recommended for children with diarrhea for the following reasons:

1) Foods in the BRAT diet are thought to act as "binders" that can reverse the diarrhea by causing constipation. However, if the diarrhea is caused by an infectious agent (such as *E. Coli* O157:H7 or *Salmonella*), the last thing you want to do is constipate the child. Infectious diarrhea should literally "run" its course—in other words, let it rip!

2) The BRAT diet is too restrictive and doesn't provide optimal nutrition.

3) There is absolutely no scientific evidence that the BRAT diet helps children recover from diarrhea. Foods rich in complex carbohydrates, lean meats, yogurt, fruits and vegetables are the preferred diet therapy. (Shapiro SD, Wallace KH, Roth TS. Rehydration and refeeding after diarrheal illness. *ADVANCE for NPs and PAs,* November 2010;35-40. King CK, et al, and Centers for Disease Control and Prevention. Managing acute gastroenteritis among children: oral rehydration, maintenance, and nutritional therapy. *MMWR Recomm Rep* 2003;52(RR-16):1–16).

HISTORICAL HIGHLIGHT

Bananas first grew in tropical Asia and were eaten by the ancient Greeks and Romans. Banana plants were transported from the Canary Islands off northwest Africa to the Americas soon after the New World was established.

Barbeque. The first recorded use of the word barbeque was in 1661. Its origin is from the Spanish word *barbacoa* which means a "framework of sticks." The original barbeque was a raised cooking device used to roast whole animals over the open fire. Today we use barbecue to refer to the backyard grill, the way in which we cook the meat, and even the sauce that we brush on the meat that we cook. The top 3 days in the U.S. for firing up the barbeque are: 1) the Fourth of July, 2) Memorial Day, and 3) Labor Day.

Bariatric surgery (Gastric bypass surgery). The World Health Organization estimates that there are one billion overweight people in the world, and that 300 million are obese (ie, have a body mass index, or BMI, of 30 or greater). In the U.S., the incidence of class 3 obesity (BMI ≥ 40) was reported at 3.1% in 2005, with the prevalence having quadrupled between 1986 and 2000 and increasing another twofold between 2000 and 2005. During those same periods, the prevalence of class 4 obesity (BMI, 50–59.9) increased fivefold and threefold, respectively. Right along with the increase in Class 3 and Class 4 obesity rates has been an increase in the number of bariatric surgery procedures performed. In 1998 there were 13,365 procedures performed; in 2007 there were 200,000 procedures performed.

Follow-up for bariatric surgery patients is essential as multiple nutritional deficiencies are expected. In one study of 379 patients scheduled for a Roux-en-Y procedure, fifty-seven percent of the patients had a micronutrient deficiency prior to the surgery. Sixty-eight percent of the patients had a vitamin D deficiency, 43.9% had an iron deficiency, 29% with a thiamin deficiency, 8.4% had a ferritin (iron storage) deficiency, and 3.2% had a calcium deficiency prior to surgery.

Suggested dosing of micronutrient supplementation after gastric bypass:

Calcium citrate 1,800 mg/d
Vitamin D 1,200–2000 IU/d
Vitamin A 4,000–25,000 IU/d
Vitamin K 0.15–0.3 mg/d
Iron 150–300 mg/d with vitamin C*
Copper 8 mg/d*
Vitamin B12 Oral: 350 mg/d or IM 1,000–3,000 μg/month
Folate 1 mg/d*
Vitamin B1 25–120 mg/d (in multivitamin)

*Please note that some of these only need to be given if there's a deficiency. (Gehrer S, et al. Obes Surg. 2010;20(4): 447–453; Condosta D. Micronutrient deficiencies after gastric bypass. Clinician Reviews. 2010;20(11):35–40)

Barley. Barley is a grain that is jam-packed with carbohydrates, high in soluble gums and pectins (fiber), and low in fat with nary a drop of cholesterol. It is also a good source of folate, the B vitamin that is seemingly good for whatever ails you. One of barley's major benefits is to lower the cholesterol via the soluble gums (something called beta-glucan) and pectins. How does that happen? Two theories on the cholesterol-lowering properties of barley are as follows: The first theory is that pectin forms a gel in your stomach that absorbs fats and literally removes them via the GI tract. The second is that the normal bacteria that inhabit the bowel feed on the beta-glucans in the barley to produce short-chain fatty acids, which in turn slow the natural production of cholesterol in your liver. In other words, you stop making your own cholesterol, which is a major contributor to serum cholesterol levels. Barley also contains tocotrienol (a member of the vitamin E family) that promotes cardiovascular health by reducing cholesterol.

After barley is harvested, the grain may be left to undergo a natural chemical process known as germination. During this process, the complex carbohydrates change into pure sugar. The grain, now called *malted* barley, is used as the base for several fermented and distilled alcohol beverages—namely beer and whiskey, and we all know about *their* benefits. If you don't, refer to Chapter A and the section on alcohol. (Ames NP, Rhymer CR. Issues surrounding health claims for barley. *The J of Nutrition* (2008);138:1237–43)

Basal flatal rate. The basal flatal rate (BFR) is the amount of gas produced as a steady state over a 24-hour period. The average BFR is 15 ml per hour, but would obviously increase exponentially after one consumes a meal. The elimination of gas is proportionate to the amount formed. Under normal circumstances, the average American passes between 500–2,000 ml of gas (flatus) per 24 hours with the average volume of per passage between 35 and 90 milliliters. (Dr. Michael Levitt, Gastroenterologist, Veteran's Administration Hospital, Minneapolis)

Following a basic standard meal, an increase from 15 ml to 100 ml is observed. This rate is referred to as the post-prandial flatal rate or PPFR. If that meal is comprised of 51% baked beans, the PPFR increases to a whopping 176 ml per hour. Finally the answer as to why baked beans are only served at outdoor picnics.

BEANS

Beans, beans, the musical fruit. Beans are seeds, packed with complex carbohydrates including starch and dietary fiber. They contain indigestible sugars, plus insoluble cellulose and lignin in the seed covering, and soluble gums and pectins in the bean. All beans are a great source of the B vitamin folate (folic acid), and a good source for both the B vitamin pyridoxine (B6) and the mineral iron.

The best beans for folate (folic acid) are as follows:
Chick-peas (1/2 cup) – 191 mcg
Black beans (1/2 cup) – 129 mcg
Pinto beans (1/2 cup) – 147 mcg
Navy beans (1/2 cup) – 128 mcg
Kidney bean (1/2 cup) – 65 mcg
(USDA Nutrient Database, 2009)

BUYING TIP FOR BEANS: Try to avoid buying dry beans in bulk. The B vitamins, especially B6, are very sensitive to light and will be destroyed when overexposed to it. If you are going to buy beans from open bins, look carefully for any holes on the bean surface. Bugs love the open bins and will burrow right through the skin and set up house. Beans in bins also may have a few stones thrown in as well as other debris, so pick your beans carefully. Make sure they are smooth-skinned, uniform in size, and evenly colored.

Beans as fiber. The flavonoids are the pigmented compounds in the coating of beans, making up 10% of the weight of the bean. Flavonoids are also the main source of fiber in navy beans, cranberry beans, mottled pintos, great white Northern beans, and black beans. A half-cup serving provides six to eight grams of fiber. The majority of this fiber (75%) is the insoluble type, thought to decrease the risk of colon cancer and other GI problems such as constipation. The other 25% is soluble fiber, which helps to lower cholesterol.

How to "de-gas" the beans. The offending agents in the beans are called oligosaccharides, which are naturally occurring carbohydrates. Our bodies lack the enzyme necessary to digest the oligosaccharides, so the bacteria in our colons perform the task for us. Unfortunately the metabolism by our friendly bacteria results in not-so-friendly fire, so to speak, and the tell-tale tail-gas is emitted as flatus.

Soaking, draining, and rinsing the beans before cooking helps to de-gas the beans. Use the quick-soak method—boil the beans in water for two minutes, then remove them from the heat with the cover on, and let them sit for two to four hours. After the allotted two to four hours, drain and discard the rinse water, rinse again, and cover with fresh cold water (in a three to one ratio of water to beans.) Finally, cook the beans one to four hours depending on the texture of the beans. Acidic foods like tomatoes should be added only after the beans are fully cooked, because acid toughens the beans.

Build up tolerance gradually. The more often you eat beans, the less likely you will suffer gas. For canned beans, drain the liquid off and rinse the beans. By rinsing canned beans several times and pouring off the water, you not only de-gas the beans but you also reduce the sodium content by 41%.

Beef, where's the lean? What are the leanest cuts of beef? This is the beef that contains the least amount of total fat and saturated fat. The grade of beef is also important—'prime' has the most marbling and therefore the most fat. Choose 'select' or 'choice' grades for a leaner cut. The leanest cuts come from the rear of the cow, literally, and include round (round steak, top round steak, bottom round roast, bottom round steak, eye round roast, eye round steak, rump roast, and tip steak), sirloin (sirloin, tenderloin/filet mignon, and top sirloin), and flank ("London broil"). Here's an example if you're still

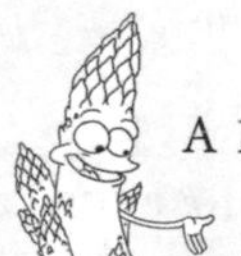

ASPARAGUS TIP

A 15-ounce can of chili beans contains 1,570 mg of sodium. Rinsing and draining the beans can reduce the sodium by 644 mg—almost 30 percent of your daily allowance of sodium.

trying to figure out what piece of beef to choose: A trimmed16-ounce prime rib has 1,000 calories and two day's worth of saturated fat. Compare that with a trimmed 12-ounce sirloin that has only 400 calories and less than half a day's saturated fat. You make the call.

The internal temperature of any cut of beef should reach a minimum of 145° F. Beef that is cooked medium or well-done should reach an internal temperature of 160° F. Remember that well-done meat is less likely to cause foodborne illness. (Probably because most people won't eat well-done meat).

BEER

Beer from yesteryear. For more than five millennia humans have treated their ailments with extraordinary creativity. For example, in 2000 B.C., Assyrian and Babylonian doctors used a salve made of frog bile and sour milk for treating infected eyes, but this concoction was considered effective only after the patient took a swig of beer chased by a slice of onion. ☺

Beer and bones. Here's a bit of research that will have all beer drinkers doing the beer barrel polka. Beer is a significant source of dietary silicon (in the form of soluble orthosilicic acid), which can increase bone mineral density. The majority of silicon in barley is in the husk, which is not greatly affected by the malting process. Pale malts have higher silicon content than the darker malts. Hops contain high levels of silicon (up to four times that found in malt) but are often used in smaller quantities than grain. The average silicon content of 100 commercial beers tested ranged from 6.4 mg/L to 56.6 mg/L. (Casey TR, Bamfort CW. *Journal of Science of Food and Agriculture,* February 9, 2010.)

BEETS

Beets and beet-red urine. Why do some individuals have 'beet-red' urine, aka "beeturia," after eating beets? It's all in the genes. A pigment in beets, betacyanin, can turn the urine beet red, but only if you have inherited both genes from your parents. The pigment can also cause feces to appear bright red. It may cause you to gasp when observing the "red" in the toilet, but it will not cause a positive fecal blood test. No worries. (And, don't tell me you don't look—everybody looks.)

Beets, the benefits. Beet greens are rich in magnesium, beta-carotene, vitamin C, and vitamin E. Beet root is rich in potassium, folic acid, and the anti-oxidant glutathione.

Belching. Taking the belch out of soda pop: If you want to lose the carbonation in your soda, pour a room temperature soft drink into a glass of ice. The radical temperature change traumatizes the carbonation ("gas") and you will lose approximately 50% of the carbonation. If you pour refrigerated soda into a chilled glass, you only lose about 10% of the carbonation. Once gas survives the initial impact of meeting the ice in the glass, it doesn't lose carbonation very quickly. Soft drinks with the most carbonation are ginger ale and lemon-lime drinks. Those with the least carbonation are soft drinks with fruit flavors (excluding lemon-lime). Colas and root beer fall in between.

Benecol. Benecol is a margarine substitute that contains plant stanol esters, a chemically altered form of a substance from pine trees. These stanol esters block the absorption of cholesterol in the digestive tract. Benecol also boosts the effects of the "statin" drugs in lowering total cholesterol (by an additional 10–12%) and lowering the LDL-cholesterol (by an additional 15–17%). (*American Journal of Cardiology* (2000);86:46–52)

Beta-carotene. Pro-vitamin A. See Chapter V.

Beverage consumption. The average American consumes over 150 gallons of liquids each year. Specifically, the average American consumes 54 gallons of soft drinks, 33 gallons of water, 23 gallons of beer, 2 gallons of wine, 20 gallons of coffee, and 19 gallons of milk.

Big Mac and super-sized fries. According to a study in *Consumer Reports on Health,* to make up for the calories in just one fast food meal composed of your basic Big Mac and super-sized fries, you would have to fast for one day and eat nary a drop of fat on the second day.

Speaking of Big Mac Attacks—three new McDonald's "fat" food restaurants come online every day. McDonald's corporate goal is to have no American more than *four* minutes from one of its restaurants. Seven percent of Americans eat at McDonald's on any given day. McDonald's corporate goal should be to have no American more than *four* minutes away from any coronary care unit.

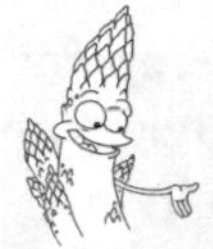

ASPARAGUS TIP

One McDonald's Big Mac and large fries is the equivalent of one cup of Crisco, or 1,040 calories and 54 grams of fat. YUCK!

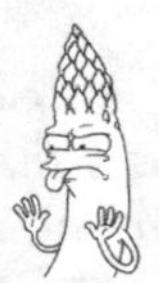

Black cohosh, visited and revisited, and visited again. Well, does it or doesn't it help hot flashes in postmenopausal women? Some studies say yes, and some studies say no. Unfortunately, conflicting studies don't tend to make reassuring data for clinical practice recommendations. To provide more definitive evidence on the effects of black cohosh on menopausal symptoms, NCCAM is funding a 12-month, randomized, placebo-controlled study to determine whether treatment with black cohosh is effective in reducing the frequency and intensity of menopausal hot flashes. The study will also assess whether black cohosh reduces the frequency of other menopausal symptoms and improves quality of life. The study will examine the possible mechanisms of action of black cohosh.

One possible mechanism of action is a presumed estrogenic activity of black cohosh. A compound recently identified in black cohosh (fukinolic acid) was shown to have estrogenic activity in the test tube. Unfortunately the evidence is contradictory. Other active compounds have also been identified.

Don't use black cohosh during pregnancy or if there is any evidence of liver disease. Women with breast cancer may want to avoid black cohosh until its effects on breast tissue are understood. Individuals who develop symptoms of liver trouble such as abdominal pain, dark urine, or jaundice while taking the supplement should discontinue use and contact their doctor. (Duke JA: Handbook of Medicinal Herbs. Boca Raton, FL: CRC Press, 2001: 120–121. Jacobson JS, Troxel AB, Evans J, et al.: Randomized trial of black cohosh for the treatment of hot flashes among women with a history of breast cancer. *Journal of Clinical Oncology* 19: 2739–2745, 2001; American College of Obstetricians and Gynecologists: Use of botanicals for management of menopausal symptoms. *ACOG Practice Bulletin* 28: 1–11, 2001)

Bilberry *(Vaccinium myrtillus.)* This blackberry is a relative of the blueberry and cranberry. It contains pectins and may be useful for your run-of-the mill basic diarrhea attack. Preliminary evidence shows that it may also be helpful in preventing and treating varicose veins, hemorrhoids, and eye conditions including diabetic retinopathy, macular degeneration, glaucoma, and cataracts. Bilberry has antioxidant properties that may contribute to its effects, especially those involving ocular conditions. As always, all botanicals/herbs should be discussed with your health care practitioner before you plunk down your hard-earned dollars.

Birdseye, Clarence. Clarence Birdseye worked for the U.S. Government as a surveyor in Labrador in 1912 and 1915. He was investigating the preservation of foods by ice when he wrote, "I saw natives catching fish in fifty-below-zero weather, which froze stiff as soon as they were taken out of the water. Months later, when they were thawed out, some of those fish were still alive." After his stint with the government, he decided to use the knowledge gained from those frozen fish and start a company that launched individually packaged boxes of peas, spinach, berries, cherries, fish, and meats. In other words, he single-handedly launched the first frozen food products in the United States.

Blueberries. When it comes to antioxidants, blueberries are one of your best choices. Blueberries placed first over more than three dozen other fruits and vegetables, including kale, strawberries, spinach, and broccoli. What is it about the blueberry that gives it that special antioxidant edge? Anthocyanin (from two Greek words meaning plant and blue) is the active ingredient that is responsible for both the blue hue of the berry and the antioxidant activity of the blueberry. Antioxidants are have been shown to play an important role in reducing DNA mutations responsible for cancer, preventing the oxidation of LDL-cholesterol that contributes to atherosclerosis and heart disease, and reduce DNA mutations responsible for aging.

Blueberries, like cranberries, can also be used as a urinary antiseptic. Blueberries also contain an unknown compound that inhibits the ability of bacteria to attach to the walls of the bladder. No attachment? No urinary tract infection.

The $64,000 question: Can eating blueberries trigger neurogenesis (the growth of new brain cells)? It appears that blueberries can trigger new neurons—but only in rats at this point. That's right! Nineteen-month-old rats that were given a blueberry enriched diet [equal to about 1 cup of blueberries per day for humans] were more skilled at navigating through mazes than rats fed the usual rat diet sans blueberries. In order to track the growth of new neurons, researchers injected a dye into rats to determine whether or not neurons were in the active phase of growth. Much to their delight, they found new brain cells in the hippocampus of the rat brain—the area of memory and learning new tasks. The next big task is determining whether or not this same effect can be observed in humans. (Tashiro A, Makino H, Gage F H. Experience-Specific Functional Modification of the Dentate Gyrus through Adult Neurogenesis: A Critical Period during an Immature Stage. *The Journal of Neuroscience*. 2007 Mar;27(13): 3252–3259.)

Blood pressure and diet. See Chapter D for the DASH diet.

Body Mass Index (BMI). The body mass index is a measure of weight relative to height, making it a crude estimate of body fat. To calculate your own BMI, multiply your weight, in pounds, by 700. Divide that number by your height in inches. Divide that number again by your height in inches. What number is staring at you from your calculator? An ideal BMI is 22. A healthy weight is a BMI of 18.5 to 25. An overweight BMI is 25 to 30. An obese BMI is 30 or higher.

What is the average American's BMI? Suffice it to say that it has changed drastically over the past 50 years. The most recent statistics from the CDC compared the height and weight of adult males and females in 1960 to the height and weight of adult males and females in 2002. The findings are discouraging to say the least.

Average Americans are about one inch taller but a whopping 25 pounds heavier than they were in 1960. This equates to an average BMI in 1960 of 25 compared to an average BMI of 28 in 2002.

Let's get gender specific, shall we? The average American woman is five-foot-four and weighs 164.3 pounds. That just happens to be a BMI of 28.1. Her optimal weight is 128 pounds, which would give her a BMI of 22. The average American man is five-feet-nine and a half and weighs 191 pounds with a BMI of 28.2. Ideally, he should weigh 150 pounds for a BMI of 22. Oh my. With 97 million Americans overweight or obese, it's tough to get a lean, mean population of perfect Americans. And it's getting tougher all the time as the weight of the average American continues to rise.

The risk of chronic diseases starts to rise with certain BMIs. Even though a BMI between 18.5 and 25 is considered to be a "healthy" number, the risk of diabetes starts to rise, especially in women, with a BMI between 22 and 25. Wow. Off we march to Weight Watchers. The risk of heart disease, stroke, and most other health problems doesn't climb until the BMI is between 25 and 27. Once you have hit a BMI of 30 or greater, the risk of all diseases skyrockets.

Children and teenagers between the age of two and nineteen have their own BMI calculator based on the CDC's BMI-for-age growth chart.

A caveat of importance: BMI is not a useful measurement for kids under the age of two, the frail elderly patient, "serious" bodybuilders, or pregnant or breast-feeding women. If you are a serious body builder the extra weight comes from muscle, not fat, and you may have a high BMI even though you're healthy. That doesn't happen to be the case for the average American, however. (*Mean Body Weight, Height and Body Mass Index (BMI) 1960–2002: United States.* Centers for Disease Control). Go to www.nhlbisupport.com/bmi/ to figure out your BMI if you're over the age of 19.

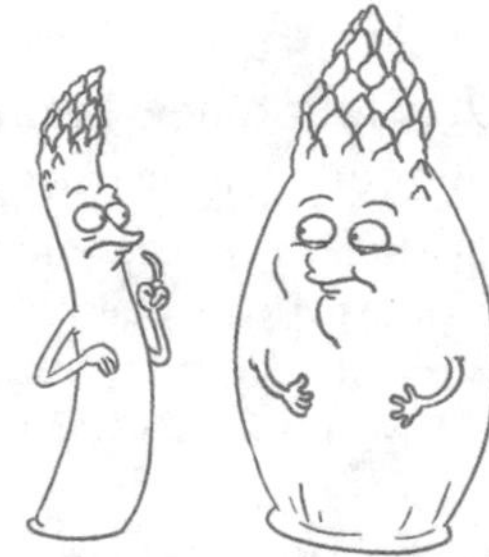

Booze. Why do we call liquor booze? One theory has it that it came from the old English term *bousen* which means to "drink deeply" or "carouse." The English used *bouse* to refer to ale or beer. The other theory is an American tale. In the mid-1800s there was a Kentucky colonel distiller named Booze who sold whiskey under his own name, Booze.

Botox. Botox is a purified, low concentrate form of botulinum toxin Q, a toxin produced by *C. botulinum,* the bacteria that cause botulism food poisoning. Botox is injected under the skin to reduce wrinkles. Toxin Q blocks a chemical that signals the muscles to contract, so the skin flattens and appears smoother. Millions of Americans have used this cosmetic to reduce wrinkles without any adverse effects. However, if used incorrectly it can be dangerous. If the toxin spreads beyond the treatment area, botulism-like symptoms may occur, including difficulty swallowing, slurred speech and breathing problems. If you are considering using Botox as a wrinkle reducer, make sure you find an experienced plastic surgeon or dermatologist to administer the toxin.

BOTULISM

Botulism. The agent of botulism food poisoning, *Clostridium botulinum,* is too small to be seen with the naked eye, yet a 12-ounce glass of the toxin it produces would kill every human being living on the face of the earth—7,052,166, 744 (7 billion, 52 million, 166 thousand, 744)—as of 1:53 p.m. July 8, 2012. Foodborne botulism results from contaminated foodstuffs in which *Clostridium botulinum* spores have been allowed to germinate in anaerobic conditions. This typically occurs in home-canned food substances and fermented uncooked dishes. Usually multiple people consume food from the same source; therefore, it is common for numerous unsuspecting individuals to be affected simultaneously. It takes 3–5 days for the symptoms to manifest after the exposure to *C. botulinum.* Symptoms of botulism include: difficulty swallowing, facial weakness, blurred vision, droopy eyelids, difficulty breathing, vomiting, abdominal cramping and paralysis. Yikes.

Botulism, honey, and infants. Infant botulism was first recognized in 1976, and is the most common form of botulism in the United States. There are 80–100 diagnosed cases of infant botulism in the United States each year with more than 90% of the cases occurring in infants younger than six months. Honey is the only known dietary reservoir of *Clostridium botulinum* spores linked to infant botulism. Eating honey in both natural and processed forms can lead to serious disease and even death in infants. Because of the environment in which it's produced, unprocessed honey often contains spores of the bacteria that cause botulism. The same can be true for processed honey. It contains *C. botulinum* spores. The spores cause no problems in children older than one and adults. Why? Because the immune systems of kids older than one and adults release binding proteins that neutralize the *C. botulinum* toxin. The GI tracts of children under one year of age are too immature to produce the proteins needed to neutralize and destroy the toxin. Once the toxin enters the bloodstream after being absorbed through the GI tract, it binds to receptors on skeletal muscle and results in paralysis. Within hours of ingesting the contaminated honey, infants become lethargic, flaccid, and can develop respiratory arrest. If the diagnosis is made early, the prognosis for a full recovery is excellent. (Sobel J. Botulism. *Clin. Infect. Dis.* 2005 (October);41 (8):1167–73. Arnon SS. Infant Botulism: In Feigin RD, CherryJ D, Demmler GJ,

Kaplan SL., eds. Textbook of Pediatric Infectious Diseases. 5th edition Philadelphia, PA: WB Saunders; 2004:1758–1766; 122;e73–e82)

Botulism and baked potatoes—a deadly combination. Contrary to popular belief, not all food poisoning from botulism is due to improper home canning. The CDC (Centers for Disease Control) reported an outbreak of botulism in April 1994 in El Paso caused by potatoes that had been baked in aluminum foil.

Potatoes, like all vegetables that are grown underground, can be easily contaminated with *Clostridium botulinum*. Washing, scrubbing, and proper cooking can usually kill the spores of *C. botulinum*. However, when potatoes are wrapped in aluminum foil, the foil reflects heat and prevents the potato from getting hot enough to kill all bacterial contaminants. Paradoxically, the heat kills off competing bacteria, making it easier for the *C. botulinum* to grow. Moreover, foil-wrapped potatoes kept at room temperature provide an oxygen-free environment needed for germination of the spores. So beware of the restaurant menu that says baked potatoes will be available after 5 p.m. This most likely means that the potato has been foil-wrapped, partially baked, un-foil-wrapped, and then microwaved right before the potato hits your plate. (Angulo FJ, et al. A large outbreak of botulism: The hazardous baked potato. *Journal of Infectious Dis* 1998;178:172–77; Baked potatoes in foil can be deadly. *Environmental Nutrition,* January 1999).

Bourbon. The manufacturers of Old Grand-Dad bourbon were able to produce their whiskey during Prohibition by labeling the beverage "For Medicinal Purposes Only." Brilliant.

BREAD

Bread. Bread comes in all shapes, sizes, colors and tastes, from banana nut to pumpernickel to rye to sourdough to whole wheat to just plain old white bread. Even ethnic groups have their own breads—notably Italian bread, French bread, and Pakistani tandoori naan. Each type of bread contains varying amounts of proteins, calories, fats, and salt.

Enriched white bread and whole wheat bread are virtually identical as far as the proteins, fats, and carbohydrates contained within; however, white bread has only half the amount of dietary fiber as whole wheat bread. All breads are high-carbohydrate foods and are considered to be good sources of B vitamins, including folate. In 1998, the Food and Drug Administration (FDA) mandated that folate be added to flour, rice, and other grain products, which include bread, to help protect against neural tube defects during pregnancy. Bread is a fairly good source of calcium, magnesium, and phosphorus; however, the amounts vary depending on the ingredients used. For example, some bread is made with milk, making the bread a great source of calcium.

HISTORICAL HIGHLIGHT

One of the superstitions of the bread world says that if bread does not rise, the devil is hiding in the oven. To protect from the devil, cooks began cutting a cross on top of their loaves to force the devil out and help the bread rise.

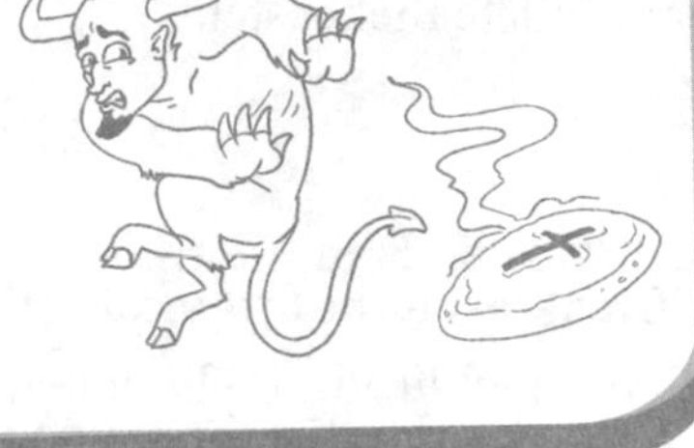

In the 1500s bread was served according to status. The working class consumed the burnt bottom of the loaf, the family ate the middle of the loaf, and the guests received the top of the loaf, or the "upper crust."

All commercially made breads are high in sodium, so if you want low sodium bread you should probably make your own. By making your own bread, you can vary the amounts of salt, sugar, fat, and fiber. One missing amino acid from bread is lysine—so it is best to serve foods with bread that contain this essential missing amino acid. And that's easy. Just add milk, cheese, eggs (how about an egg salad sandwich?), meat, fish, or poultry.

Food was a very big factor in Christianity. What would the miracle of the loaves and fishes be without it? And the Last Supper— how effective would that have been? —Fran Leibowitz

---

One amino acid that is abundant in bread is tryptophan. When you mix the high carbohydrate content of bread with the tryptophan, you get a naturally occurring calming effect in the brain. The amino acid tryptophan is the major precursor to serotonin in the brain. The carbohydrate helps to "carry" the tryptophan into the brain where it is converted into serotonin, the calming neurotransmitter. This calmness translates to "comfort," so many folks, especially women, will eat lots of bread when they need to be "comforted."

Bread and the Maillard reaction. Impress every one of your friends by telling them that you will be performing a chemical reaction in the kitchen known as the Maillard reaction, named after the French chemist who first identified it. As the drum rolls, the suspense heightens, the group waits with bated breath, two pieces of toast will pop out of the toaster and you will exclaim Voilà! Zee Maillard reaction!!

Yes, the Maillard reaction is also known as toasting bread. It is a chemical process by which the sugars and amino acids are caramelized on the surface of the bread, turning it golden brown. One of the side effects of toasting is a change in the nutrient value of bread. The proteins are inactivated and the sugars turn into fiber. However, it remains to be seen as to whether or not the fiber produced by the toasting process has any nutritional value. Some experts are concerned about the carcinogenic potential of toasted bread. Get over it. This risk is a non-issue and should not make you race to the kitchen to annihilate the toaster.

BREAKFAST

Breakfast is the first meal of the day, consumed in the morning. The word is a compound of "break" and "fast," referring to the conclusion of fasting since the last meal of the previous day.

Breakfast…what drugs should be taken PRIOR to breakfast? Certain drugs are best taken before "breaking the fast." For example, the drugs taken for osteoporosis, drugs taken for GERD, drugs taken for diabetes, and drugs taken for hypothyroidism should all be taken prior to a meal, and most should be taken prior to breakfast. The reasons are many, and each drug has its own reason.

The bisphosphonates, aka the "dronates," are prescribed for the prevention and treatment of osteoporosis. Their brand names are familiar to one and all—Fosamax (alendronate), Actonel (risedronate), and Boniva (ibandronate), quickly come to mind.

These drugs are highly erosive to the esophagus and need to be taken with a full glass of water (not tea, not coffee, not milk, not prune juice) 30 to 60 minutes before breakfast. Not only must one take this class of pills with water 30 to 60 minutes prior to breakfast, one must also remain in an upright position so that the pill can zip quickly through the esophagus and land unceremoniously in the stomach. If any one of these pills remains in the esophagus for a lengthy period of time, the pill may cause esophageal erosion (or ulceration). The erosion may lead to a ruptured esophagus. Ouch.

The proton pump inhibitors, or the "prazoles," also known as the drugs taken for gastroesophageal reflux disease (GERD), must also be taken 30 to 60 minutes prior to breakfast. Who are the "prazoles"? Omeprazole (Prilosec), lansoprazole (Prevacid), esomeprazole (Nexium), pantoprazole (Protonix), dexlansoprazole (Dexilant) and rabeprazole (Aciphex). The rationale is completely different from the osteoporosis drugs, but equally important. The "prazoles" inhibit an active proton pump in the stomach that pumps acid into the lumen of the stomach immediately after a meal. Taking the pill 30 to 60 minutes prior to the meal ensures that the peak serum concentration of the drug coincides with maximal acid secretion. Acid just so happens to be the culprit that causes the burning in the esophagus. No acid? No GERD. It's as simple as that. It usually takes 3 to 4 days of daily medication before the PPIs exhibit their full benefit. So why do hospitals give the proton pump inhibitors at 9 a.m., two hours after breakfast? Beats me, but that's why patients complain that the drug is "not working." Timing is *everything.* (Hatlebakk JG, Katz PO, Camacho-Lobato L, Castell DO. Proton pump inhibitors: better acid suppression when taken before a meal than without a meal. *Aliment Pharmacol Ther* 2000;14:1267–72; Sachs G, Shin JM, Howden CW. Review article: The clinical pharmacology of proton pump inhibitors. *Aliment Pharmacol Ther* 2006;23(Suppl 2):2–8)

Individuals with hypothyroidism are encouraged to take their thyroid replacement pill, usually levothyroxine (generic) or brand names, Levothroid, Levoxyl, Synthroid, or Unithroid in the morning before breakfast. Thyroid hormone is best absorbed on an empty stomach with a full glass of water 30 minutes prior to food intake. So, can you take the thyroid replacement pill before dinner? Sure...however, with thyroid replacement therapy, remember that consistency is the best policy. If you feel better taking it prior to supper and you can remain consistent with this regimen, by all means do so. Even though timing is important, the thyroid replacement pill should also be taken alone—in other words, no other drugs, no supplements such as calcium and iron, and certain foods (soy, fiber, coffee) may affect the absorption or interfere with the metabolism of levothyroxine. (Treatment Guidelines for the Medical Letter 2009 (August);7(84):58)

Insulin is another drug that should be administered prior to meals. Insulin requirements vary according to the patient's weight, time of day, amount of carbohydrates, and length of time the patient has had diabetes. As a general rule of thumb, patients need to inject rapid-acting insulin (Lyspro/Aspart/Glulisine) 5 to 15 minutes prior to the meal and regular insulin 30 to 60 minutes prior to a meal. The other rule of thumb is the carbohydrate to unit ratio. Generally, one unit of rapid-acting insulin will dispose of 12 to 15 grams of carbohydrate. This range can vary from 6 to 30 grams or more of carbohydrate depending on an individual's sensitivity to insulin.

Breakfast, don't skip it ladies. Researchers from the University of Nottingham fed 10 healthy women, ages 19–38, breakfast for two weeks. They skipped breakfast for the next two weeks, while the researchers monitored their daily calorie intakes, lipid profiles and insulin levels. They found that when women skipped breakfast, they ate an average of 100 more calories per day, had 10% higher levels of circulating insulin, 9% higher total cholesterol, and 17% higher LDL-cholesterol. YIKES. Eat breakfast! (*Am J Clin Nutr,* February 2005)

Breakfast and cognition in school-aged children. Wouldn't it be nice if something as simple as breakfast would save our ailing educational system and flagging student performances? Previous studies have demonstrated that increases in serum glucose improve learning and memory in humans and rodents. The converse is also true in that the lack of nourishment has been shown to adversely affect the cognitive function in school-aged children. A study in the October 1996 *Archives of Pediatric and Adolescent Medicine* examined the effects of breakfast on short-term cognitive function in children.

The study included approximately 500 Israeli children, aged 11–13, from varying socioeconomic backgrounds. Two-thirds of the children received a bowl of sugared flakes and a glass of whole milk at school for two weeks, while the remaining children ate their usual breakfast at home or skipped breakfast. Both groups were given a battery of cognitive tests at baseline and after the two-week trial period.

After the two-week trial period, children who ate breakfast at school and tested shortly after scored significantly higher on almost all the tests than children who missed breakfast or who ate breakfast at home one to two hours before the test. There were no differences in test scores between the children who missed breakfast and the children who ate breakfast at home.

It appears as if a burst of glucose shortly before cognitive testing improves intellectual performance. Further studies are needed to evaluate the relative effects of meal content and timing on performance. (Vaisaman N, et al. Effect of breakfast timing on cognitive functions of elementary school students. *Archives of Pediatrics and Adolescent Medicine* 1996 (October);150 (10):1089–1092; Ramperaud GC et al. Breakfast habits, nutritional status, body weight, and academic performance in children and adolescents. *J Am Diet Assoc* 2005;105:743–760.)

Continental breakfasts are very sparse. My advice is to go right to lunch without pausing. —Miss Piggy

---

Breakfast of champions. After a good night's sleep, you should "break the fast" with a nutritious and delicious high-powered breakfast to start your day. The best combination to fuel your brain and body is a breakfast consisting of complex carbohydrates (whole grains, fruit), protein (lean meat and dairy), and some fat (margarine, nuts). This combination keeps your blood sugar from skyrocketing and then falling precipitously, and gives you long-lasting energy needed to make it through the hectic morning. Try one or more of these tasty combinations:

1) Whole grain cereal with skim milk and a big 'ol banana with a smidgen of peanut butter, or
2) A whole wheat pita stuffed with tomato slices and low fat mozzarella cheese zapped in the microwave, or
3) Whole grain oatmeal made with low-fat milk and topped with a sprinkling of chopped dates and walnuts.

Any of the above three taste treats will jump start your morning and have a lasting effect until lunchtime. (Joan Salge Blake, M.S., R.D.)

Breakfast and the blues. Having breakfast on a daily basis helps to keep depression away. Researchers reporting in the *International Journal of Food Sciences and Nutrition* found that adults 20–79 years of age who eat breakfast daily tend to feel less depressed, less stressed, and have lower levels of emotional distress than people who don't eat breakfast every day. In addition, the research showed that persons who eat breakfast also tend not to smoke, drink less alcohol, and follow a healthier diet. (Smith AP. Breakfast and mental health. *Intl J of Food Sciences and Nutr* 1998 (September);6:397)

Breakfast and weight gain. Study after study has correlated skipping breakfast with weight gain not only in children but also adolescents and adults. BMIs were found to be higher in all groups if breakfast was deleted from the daily meals. So if you're trying to lose weight, don't skip breakfast! (Purslow LR, et al. Energy intake at breakfast and weight change: Prospective study of 6,764 middle-aged men and women. *Am J of Epidem* 2004;167(2):188–92; Affenito SG. Breakfast: a missed opportunity. *Journal of the American Dietetic Association* 2007;107 (4):565–569)

Breast milk fatty acids and IQ tests in infants. Babies fed formula enriched with two fatty acids found in breast milk—DHA (docosahexanoic acid, an omega-3 fatty acid) and arachidonic acid—performed better on tests of mental development than babies fed plain formula. The test used was similar to the IQ test with 100 points being the average score. The mean result for babies fed with the supplemented formula was 105 compared to a score of 98 for the babies fed plain formula. The spread of scores was also an eye-opener: 26% of the infants on the "breast milk formula" scored over 115, compared to only 5% of those on plain formula. Ten percent of the babies on plain formula scored below 85; none in the enriched formula group scored this low. (*Developmental Medicine and Child Neurology,* March 2000)

Brewer's yeast. As the name implies, brewer's yeast was originally identified as a primary ingredient in the beer-making process. Brewer's yeast is a single-celled fungi *(Saccharomyces cerevisiae)* specifically grown as a nutritional supplement rich in chromium, selenium, proteins, and B-complex vitamins. Vegetarians are well-aware of the B12 component of brewer's yeast, as it is one of the important non meat sources of B12.

Brewer's yeast is a probiotic, living naturally in the digestive tract. As a dietary supplement, brewer's yeast is a non-living dried product with numerous benefits. The substantial amount of chromium in brewer's yeast contributes to decreasing insulin resistance, potentiating insulin receptors, and increasing beta-cell function of the pancreas. Does this mean brewer's yeast can be substituted for the pills used to treat type 2 diabetes or insulin? No, not at all. However, it does mean that a diabetic should be careful when taking brewer's yeast as the blood sugar may drop to hypoglycemic levels.

Other functions of brewer's yeast include boosting the immune system, reducing the symptoms of PMS, and triggering apoptosis in metastatic breast cancer cells. Combining brewer's yeast with antibiotics for the treatment of *Clostridium difficile* antibiotic-associated diarrhea has been shown to reduce the duration of symptoms as well as the rate of infection recurrence.

If you're interested in taking a brewer's yeast supplement, the daily dose is 500 mg. It comes in tablets, flakes, powders, and liquids. Consult your healthcare practitioner before starting brewer's yeast—you may be taking a prescription drug that will interact with this supplement. (Kovacs DJ, Berk T. Recurrent *Clostridium difficile*-associated diarrhea and colitis treated with *Saccharomyces cerevisiae* in combination with antibiotic therapy: a case report. *J Am Board Fam Pract.* 2000;13:138–140; Sego S. Brewer's yeast. *The Clinical Advisor.* August, 2011;116–18)

BROCCOLI

Broccoli. The word "broccoli" derives from the Latin word brachium, meaning "branch" or "arm."

Italians brought broccoli to New York City in the 1920s and it has taken on a life of its own in this country. The average American today consumes *900* percent (no, this is not a typing error) more broccoli than the average American consumed in 1980. Broccoli is a potent anti-cancer agent in that its phytochemicals neutralize carcinogens. Broccoli is an excellent source of fiber, vitamin C, potassium, and folic acid. And, it only has 45 calories to boot. Sound too good to be true? Well, it's not. Broccoli packs a powerful nutritious punch.

If you are planning to get your daily calcium intake from devouring broccoli florets, you had better think again. One cup of cooked broccoli (stems and florets) has 70 mg of calcium. Assuming that you are planning on getting all of your calcium from broccoli, you would need to consume approximately 17 cups of broccoli per day. You can cut this number considerably if you skip the stems and only eat the floret part of the broccoli. The florets contain 7–8 times more calcium than the stems. You eat the florets, give the stems to your children.

Even though broccoli isn't your best bet for calcium, the other benefits of broccoli are numerous. One cup of broccoli is an excellent source of fiber (5 grams), vitamin A (50% of Daily Value), folate (23% of Daily Value), vitamin C (170% of Daily Value), and potassium (505 mg or 8% of Daily Value). It also has a smidgen of vitamins E and K and hardly any calories (44 calories in that one cup). Lutein and beta carotene are abundant and help to prevent the "wet" type of macular degeneration.

ASPARAGUS TIP

A March 2007 study in the Journal of Food Science examined the effects of boiling, steaming, microwaving and pressure cooking on the nutrients in broccoli. Steaming and boiling caused a 22 percent to 34 percent loss of vitamin C. Microwaved vegetables and pressure-cooked vegetables retained 90 percent of their vitamin C.

To benefit from all the vitamins and minerals contained in broccoli, make sure you eat it raw, since raw broccoli has up to 40% more vitamin C than broccoli that has been cooked or frozen. Another way to save the goodies in broccoli is to let the water boil for 60 seconds prior to putting it in the pot. Broccoli will lose large amounts of vitamin C if you start cooking it in cold water. You can also zap it in the microwave to retain the health benefits. One other note, cooking makes the beta carotene and lutein more readily available to protect the eyes. Perhaps rotating raw broccoli with the cooked broccoli might be the way to go.

The American Cancer Society claims that certain phytochemicals (phyto=plant) in broccoli are thought to have anti-cancer properties. Other compounds, isothiocyanates, including sulforaphane and indole-3-carbinol (I3C), have been shown to be potent antioxidants and to possibly have anti-cancer properties as well. A 2005 European study found that people who ate cruciferous vegetables at least weekly were 72% less at risk for lung cancer (broccoli belongs to the group of "cruciferous" vegetables named for their cross-shaped flowers). An April 2008 study by the Roswell Park Cancer Institute also found a protective benefit against bladder cancer from raw cruciferous vegetables.

For the record, it's the sulforaphanes that give broccoli its sulfa-smelling, flatus/gas-producing properties.

In addition to their foul-smelling properties, the sulforaphanes have been shown to inhibit the growth of *Helicobacter pylori,* the bacteria responsible for stomach and duodenal ulcers and the culprit in stomach cancer. This compound was shown to kill the bacteria inside the gastric cells, where antibiotics may not be able to reach. The researchers suggested that eating broccoli along with taking antibiotics to eradicate *H. pylori* might have a synergistic effect in patients who don't respond to antibiotics alone. (*Proceedings from the National Academy of Science,* May 28, 2002)

If you are a broccoli fan, give a shout-out to California. California produces 90% of all broccoli consumed in the United States. (American Cancer Society, 2010)

If broccoli is sooooooooo perfect, why doesn't everyone like it? The most famous person to dislike broccoli was none other than George H. W. Bush, the 41st President of the U.S., when he famously proclaimed: "I do not like broccoli. And I haven't like it since I was a little kid and my mother made me eat it. And I'm the President of the United States and I'm not going to eat any more broccoli."

OK, OK, OK! How about trying a few of broccoli's closest relatives? Of course, just the botanical names might scrunch your nose up—broccoflower is a hybrid that obviously blends broccoli and cauliflower; broccolini is another hybrid with broccoli and Chinese kale—looks like broccoli that has been put on the rack and stretched; broccoli rabe—a nutty, bitter green that has a very distant relationship to broccoli—kind of like a cousin ten-times removed; Chinese kale is known as Chinese broccoli and is sweeter than broccoli, but has a similar taste; Romanesca is also known as "Romanesca cauliflower" or Romanesca broccoli" and some describe it as a blend of tastes of sweet corn, green beans and cauliflower. Hmmmmm…interested, George?

Brussels sprouts. Another member of the cruciferous family, Brussels sprouts has the distinct pleasure of being the most hated food in the U.S. according to a 2008 survey. If, however, you love your Brussels sprouts, be assured that they are packed with lutein (for the eyes), and vitamins C and K, and they only have 60 calories per cup.

"Yuck," you say, "they have a bitter taste." Ah, but they don't if you buy dark, tightly closed sprouts about an inch in diameter with no yellow or brown spots. Don't let them hang out in the refrigerator either…eat them within in a day or two of purchase and you'll be surprised at how tasty they can be.

Buffet. For the cafeterias and buffet restaurants around the world, we have Pierre Buffet to thank. The seventeenth-century Parisian gambler allowed his guests to serve themselves food from a side table. With that, the food self-service concept was born and Pierre's name would forever be associated with it.

Bulimia Nervosa. ("Hunger like an ox due to a mental disorder.") Bulimia nervosa is an eating disorder characterized by episodic patterns of binge or compulsive eating, frequently followed by purging (self-induced vomiting) or other efforts to control body weight such as the use of laxatives and diuretics, and periods of fasting and excessive exercise. Ninety percent of bulimics are females, most often between the ages of 13 and 25. High-risk individuals include teenage girls with poor self-images who come from a relatively high socioeconomic class. Individuals with bulimia are afraid of becoming fat; however, they will consume huge quantities of calories (5,000 to 20,000) during a single binge. Most of the foods consumed are "comfort foods": sweet foods high in calories, or smooth, soft foods like ice cream, cake, mashed potatoes, pasta, and pastry.

The binge is followed by the purge or by using 20 or more laxatives per day. Patients with bulimia may have problems with dehydration or depletion of essential electrolytes such as hydrogen and chloride from the vomiting, or depletion of sodium and potassium from the diuretic and laxative abuse. Tooth decay and erosion of the enamel are common and are caused by regurgitated stomach acid. Excoriation of the back of the first two fingers on the dominant hand is also common due to the self-induced vomiting. Other common findings in bulimics include depression, anxiety, social phobias, or panic disorder. In addition, bulimics tend to engage in other addictive behaviors such as drug or alcohol abuse. Be especially wary of the type 1 diabetic female who presents with wide swings in glycemic control. Some studies have indicated as many as 33–77% are bulimic. These young girls will deliberately withhold their insulin to induce weight loss, resulting in hyperglycemia and diabetic ketoacidosis. Or, they will take their insulin, eat, and purge. The result is excess insulin for the amount of food absorbed, resulting in very low blood sugar, or hypoglycemia. (Rosenthal, M.S. The Gastrointestinal Sourcebook. Los Angeles: The Lowell House, 1997.)

You know, I know everybody, um...has kind of nicknamed me the butter queen. —Paula Deen, "The Butter Queen"

Butter bits.

...it takes 21 pounds of milk to make one pound of butter.

...the U.S. produces more than 1.2 billion pounds of butter per year.

...the Average American consumes more than 4 pounds of butter per person per year.

...1 tablespoon of butter is 100 calories; 99% of the calories come from saturated fat.

...butter in the refrigerator stays fresh for one month.

...butter stored in the freezer stays fresh for four months.

Butterbur for migraine prevention. Guidelines recently published by the American Academy of Neurology have recommended the herbal product Petasites (butterbur) for the prevention of migraine headaches. (AAN Guidelines, www.aan.com April 12, 2012)

CHAPTER C

Only Irish coffee provides in a single glass all four essential food groups: alcohol, caffeine, sugar, and fat.

—Anonymous

CABBAGE

Cabbage and arthritis. Peel off two of the large outer leaves of a green cabbage and use a rolling pin to bruise them. Warm the leaves in a microwave, steamer, or oven. Wrap the leaves around the painful joints for 15 minutes and repeat the process 2–3 times per day. A similar process can be used for back pain—make a compress with the bruised cabbage leaves and apply it to the painful area of the back for one hour (do not warm the leaves for the back application). (Michael Van Straten, DN)

Cabbage and breast inflammation (mastitis). Well, if cabbage can do the trick for an "itis" of the joints, it can also do the trick for an "itis" of the breasts. Head back to the produce department for another head of green cabbage. There's nothing like using a head of green cabbage to alleviate the pain and swelling of mastitis in breast-feeding moms. One small randomized trial in the June 1993 issue of *Birth* suggests that the use of cool cabbage leaves reduces the perception of engorgement and more than doubles the likelihood that a patient will continue to breast-feed up to eight weeks postpartum. Lactation experts recommend using a partially frozen cabbage and peeling the leaves off to wrap around the breast. The leaves are held in place with a brassiere and changed for cooler leaves when necessary. (Cheryl V, et al. Do cabbage leaves prevent breast engorgement? A randomized, controlled study. *Birth* 20;1993 (June):61–64)

Cabbage, the Chinese way. Tired of cauliflower and broccoli? Try a few of the delicious Chinese cabbage varieties. There are numerous varieties of Chinese cabbages and they all have the same health benefits as their cousins in the cruciferous vegetable family. To add a bit of variety to your plate, pick up Bok Choy, Chinese Oil Vegetable Cabbage, Napa Cabbage, Shanghai Bok

Choy, or Tientsin Cabbage. A personal favorite is Bok Choy, sprayed with a bit of olive oil, add a dash of sea salt, and toss on the grill for a few minutes. Delicious and nutritious.

CAFFEINE

Caffeine. Caffeine is a stimulant that influences the activity of pathways in the central and peripheral nervous systems. Caffeine is defined as an ergogenic compound that raises the heart rate and blood pressure. Ergogenic is defined as an external influence that enhances performance. Caffeine has been shown to be an effective ergogenic compound for athletes when ingested before or during exercise in moderate quantities. To obtain maximum effects on exercise performance, abstain from all caffeine for 7 days prior to the big event. On the day of the event, consuming caffeine at a dose of 3–6 mg/kg, will enhance the performance. Think twice before you do this if you are training for an Olympic event. Yeah right, but if you are…caffeine is on the list of banned substances by the International Olympic Committee.

Caffeine in a cuppa joe. Each year Americans drink about 127 billion cups of coffee. Twenty-five percent of those cups are decaffeinated. *Here's the scoop:*

- Drip coffee contains 150 mg of caffeine per 5-ounce cup
- Percolated coffee contains 100 mg of caffeine per 5-ounce cup
- Decaffeinated coffee contains 3 mg of caffeine per 5-ounce cup

Caffeine as a diuretic—the myth. Caffeinated drinks do not dehydrate you. This myth has been propagated for years in the literature and on the Internet. A 2006 study from the Institute of Medicine debunked this myth. (Journal of the American College of Nutrition. 2006; 9:59)

Caffeine Quips.

- Most adults can safely consume up to 400 mg/day of caffeine…about three 8 ounce cups of coffee.
- Keep caffeine amounts under 45 mg/day for kids around 4 years old and 85 mg per day for 12 year-olds.
- Studies suggest that extroverted people are less sensitive to caffeine's effects than introverts.
- Pain relievers fortified with caffeine have proven to be more effective than pain relievers without caffeine. Excedrin Extra Strength, two tablets, has 130 mg of caffeine, about the same amount in a 16-ounce Starbucks Vanilla Latte (Grande), or a 16-ounce Full Throttle energy drink, or two cans of Mountain Dew.
- The robusta coffee beans used in less expensive brands of coffee contain almost twice as much caffeine as the arabica beans preferred by coffee

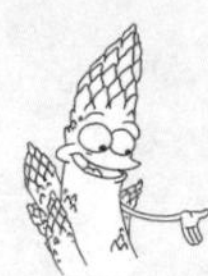

ASPARAGUS TIP

When drinking a cup of caffeinated coffee the maximum peak plasma concentration occurs in exactly 29.8 minutes.

connoisseurs. In other words, cheap coffee gives you a bigger buzz than your $5.00 grande mucho dinero coffee.

- Military studies of subjects who hadn't slept for 48 hours showed that 600 mg of caffeine improved alertness and mood as much as 20 mg of amphetamine.
- Going without caffeine for a day and a half increases blood flow to the brain (cerebral vasodilation), which may explain caffeine-deprived pounding headaches.
- Caffeine might wake you up but it won't make you sober. Actually it might make you think you are sober. Researchers from Temple University found that caffeine given to mice (the equivalent of between one and eight cups of coffee for humans) made the mice more alert but did nothing to reverse the cognitive impairment caused by the alcohol.
- Four days after quitting smoking, a smoker retains 46 per cent more caffeine from a cup of coffee. Why? By-products of cigarette smoke speed the breakdown of caffeine in the blood. Smokers clear caffeine much faster than nonsmokers. This just means that smokers need to drink more coffee to maintain their caffeine high.
- Pharmaceutical companies have to label the amount of caffeine in their offerings, but food and beverage companies do not. The following are a few familiar products and the approximate amount of caffeine contained in the specified amount:

Hershey's milk chocolate almond bar, 6 ounces	25 mg
Expresso, 1-oz shot	40 mg
Brewed tea, 8-oz cup	50 mg
Coca-Cola, 20 oz. bottle	57 mg
Wal-Mart's Sam's cola, 12 oz. can	13 mg
Red Bull energy drink, 8.3 oz. can	80 mg
Excedrin pain reliever, 2 tablets	130 mg
Brewed coffee, 12-oz cup	200 mg
Mountain Dew 64-oz Double Big Gulp	294 mg

CALCIUM

Calcium-containing foods. By now everyone should know that eating foods containing calcium is much more beneficial and most likely safer than taking calcium in supplements (more on that topic in a moment). Keep the following list handy when your nagging nurse practitioner tells you to eat more calcium-containing foods…Ok…Ok…Ok…

DAIRY products

Food	Calcium
Part skim ricotta cheese 1 cup	669 mg
Plain, low-fat yogurt 8 oz.	415 mg
Low- or non-fat milk 1 cup	305 mg
Swiss cheese 1 oz.	272 mg
Low-fat cottage cheese 1 cup	207 mg
Part-skim mozzarella 1 oz.	207 mg
Provolone cheese 1 oz.	210 mg
Cheddar cheese 1 oz.	204 mg

So, you can't eat dairy products because of a condition known as lactose intolerance? Try some of the following:

GRAINS and NUTS

Food	Calcium
Almonds 1 ounce	75 mg
Total brand Raisin Bran 1 cup	238 mg
Corn Flakes 1 cup	237 mg

VEGETABLES

Food	Calcium
Black-eyed peas 1 cup	211 mg
Broccoli 1 cup	62 mg
Collard greens 1 cup	357 mg
Spinach, frozen 1 cup	277 mg
Soybeans, green (edamame)1 cup	261 mg
White beans 1 cup	191 mg

FISH

Food	Calcium
Ocean perch 3 ounces	116 mg
Salmon 3 ounces	181 mg

(ods.od.nih.gov/factsheets/calcium.asp)

Can eating calcium-containing foods or supplements trigger weight loss? The March 2009 *British Journal of Nutrition* reported that adding calcium supplements to the diets of obese women with low calcium intake helped to curtail their appetites. Among the women with the lowest calcium intake to start with—600 mg daily—those taking the calcium supplement lost an average of more than 13 pounds compared to about 2 pounds for the placebo group. The researchers hypothesize that the brain detects a lack of calcium and ramps up the hunger signal to increase food intake. However, if there is enough calcium on board, so to speak, the brain says that it's not necessary to scarf down more food. Hunger pangs will subsequently dissipate along with the weight. Yeah, when pigs fly.

A study by Zemel et al. reported another possible mechanism for weight loss. Apparently calcium discourages fat storage and encourages fat breakdown. Got skim milk? (Zemel MB et al. Regulation of adiposity by dietary calcium. *Federation of the American Society of Experimental Biology,* 2000 (June);14:1132–38)

Calcium and colon/breast cancer prevention. "Dairy food, which is relatively high in potentially anticarcinogenic ('against cancer') nutrients such as calcium, vitamin D, and conjugated linoleic acid, has been postulated to protect against the development of colorectal and breast cancer." (Yikyung Park, ScD, National Cancer Institute. *Archives of Internal Medicine,* February 23, 2009)

Calcium supplements. If you decide to take calcium supplements instead of eating foods high in calcium, what type of supplements should you take? Dr. Robert Heaney from Creighton University in Omaha, NE, states that the type of calcium is not that important. He wants you to make sure that you get *enough* calcium. Other experts challenge his opinion and prefer that you choose a specific type of calcium supplements based on certain variables. Read on.

In other words, is calcium citrate better than calcium carbonate? Is calcium carbonate better than calcium lactate but not as good as calcium phosphate? Jeez. Each type of calcium supplement has varying amounts of elemental calcium. So, when choosing a calcium supplement, *read the label.* Look for the term elemental calcium on the label. The number next to this phrase tells you how much calcium your body will absorb from each pill.

Here's the scoop. Calcium is always bound to another substance. In other words, you can bind calcium to carbonate, lactate, citrate, or phosphate. Calcium carbonate has a higher amount of elemental calcium than calcium citrate, which in turn has a higher amount of elemental calcium than calcium lactate. Calcium carbonate has 40% elemental calcium whereas calcium citrate has 20% elemental calcium. Let's do the math. A 500 mg pill of calcium carbonate has 40% elemental calcium or 200 mg of elemental calcium per pill (40% x 500 mg = 200 mg); a 500 mg pill of calcium citrate has 20% elemental calcium or 100 mg of elemental calcium per pill (20% x 500 = 100 mg). You will have to take twice as many calcium citrate pills to get the same amount of elemental calcium that you get from a calcium carbonate pill. So, we're back to the age-old advice—*read the label.*

The following are some rules about calcium consumption:

1) If at all possible, rely on calcium-rich foods as your major source of calcium: one cup of frozen yogurt (900 mg); one cup of calcium-fortified Lactaid nonfat milk (500 mg); one cup of yogurt, non-fat plain (350-400 mg); 1 cup of fat-free or 1% milk (300 mg) are all excellent choices. Even a cup of spinach contains 277 mg of calcium.

2) Avoid natural sources of calcium like bone meal, dolomite, and oyster shell that don't have the USP label*. These may contain toxic amounts of lead, which, over time, can lead to cognitive impairment. In other words, you have strong bones—but you are clueless as to how you got them.

3) The body best absorbs calcium when it is taken several times a day in amounts of not more than 500 mg. If you can only take it once a day, then

taking it all at once is better than not taking it at all. Calcium supplements must be taken at least 6 days a week or the full benefits will not be received.

4) Calcium carbonate is best taken with food whereas calcium citrate can be taken on a full stomach or an empty stomach.

5) Calcium citrate is less constipating than calcium carbonate.

6) Another type of calcium supplement is called chelated calcium. It is well-absorbed and it is not associated with constipation, but is more expensive and twice the size of calcium carbonate. It also requires a high pill count to achieve the same dose, so compliance flies right out the window.

ASPARAGUS TIP

Products with the USP designation meet the standards of manufacture, including dissolvability, set by the United States Pharmacopoeia (USP), an independent, not-for-profit group.

What does dissolvability mean? Place your calcium supplement in a small amount of warm water for 30 minutes and stir occasionally. If it hasn't dissolved within 30 minutes, it will most likely not dissolve in your stomach. Chewable and liquid calcium supplements dissolve well because they are broken down before entering the stomach.

Calcium supplements and postmenopausal females. Most experts say that calcium citrate may best be suited for older women. As mentioned above, it may be taken on a full or empty stomach and can be absorbed with or without gastric acid. Calcium citrate is best absorbed in a low acid state as compared to calcium carbonate. As we age we have a tendency to have less acid in our stomach. This is controversial but since we don't have a cheap way of measuring acid in the stomach it's best to assume a low calcium state and take calcium citrate.

Calcium supplements and proton pump inhibitors. Proton pump inhibitors inhibit 90-100% of the acid produced in the stomach within 7 to 10 days. This is the desired effect if you have gastroesophageal reflux disease, or GERD. The proton pump inhibitors include: omeprazole/Prilosec/Losec, rabeprazole/Aciphex/Pariet, lansoprazole/Prevacid, dexlansoprazole/Dexilant, pantoprazole/Protonix/Pantoloc, or esomeprazole/Nexium, also known as the "purple pill"). One of the problems with inhibiting most of the acid produced by the stomach is the lack of the absorption of calcium from dietary sources. Long term use of the proton pump inhibitors can lead to osteopenia (low calcium in the bones) and possibly osteoporosis (extremely low calcium with an associated high risk for fractures), especially in smokers. Calcium citrate supplements are recommended for patients on proton pump inhibitors, as this the best calcium supplement for a low stomach acid state. (Messinger-Rapport BJ, Thacker HL. A practical guide to prevention and treatment of osteoporosis. (*Geriatrics* 2002;57(April): 16–24)

Calcium supplements and cancer risk reduction in postmenopausal females. A study in the *American Journal of Nutrition* followed 1179 healthy post-menopausal women randomly assigned to receive 1400 mg to 1500 mg of supplemental calcium alone, supplemental calcium plus 1110 IU vitamin D3, or placebo. After all of the fancy statistical regression studies, the study concluded that calcium and vitamin D reduces all cancer risks in postmenopausal women. (Lappe JM et al. Vitamin D and calcium supplementation reduces cancer risk: results of a randomized trial. *Am J of Clin Nutr* 2007;(85): 1586–1591)

Calcium supplements and cardiovascular disease risk. A study published in the April 19, 2011 *British Medical Journal* reported a modest increase in the risk of cardiovascular events in women taking calcium supplements with or without vitamin D. The relationship between taking calcium supplements was especially true for a myocardial infarction (in lay terms—a heart attack). After looking at all of the other studies with calcium and vitamin D with cardiovascular events, researchers concluded that there's still no solid evidence of a cause-and-effect relationship and that the study should not, in any way, scare women away from supplementing with calcium up to the recommended daily level.

Calcium supplements, brassica vegetables, soy, and levothyroxine (thyroid hormone). Calcium supplements are among the top 25 over-the-counter products sold in the U.S. Calcium supplements are taken not only to prevent osteoporosis but to also treat patients with osteopenia (low bone density) and established osteoporosis. Unfortunately, calcium supplements can interfere with drugs taken for hypothyroidism, including the top selling levothyroxine (Synthroid, Levothroid, Levoxyl, and others). Calcium carbonate supplements can reduce the utilization of thyroid hormone, especially when taken in high doses and within four hour of the thyroid supplement. (Milner M. Hypothyroidism: optimizing medication with slow-release compounded thyroid replacement. *International J of Pharma Compounding* (July/August 2005)

Levothyroxine is best absorbed on an empty stomach taken in the morning one hour prior to breakfast. In order to minimize the interaction between calcium carbonate and levothyroxine, separate the doses by at least four hours. Taking 500 mg of calcium at lunch and dinner minimizes any impairment of utilization of thyroid hormone taken in the morning. (Schneyer C. Calcium carbonate and reduction in levothyroxine efficacy. *JAMA* 1998;279:750)

High amounts of soy in the diet can also inhibit thyroid hormone synthesis, especially if the patient also has low iodine levels. Advise your patient to eat soy in small amounts in the evening meal. Consuming large amounts of "the really good for you" brassica vegetables (broccoli, cauliflower, and Brus-

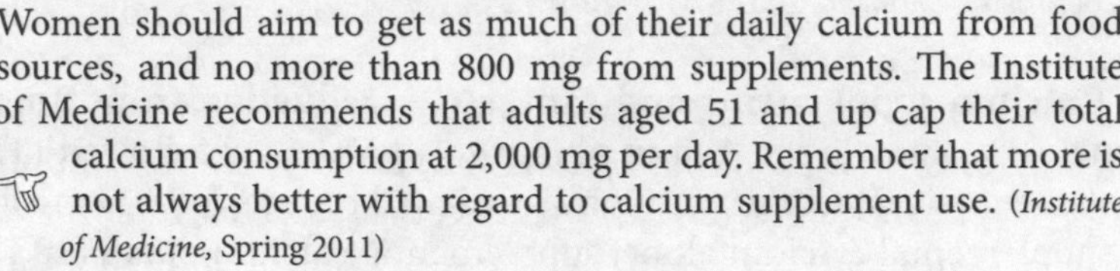

ASPARAGUS TIP

Women should aim to get as much of their daily calcium from food sources, and no more than 800 mg from supplements. The Institute of Medicine recommends that adults aged 51 and up cap their total calcium consumption at 2,000 mg per day. Remember that more is not always better with regard to calcium supplement use. (*Institute of Medicine*, Spring 2011)

sels sprouts) can also reduce the utilization of thyroid hormone. (Wold RS, Lopez ST, Yau LY, et al. Increasing trends in elderly persons' use of nonvitamin, nonmineral dietary supplements and concurrent use of medications. *J Am Dietetic Assoc* 2005;105(1). Bonakdar, R. Herb-drug interactions. *Patient Care* 2003;January: 58–69)

Calcium supplements and kidney stones. A study published in the July 2011 issue of the *American Journal of Clinical Nutrition* found that women whose daily calcium intake was 1,800 mg or higher had a 17 percent increase of kidney stone formation over a seven year period. However, if the majority of the calcium intake was from food sources, the risk was much lower. The study also found that supplements are more likely to cause hypercalcemia (too much calcium in the blood) than dietary sources.

Calcium supplements and/or calcium in foods and the DASH (Dietary Approaches to Stopping Hypertension) diet. Food as the source of calcium is two times better than calcium supplements when used as a component of the DASH diet to lower blood pressure. Following the DASH diet, which includes two to three servings of low-fat or nonfat dairy foods per day, is equal to or better than single-drug therapy for hypertension. (See Chapter D for the complete DASH diet recommendations)

Calcium as a component of multivitamins. When purchasing a multivitamin, check out the phosphorus content—the less phosphorus the better. Greater than 100 mg of phosphorus will impair the absorption of calcium and wreak havoc with bone mineralization. These two minerals have an inverse relationship with one another. As one goes UP the other goes DOWN.

The explanation. Calcium and phosphorus compete with each other for excretion by the kidney. When serum phosphorus is high, calcium is excreted from the kidneys. Where does that calcium come from? Calcium is removed from bones to help offset the extra excretion from the kidneys leading to osteopenia (low bone density). It's not just multivitamins that can be high in phosphorus. Certain food that are high in phosphorus also increase calcium excretion. Red meat, soft drinks, hard cheeses, and chocolate are also high in phosphorus. Consuming copious amounts of these foods over the years can contribute to diminished bone density and osteopenia.

Calcium supplementation and muscle cramps during pregnancy. Nighttime muscle cramps are common during the second half of pregnancy. In a small study in the *International Journal of Gynecology and Obstetrics,* Iranian women were treated with calcium carbonate (500 mg once a day), magnesium aspartate (7.5 mmol twice a day), thiamine (B1) (100 mg once a day) plus pyridoxine (B6) (40 mg once a day) for two weeks or no treatment for two weeks. A complete absence of cramps was found in the B1 plus B6 group in 72% of the patients compared to only 52% of the patients in the calcium group and only 29% in the magnesium group. Only 9% of the no-treatment controls had an absolute improvement or the complete absence of cramps. Why not give it a whirl? All of the above supplements have been shown to be safe during pregnancy so perhaps start with the B vitamins in your patients. (Sohrabvand F et al. Vitamin B supplementation for leg cramps during pregnancy. *Int J Gynaecol Obstet* 2006 Oct;95:48–49)

Calcium, calcium supplements, and osteoporosis. The typical American diet provides less than 600 mg of calcium per day. The amount of calcium recommended per day to prevent osteoporosis is 1,000 mg if you are between the ages of 19 and 50; 1,200 mg if you are between 51 and 70; and 1,500 mg if you are more than 70 years of age. If you don't plan on consuming 3 to 4 servings of low-fat milk, yogurt, or cheese every day, or other foods listed earlier to provide an adequate intake of calcium, then take calcium supplements to provide the additional calcium needed. (Zip over to Chapter V to learn more about vitamin D)

Calcium supplements and PMS (premenstrual syndrome) or PMDD (premenstrual dysphoric disorder). First of all, what are PMS and PMDD? Both are syndromes that occur a week before a woman's menstrual period and resolve within a few days of the onset of her period. The only actual difference between the two is the severity of the symptoms. PMS symptoms are primarily irritability, moodiness and premenstrual depression, whereas women with PMDD tend to have more severe symptoms that interfere with work, school, social activities, or relationships. In other words, women with PMDD need absolutely *no* encouragement to pull out an AK-47 and mow down everyone who happens to annoy them at any given moment in the day. Both conditions may have an underlying abnormality in calcium metabolism unmasked by fluctuating hormones. Taking 500 mg of any type of calcium supplement twice a day as a supplement was shown by Ghanbari and others to reduce the symptoms of PMS in a group of college students. Khajehel demonstrated a 4.20% reduction in symptom severity with 500 mg of calcium plus 200 mg of vitamin D twice a day during the 15th to the 24th day of the menstrual cycle.

So, for those of you with PMS, why not give it a try? It certainly couldn't hurt and the extra benefits of calcium for numerous other conditions would

ASPARAGUS TIP

If all Americans who are enrolled in Medicare took calcium with vitamin D daily, it could result in 776,000 fewer hospitalizations for hip fractures over five years. (The Health Impact Study IV commissioned by the Dietary Supplement Education Alliance September, 2009)

be beneficial. For those of you with PMDD stay away from AK-47s—and take calcium supplements. For everyone—don't exceed 2,000 mg of calcium per day from food and supplements combined. (Ghanbari Z, et al. Effects of calcium supplement therapy in women with premenstrual syndrome. *Taiwanese J of OB-GYN* 2009 (June);48:124–29; Khajehel M, et al. Effect of treatment with dydrogesterone or calcium plus vitamin D on the severity of premenstrual syndrome. *International Journal of OB & GYN* 2009 May);105:158–61)

CALORIES

Calories. Calories are simply a way of measuring the amount of energy supplied to you by the foods you eat and the liquids you drink. The French scientist Lavoisier invented the first method of calculating calories in the nineteenth century. A calorie is the amount of heat required to raise 4 pounds of water one degree Fahrenheit (or the amount needed to raise 1 quart of water one degree Celsius). Calorie counting should become a national pastime for the average American. In fact, calorie counting is a necessity for the millions of Americans who must watch their weight. Most dieticians eschew the plethora of fad diets today—the Atkins diet, The Modified Atkins Diet, The South Beach Diet, The Modified South Beach Diet, The Zone, Sugar-busters, The Maker's Diet, The LA Diet, The Diet to End All Diets, The Dean Ornish Diet, The Apple Cider Vinegar Diet, The Diet from Hell, The French Paradox Diet, etc. The best way to lose weight, most dieticians advise, is to cut calories. Of course, a bit of exercise helps you burn the calories that you consume, but the majority of weight loss centers around a reduction in calories. In fact, any calories that we don't use to raise that 4 pounds of water 1° F turns to adipose tissue, a fancy way of saying fat tissue. One measly pound of fat equals 3,500 calories. And yes, you can do the math. That means in order to lose one single pound on the scale you need to subtract 3,500 calories from your diet or burn it off on the treadmill.

Calories. Just how many calories does the average American need? A person's daily caloric needs depend on many factors, including age, height, weight, and activity level. The average goal for most active women, teenage girls, and sedentary men is 2,200 per day. If you are a woman and a couch potato, subtract 300–400 calories. As we age we need fewer calories. Caloric needs decrease 2% per decade for an adult. Older adults and sedentary women need approximately 1,600 calories per day. In other words, at age twenty, a cheeseburger and fries doesn't equate to thunder thighs. At fifty, the cheeseburger and fries make a beeline for the belly. If you are an extremely active male or female, you will need more calories.

You can find weight charts in just about every diet book, and, of course, on the internet. BUTT…and that's a big BUTT*…if you want to lose one pound per week, subtract 500 from your daily caloric needs. And, of course, the opposite would be true. If you choose to gain one pound per week, add 500 calories to your daily caloric needs.

*By the way, if you are an average American your butt is 15 inches long. The width has not yet been determined for the average American butt.

If you want an actual chart, the Institute of Medicine has conveniently put together a chart for your gender, your age, and your activity level. Go to www.iom.edu for your individualized caloric needs.

In two decades I've lost a total of 789 pounds. I should be hanging from a charm bracelet. —Erma Bombeck

---

Calorie consumption—gender differences. American women are consuming 335 more calories a day than they did 30 years ago, and men have increased their consumption by 170 calories more per day. And, most of those

ASPARAGUS TIP TO CUT CALORIES:

- Drink five fewer beers per week and reduce your weekly calorie intake by 700.
- Use two teaspoons of mustard instead of one tablespoon of mayonnaise on your sandwich once a week and save 90 calories.
- Have one cup of pretzels over the course of one week instead of one cup of nuts and cut 620 calories.
- Use two ounces of fat-free salad dressing instead of two ounces of regular salad dressing (one ounce = two teaspoons) five times per week and save 1,200 calories.
- Use non-stick spray instead of one tablespoon of oil in cooking three times per week and save 330 calories.
- Have a medium piece of fruit instead of two gourmet cookies three times a week and save 1,170 calories.
- As mentioned, a pound is 3,500 calories no matter how you weigh it. Overeat or under-exercise by 200 calories per day and in 17 days you have gained one pound. And the reverse is true. Eat 200 fewer calories per day or burn 200 extra calories per day and you will lose one pound in 17 days. "Seventeen days?" you shriek. "I need to lose 10 pounds by the weekend!!!" Not gonna happen.

extra calories come in the form of high-carbohydrate foods such as cookies, ice cream and soft drinks. No wonder the obesity rate has skyrocketed since the 1970s in the U.S.

Calorie facts.

- It takes just *one* minute to eat 250 calories in the form of cakes, biscuits, chocolate, fast food, and junk food. It takes five minutes to eat the same number of calories in "slow" foods, such as a serving of whole grain pasta or whole grain cereal.
- Stand up while yammering on the phone. If you stand during a 15-minute chat you will burn 25 calories. If you sit during that same 15-minute chat you will only burn 10 calories.
- You can boost the number of calories you burn each day by 15 percent with three 30-minute sessions of strength-training exercises each week. Log on to www.strongwomen.com for strength training exercises you can do in the privacy of your own home.
- It takes one week of eating 700 fewer calories and walking for one hour each day to burn two pounds of body fat. Walking for 30 minutes just twice a day burns 320 calories. Do this daily for 60 days and you will have walked off 19,200 calories—the equivalent of almost 6 pounds of fat.
- Cutting out all processed food as well as added salt from your diet reduces salt intake to around one-tenth of an ounce a day. Do this for 5 days and your body can release up to two-and-a-half pints of excess water stored in tissues, which can lead to a weight loss of nearly three pounds.
- How hungry are you? The next time you feel a wee bit puckish between meals, grab a glass of water and sip it slowly. Wait for 10 minutes. If you still feel hungry, eat something. If you don't feel hungry you are experiencing 'faux hunger' and it will pass with the consumption of water. The 10-minute rule also applies to dessert. Wait 10 minutes after finishing dinner before making a decision on that bowl of vanilla ice cream smothered in hot fudge. This crucial 10-minute pause gives the receptors in your stomach time to register how full you really are—usually the decision will be to forego that dessert. Yeah, right.
- So you have had too much to drink last night and you have the desire to eat everything within a 20-mile radius for the next 36 hours? Especially a double cheeseburger and large order of French fries. Alcohol makes the blood sugar dip for up to 36 hours after your last drink. When you wake up after a wild night-on-the-town, take small sips of orange juice to slowly increase blood sugar and boost energy. This will also help to curb the overeating urge and reduce the 1500-calorie load that a double cheeseburger and large order of fries can pile on.
- Leave 10% of each meal on your plate. For the average American, leaving just 10 percent behind at each meal every single day—about 89,930 calories per year, or the amount in 300 candy bars—is the equivalent to

a 10 pound weight loss over a year's time. (Cynthia Sass, author, Cinch! Conquer Cravings, Drop Pounds and lose Inches)

Calorie burning and various forms of exercise...
.....20 minutes of bicycling will burn 2 chocolate truffles (100 calories each)
.....40 minutes of swimming laps will burn the 20 oz. caffè mocha with whipped cream (400 calories) you drank on the way to the pool
.....70 minutes of playing tennis will burn off the 650 calorie slice of cheese pan pizza you had for lunch
.....40 minutes on the Stairmaster will take care of that 400 calorie chocolate chip cookie you picked up at the airport kiosk
.....two hours and 30 minutes of ballroom dancing wipes out your morning bagel with cream cheese (500 calories)
.....30 minutes of raking leaves burns a 120 calorie teaspoon of olive oil
.....two hours and 40 minutes of brisk walking negates the 700 calorie creamy slice of New York style cheesecake from the Cheesecake Factory
.....60 minutes of jogging for the 450 calorie blueberry muffin from Starbucks

Think before you devour.

Calories, cucumbers, and celery. How many times have you heard the myth that you burn more calories digesting cucumber or celery than you get from eating them? True or not true? NOT true. A 10-inch stalk of celery and a half a cup of cucumber slices contain about 8 calories each, but they're also very easy to digest. In other words, cucumber slices don't possess "negative calories." Celery is primarily cellulose, an indigestible complex carbohydrate that zips right through the digestive system. Cucumbers are practically all water. Since we need to eat or drink between 1800 and 2400 calories per day depending on our weight, gender, and lifestyle, we would have to eat between 18 and 24 pounds of celery, or 35 to 48 pounds of cucumber to cover our daily needs. HAHAHAHA… (*Science Illustrated* September/October 2008)

Caloric intake and the ability to concentrate. The amount that one eats may influence his/her ability to concentrate. People make more mistakes on tasks that demand sustained attention, such as proofreading, after eating a 1,000-calorie meal compared to a 300-calorie meal, according to research by Angus Craig of the University of Sussex in Brighton, England. Having more or less food than usual also increased errors, although those who ate large meals did much worse as a group. Skipping lunch was not a solution. On an empty stomach, performance fell even lower. People who skipped a meal also felt more tense and anxious. (Lamberg L. Bodyrhythms. New York: William Morrow and Company, Inc., 1994.)

Caloric intake and gastric bacteria. People with weight problems may have the wrong kind of bacteria in their guts. There are two major types of bacteria that help us digest our food: *Bacteriodetes* and *Firmicutes.* Every stomach contains both types; however, the stomach of obese individuals contains much larger proportions of *Firmicutes* than the stomachs of lean individuals. A separate study found that *Firmicutes* bacteria extract more calories from a given food. In fact, when *Firmicutes* bacteria from obese mice were transplanted into the guts of normal mice, they gained 20 percent more weight than those who received bacteria from thin mice. Another study found that populations of these two bacteria shift as people lose weight, from more to less efficient calorie-absorbing bacteria types. Lean people also have more bacterial diversity than obese people in their gut microbes. These results mean that the obesity epidemic cannot be entirely blamed on your parents (genetics) or even the couch—the other dynamic factor may just be the type of bacteria that you have in your belly. Stay tuned—this is a fascinating area of research. Weight loss just might be a microbe or two away. (Gebel E. *Diabetes Forecast* 2011 (February): 36–39)

***Campylobacter jejuni* as a foodborne illness.** The most common cause of food-borne illness in the U.S. is not *E.Coli* O157:H7, nor is it *Salmonella* or *Shigella*. It is none other than *Campylobacter jejuni,* the ubiquitous bacteria found in the intestines of poultry, turkeys, and other birds. These bacteria are shed in "fowl feces" and proceed to cause misery in those who consume undercooked contaminated poultry products. Bloody diarrhea, fever, and abdominal pain are the most common symptoms. Approximately four million Americans acquire this foodborne pathogen every year in the United States. Deaths are relatively rare, between 200 and 1,000 per year, and mostly in the elderly or immunocompromised patients.

In about 1 per 1,000 cases, exposure to *Campylobacter jejuni* can trigger the development of Guillain-Barre syndrome, a demyelinating peripheral neuropathy that strips the longest nerves of their myelin. The patient experiences an ascending paralysis starting with the feet and moving up the trunk involving the muscles of respiration. Patients will usually recover; however, full recovery depends on a number of factors. It is estimated that 40% of all Guillain-Barre cases are preceded by eating contaminated chicken one to three weeks prior to the symptoms.

Freezing chicken will reduce the levels of *Campylobacter jejuni* contamination, and cooking poultry all of the way through will destroy it completely. White meat should be cooked to 170° F and dark meat should be cooked to 180° F. *Campylobacter jejuni* does not multiply or spread rapidly, and it cannot spread from one infected person to another. Most people, who get *Campylobacteriosis* as the infection is called, recover after about a week without treatment and without long-term consequences.

Cancer and diet. The estimated number of new cancer cases in the U.S. for 2010 was 1,529,560. Experts estimate that eating healthier foods and getting up off this couch that I'm sitting on can prevent 30% to 40% of cancers in the U.S. and around the world. Eating more fruits and vegetables alone could eliminate 20%. (Food, Nutrition, Physical Activity and the Prevention of Cancer: a Global Perspective. November 2007. http://www.aicr.org) (AmericanCancer Society, 2010)

Findings linking nutrition and cancer include:

- A strong link between excessive calorie intake and increased cancer risk
- Folate is needed to repair and manufacture DNA; without it, broken and abnormal DNA increases, raising the chances of getting cancer.
- Several studies have linked low dietary levels of folate to a higher risk of cancer. People with the highest folate intakes have about a 40 percent less risk of colon cancer than those with the lowest folate intakes.
- Over supplementing with folate (10 times the recommend RDA) can actually promote cancer—so don't overdo it.
- Excessive caloric intake has been linked to skin cancer. High fat diets have been linked to skin cancer. The plant or phytonutrient genistein, found primarily in soy foods, has consistently shown to have a protective effect against skin cancer.
- Excess weight accounts for 14 percent of all cancer deaths in men and 20 percent of all cancer deaths in women.
- Insulin levels and insulin-like growth factor increase as body weight increases. Women with the highest circulating insulin are 2½ times more likely to be diagnosed with breast cancer than those with the lowest levels of circulating insulin. (*Journal of the National Cancer Institute* 2009;101:48)
- Cranberries may protect against prostate cancer, but the findings are preliminary.
- Lycopene may be a potent inhibitor of lung cancer.
- Calcium continues to be an anti-colon cancer nutrient. In a landmark clinical trial, calcium supplements (1,000 mg a day) lowered the risk of new precancerous colon polyps in people who had already had one. (*Journal of the National Cancer* Institute 2007;99:129)
- Red meat and processed meats are convincingly associated with an increased risk of colon cancer. The heme iron content in red meat may act as a catalyst in the gut and generate free radicals that damage DNA. There's also a concern about carcinogens formed during high-heat cooking. And, processed meats may have more nitrites that turn into carcinogens called nitrosamines. (The International Research Conference on Food, Nutrition and Cancer was held in July 17–18, 2003, in Washington, D.C.)

Cancer and diet—part 2. A report released in May 2011 by The World Cancer Research Fund/American Institute for Cancer Research's Continuous Update Project (CUP) Expert Panel (really?), provides more evidence that foods have protective effects and promoting effects. Red meat and processed meats continue to get the thumbs down when it comes to colon cancer, but you can reduce the risk of colon cancer you consume foods high in fiber and limit your intake of red meat to a total of 18 ounces per week (5 to 6 medium portions). Nix processed meats completely.

High-fat foods are also on the thumbs down list—limit your intake of cheese, whole-milk products, and, of course, fatty meats. Products with higher fat content are more likely to have cancer-promoting dioxins. For this reason, skim milk and leaner cuts of meat are better for you. See Chapter D for more on dioxin.

White sugar and white flour have a high glycemic index. So what? Foods with high glycemic indexes trigger the production of insulin and insulin-like growth factors—both of which have been implicated as tumor promoters for breast, colon, and prostate cancer. Choose foods that have lower glycemic indexes, such as brown rice, sweet potatoes, and whole grain pasta. See Chapter G for a more complete list of low-glycemic index foods.

The good-for-you-foods are cruciferous vegetables (broccoli, Brussels sprouts, cauliflower, cabbage, and broccoli rabe) that contain all sorts of cancer-fighting compounds. Sulforaphane, found in copious amounts in broccoli, activates cancer-fighting detoxifying enzymes. We all have a certain amount detoxifying enzymes that we have inherited, but adding a helping of broccoli two or three times a week can provide increased protection. The body's first line of defense against nasty environmental carcinogens such as dioxin, is to be able to excrete them, and detoxifying enzymes are just the ticket for excretion of these carcinogens. Cruciferous vegetable also contain compounds called indoles. One in particular, indole-3-carbinol, is especially important in preventing prostate, breast, and cervical cancer.

Fish high in omega-3 fatty acids also increase the body's production of detoxifying enzymes. Salmon is the obvious choice here as it has the highest omega-3 fatty acids in the fish world, but many other fish contain omega-3 fatty acids as well. (See Chapter O for a complete list of foods high in omega-3 fatty acids.)

Ok, so you're whining about the fact that you don't like fish…whine, whine, whine. Zip over to the seed aisle and grab a package of flaxseeds, chia seeds, and/or pumpkin seeds—all contain the vegetable form of omega-3 fatty acids known as alpha linolenic acid. Grind up the flaxseeds to get the

ASPARAGUS TIP

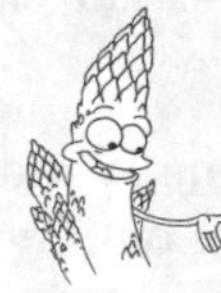

Of the 571,950 cancer deaths that occurred in 2011 in the U.S., the American Cancer Society estimates that 33% would never have happened if no one smoked. And another third could have been prevented with weight loss, exercise, and healthier eating.

omega-3 benefits—whole flaxseeds just end up in the toilet unchanged but at least you have the benefit of regularity. FYI—sunflower and sesame seeds don't have the same benefits as pumpkin seeds, flaxseeds, or chia seeds.

Red grapes and red wine contain resveratrol, another detoxifying compound that increases the amount of detoxifying enzymes.

Berries, berries and more berries have also been shown to slow breast and esophageal cancers. And the berries don't have to be the exotic acai berries, golgi berries, and noni berries. Good ol' blueberries, blackberries, red raspberries, and black raspberries do the trick.

Spices can also provide protection against cancer. These include turmeric, garlic, and rosemary—all of which contain compounds that increase detoxifying enzymes.

Candy. Yummy but with lots of sugar, lots of calories, and not a lot of health benefits. Here are a few secrets about how to choose between various candies when you're in the movie theatre concession. If you are contemplating the choice of a York Peppermint Pattie or a bar of Ghirardelli Pure Milk Chocolate, you might want to choose the Peppermint Pattie. It has 170 calories and the Ghirardelli Pure Milk Chocolate bar has 580 calories. Willi-Nilli, drop the Ghirardelli. The difference between a 1.7-ounce bag of Peanut M &Ms and a 1.7-ounce bag of Plain M&Ms is 10 calories—not enough to spend days agonizing over the choice. Get the peanut bag if you're not allergic to peanuts, as peanuts give you a wee bit of cardiac protection—not a lot but a wee bit is better than zero. A 4-ounce box of Milk Duds during a two hour movie will set you back 490 calories. Don't even think about substituting the Milk Duds for Junior Mints. The 5.5-ounce box of Junior Mints is 620 calories. Sure it's more ounces for that 620 calories but rest assured you will eat the entire box.

So you say, I'll only have the movie popcorn and forget about the candy afterwards. The small popcorn without butter has 400 calories, but since it's been popped in coconut oil you have just wiped out a day's worth of saturated fats. Consuming a large bucket of movie popcorn will add 1,150 calories, without butter, to your daily calorie consumption and if you choose the butter, add an additional 500 calories to that 1,150 and more than three day's worth of saturated fat. Hmmmm…what to choose? Bring your own air-popped popcorn or choose a store-bought popcorn that is 94% fat-free.

Canker sores. The medically correct term for canker sores is aphthous ulcers. These benign painful ulcers typically occur in the inner surface of the cheeks and lips, but can appear anywhere in the mouth including the tongue, gums, and soft palate. Approximately 20% of average Americans suffer from occasional canker sores, and women are more prone to them than men. The sores usually last between 5 and 14 days.

What causes canker sores? Who knows? Hypotheses abound; however, the definitive cause remains elusive. Some postulated causes include mouth trauma (hard toothbrushes, dental work, and an accidental chomp to the inside of the cheek), food allergies (citrus and chocolate), nutritional deficiencies (B12, folate, iron, zinc), hormonal changes (the ups and downs of estrogen and the menstrual cycle), and immune system impairment. One additional cause discussed in the dental literature is an ingredient found in toothpaste known as SLS, or sodium lauryl sulfate. Another very important cause of canker sores is celiac disease. Consider this possibility in kids or adults with gastrointestinal problems such as bloating and diarrhea.

From the preceding list it would seem that prevention would focus on eliminating citrus and chocolate from the diet, correcting nutritional deficiencies with multivitamin therapy, remove the ovaries, begin a gluten-free diet, and switch to toothpaste that lacks SLS. After completing that checklist of things to do for prevention, what can you do to treat the existing canker sores? Here are a few helpful hints for soothing the discomfort of the cantankerous canker sore:

- Squeeze a vitamin E capsule onto a cotton swab and apply to the sore for 10 minutes, as needed, to make eating more comfortable.
- Apply licorice in a tincture, powder, or tablet of deglycyrrhizinated (DGL) licorice directly to the canker sore.
- Avoid spicy, acidic, and abrasive foods.
- Rinse the mouth with salt water and continue good oral hygiene procedures *even if pain makes it uncomfortable.*
- Over-the-counter topical salves like Anbesol can numb the area temporarily and provide relief for the immediate consumption of a meal.

Canola oil. One of the internet-generated myths about this heart-healthy oil is that it contains toxins and should not be consumed. Actually, canola oil contains monounsaturated fats and is lower in saturated fats than any other oil except olive oil.

So, how did this myth originate? The myth originates from the fact that canola oil has its origins from a rape plant, a member of the mustard family whose seed oil contains a toxin known as erucic acid. Rapeseed oil is banned in the U.S. because it contains 30–60% erucic acid which can be toxic when used for cooking.

Thirty years ago, Canadian scientists developed a rape plant whose seed oil contained less than 2% erucic acid. This was obviously quite an improvement from the 30–60% found in the older version of the rape plant. They named this plant variety "canola" as a combination of two words—"can" for Canada and "ola" for oil. Current erucic acid levels in canola range from 0.5% to 1%, well under the 2% limit set by our government food police as a safety precaution.

Cantaloupe. The cantaloupe was named after the Italian papal village of Cantalup, where it was cultivated around 1700 A.D. Leave it to the Italians to take the credit, but the true cantaloupe was native to Persia (present day Iran) around 500 A.D. And, interestingly, the cantaloupe grown in the U.S. is not a true cantaloupe (found mostly in Europe and the Middle East), but is a melon in the muskmelon family. Honeydew melons are in the same family of melons as the cantaloupe.

So the question begs to be asked…how do you tell the difference between a "true" cantaloupe from Europe and the Middle East vs. the commercial cantaloupes that come from California, Texas, and Arizona. Easy. Look at the surface of the cantaloupe—the true cantaloupes have a rough, pebble surface, but no "netting" as is characteristic of the muskmelon cantaloupe grown in the U.S.

The beautiful orange color is the result of beta-carotene, the potent antioxidant that converts to vitamin A in the body. Cantaloupe provides more than 100% of the Daily Value for vitamins A and C, as well as significant amounts of potassium, folate and fiber.

One cup of cantaloupe contains only 60 calories and is packed, and I do mean packed, with 5,987 IUs of vitamin A (mostly beta-carotene, the precursor to vitamin A); 65 mg of vitamin C, 37 micrograms of folate, 473 mg of potassium, and 1.6 grams of fiber.

Best time to buy? Peak season is June through August. A ripe melon feels heavy for its size and the rind is mostly yellow to cream colored. Don't choose one that has green on the rind. Push the stem end with your index finger—if soft, but not mushy, it's perfect. Cut the melon into halves or quarters, but don't scoop out the seeds until you're ready to indulge in the sweet, delicious, and juicy taste of the cantaloupe.

HISTORICAL HIGHLIGHT

Cantaloupe's claim to pharmaceutical fame. Even though Alexander Fleming discovered penicillin in 1928, it wasn't mass produced until the late 1940s. The problem was cultivating a strain that grew quickly enough. The major breakthrough happened by accident in 1943 when Mary Hunt, a lab worker in Peoria, Illinois, brought in some moldy cantaloupes from the local market. They were infected with a "pretty, golden mold," *Penicillium chrysogenum,* which yielded two times more penicillin than Fleming's original mold. Dr. Elizabeth McCoy (1903–1978), a bacteriologist in Wisconsin, took it one step further. Dr. McCoy discovered that by irradiating this "pretty, golden mold," she could produce a mutant strain, X1612, which was a thousand times more productive and paved the way for the commercial production of all antibiotic drugs.

Scrub the outer surface under running water before cutting into the melon. This removes bacteria from the surface, preventing its transfer to the flesh when you cut into it. Melons carry microbes on their surface because they sit on the ground while growing. Salmonella outbreaks and a recent Listeria outbreak have been traced back to cantaloupes.

CAPSAICIN

Capsaicin—some like it HOT. Capsaicin (cap-SAY-son) is a nutrient that stimulates neurons in the substance P (think P for PAIN) system, responsible for evoking the sensation of heat associated with spicy food. The belief that spicy foods contribute to heartburn after a meal is widespread but at this point, erroneous. In other words, evidence in the medical literature doesn't support this fact. One small study demonstrated a reduction in time from the spicy food intake to the symptoms associated with heartburn, but there was no clear cause and effect. That being said, individuals with heartburn respond differently to spicy foods. So the blanket statement that spicy foods don't trigger heartburn is individually-based. (Rodriguez-Stanley S, Collings KL, et al. The effects of capsaicin on reflux, gastric emptying and dyspepsia. *Aliment Pharmacolo Ther* 2000;14:129)

Capsaicin and non-allergic nasal stuffiness. Researchers at Johns Hopkins Asthma and Allergy Center are experimenting with capsaicin, the chemical that gives hot peppers their zing, as a treatment for chronic, non-allergic nasal stuffiness. Repeated doses appear to clear up nasal passages without permanent damage. One annoying problem—the first few snorts, given ten minutes apart, burned just a tad, and made both the nose and eyes run. (Philip G, et al. The human nasal response to capsaicin. *J of Allergy and Clin Immun* 1994;94:1035–1045)

Capsaicin and oral ulcers from chemotherapy. History once again gives us a lesson or two in the treatment of various ailments. In the 1400s, the Aztecs mixed powdered chilies with honey to treat lacerations of the mouth. Oncologists are now capitalizing on this therapy to treat painful oral ulcers caused by chemotherapy or radiation therapy in 40 to 70 percent of the patients receiving cancer treatment. Ann Berger of the Yale Cancer Center has mixed a taffy-like candy made with capsaicin. When Dr. Berger gave capsaicin-laced candies to 17 patients, 12 of them reported significant pain relief. On a scale from 1 to 10, with 1 being the least pain and 10 being the most pain, ten of the patients rated their pain a 2 as compared to a 6 prior to the candy mixture. (Berger A. *J of Pain and Symptom Management,* 1995)

Capsaicin—as a drug for pain management. A pharmaceutical preparation of purified capsaicin(brand name Zostrix) may be best known for its ability to provide topical pain relief for patients with osteoarthritis or the pain of peripheral neuropathy, specifically shingles. When capsaicin is applied, it causes the body to release a chemical pain messenger called substance P. The supply of substance P decreases each time the capsaicin is applied until the area of the body becomes numb to the pain sensation. As a result, repeatedly applying capsaicin cream to an area of injury (three to five times a day) is necessary to derive benefits from its use.With the use of capsaicin cream, a local stinging or burning sensation is common; however, this sensation dissipates after several days of therapy. Capsaicin cream has no known systemic side effects or drug interactions. So be sure to follow the instructions and apply it regularly and consistently for the best relief for your arthritis or neuropathy. (www.zostrix.com)

*One of my seminar participants told me an amusing story about capsaicin and her osteoarthritic hands. She had just completed applying capsaicin to her fingers, hands, and wrists when her husband decided that the "moment was right." She was moving her hands in all of the usual places when he suddenly jumped out of bed, ran from the bedroom clutching his private parts for dear life and yelping about the severe burning sensation caused by her gentle, capsaicin-tainted touch. Obviously there should be a "lag-time" between application on one's hands and the subsequent inadvertent "application" on the private parts of a partner.

Capsaicin and prostate cancer. Chili peppers contain the spicy chemical capsaicin, which may have the power to destroy cancer cells—at least in mice. When researchers gave capsaicin to mice with prostate cancer, their tumors regressed to one-fifth their original size. Of course the prostate shriveled—you not only would have to have a cast-iron stomach to consume the amount of capsaicin the scientists gave the mice but the amount of "burn" on the way out most likely fried the prostate and reduced it to the size of a sesame seed. The weekly dose per mouse was the equivalent of about 600 jalapeños. It's doubtful that this will translate into the newest treatment for prostate cancer in humans.

ASPARAGUS TIP

After rubbing capsaicin cream onto affected skin and/or joints, wash your hands thoroughly. Touching other body parts (yours or someone else's) can cause pain and burning, so be careful where you touch—eyes, nose, or "private parts"—all can burn "like the dickens" if you're not careful. (Deal CL, et al. Treatment of arthritis with topical capsaicin: A double-blind trial. *Clinical Therapeutics* 1991;13(3):383–395.

Carbohydrate ("carb") counting and diabetes. Carbohydrates have the greatest impact on postprandial (after a meal) blood glucose levels. All diabetics need to understand which foods have carbohydrates (starches, fruit, starchy vegetables, milk, cookies and other sweets), what an average serving size is, and how many servings to select for meals and snacks. Evidence shows that it is the total carbohydrate consumed—rather than the source or type of carbohydrate—that matters for blood-sugar control*. (Szerlong H, Daitch L, Stallings J. Nutrition therapy for new diabetes patients. *Clinical Advisor.* 2011. June: 60–66)

(*Controversy swirls in the world of nutrition. Are there good carbs and bad carbs? Do carbs with high glycemic indexes wreak more havoc than foods with low glycemic indexes? At the moment, as stated above, all carbohydrates influence blood sugar control…if you want more on low glycemic index carbs vs. high glycemic index carbs, zip over to the G chapter and check out Glycemic Index.)

Carbohydrate counting is actually more important than reading the label for sugar content. Forget the sugar amount on the label and look at the serving size and the total grams of carbohydrate per serving size. A carbohydrate choice is a serving that equals 15 grams of carbohydrate. For example, *Sunshine Vanilla Wafers* contain 21 grams of carbohydrate in a serving size of 7 cookies. Oops, that's too many carbs for the 15 grams mentioned as a carbohydrate choice. Soo…if you insist on *Sunshine Vanilla Wafers* at that very moment, you have to cut back on the number of cookies for your serving size. Five cookies, not seven, would be about 15 grams of carbohydrate. Shove those other two Vanilla Wafers back in the box for another time.

A consult with registered dietician (RD) is an absolute must if you have diabetes, or if you are just interested in learning more about healthy eating. He/she can go over choices with you, explain serving sizes, portion sizes, dress sizes, shoe sizes, the number of allowable carbohydrate choices, caloric needs for your specific lifestyle, and a myriad of other topics related to health and nutrition.

The following are examples of foods and the number of carbohydrate grams:

Bread per *one* slice:

Thin slice	13 grams
Extra thin	10 grams
Light thin	7.5 grams
Toasting slice	16 grams
Thick slice	20 grams
½ cup of oat bran	11 grams
3 Oreo cookies	24 grams
1 plain baked potato with the skin	56 grams
1 plain baked potato without the skin	34 grams
McDonald's *small* French fries (2.4 ounces)	28 grams

Cheese, cottage, low-fat, 1 cup .... 8 grams
Carrots, cooked, 1 cup .... 13 grams
Yogurt, plain, low-fat, 8 ounces .... 16 grams
Apple, with skin, 1 medium .... 17 grams
Banana, 1 medium .... 25 grams
Beans, black, cooked, ½ cup .... 20 grams
Corn, yellow, cooked, ½ cup .... 20 grams
White or brown rice, cooked, ½ cup .... 22 grams
Spaghetti, cooked, 1 cup .... 43 grams

How about beverages?
1 cola beverage, 12 ounces .... 35 grams
Cranberry juice cocktail, 8 ounces .... 34 grams
Orange juice, 8 ounces .... 26 grams
Tonic water, 6 ounces .... 16 grams
Beer, regular, 12 ounces .... 13 grams
Milk, 2-percent, 8 ounces .... 11 grams
Tomato juice, 8 ounces .... 10 grams
Beer, light, 12 ounces .... 6 grams
Wine, red or white, 3.5 ounces .... 3 grams
Club soda, liquor, water .... 0, zippo, zilch, nada

Carbohydrates, complex. Complex carbohydrates include starchy vegetables, whole grains, and legumes. Of course your registered dietician would prefer that the carbs you choose would be whole grains, sweet potatoes, and beans, but all types of fruits and vegetables are good for you.

Carbohydrates and mood. The role of carbohydrates in promoting relaxation—at least in part by enhancing serotonin levels— suggests that complex carbohydrates such as whole grains can be good for your mood. So, the question is: Do dieters that cut back on carbs lose their sunny disposition along with the pounds? Australian researchers decided to test this question and the results are surprising. They tested 106 overweight and obese participants, average age 50. While cutting calories equally, one group followed a very low-carbohydrate, high-fat diet, and the rest ate a high-carb, low-fat diet. After one year, both groups averaged about a 30-pound weight loss. But their moods differed as the study continued.

Initially, after the first eight weeks, both groups experienced an improvement in mood as measured by scores on three standard tests. However, only the high-carb group demonstrated lasting improvement on most measurements of mood, including hostility, confusion, depression and overall bad mood. Those on the low-carb diet returned to their baseline, and more negative moods. The difficulty sticking to a low-carb diet may be a factor in the group's negative moods. But low serotonin and the lack of proteins affecting neurons may also play a major role in the grouchy factor. (Brinkworth GD. *Archives of Internal Med.* 2009 Nov 9)

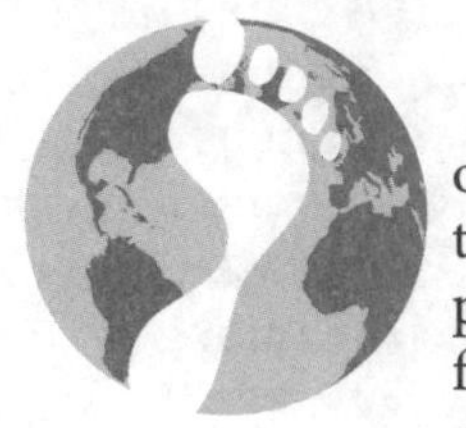

Carbon footprint. A carbon footprint is the measure of the impact of human activities on the environment in terms of the amount of greenhouse gas (GHG) emissions produced. The way we eat has significant impact because food production, packaging, transportation, preparation and waste account for 1/3 of GHG emissions produced. Minimizing carbon dioxide and other GHG emissions associated with climate change reduces your carbon footprint.

Choosing a plant-based diet has the biggest impact on lowering your carbon footprint. Meat requires many more pounds that its weight in grain feed. Grain feed has to be grown, irrigated, processed, packaged and shipped. In addition to adding a significant amount to the carbon footprint by consuming grain, the cattle that are grain-fed release GHG emissions in the form of methane and nitrous oxide, both of which can trap heat and add to climate change.

Lamb, beef, cheese, pork and farmed salmon generate the highest GHG emissions, use the most resources to produce, and are most damaging to the environment. Organically grown products have less impact on the environment because fewer chemicals are used.

The carbon footprints of common foods are listed below based on the equivalency in carbon emissions for car miles driven per four ounces of food consumed.

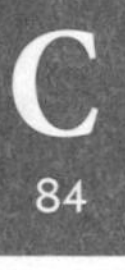

CARBON FOOTPRINT of common foods
Lentils and tomatoes less than ¼ of a mile
2% milk—less than 1 half mile
Chicken—less than 2 miles
Salmon, pork—less than 3 miles
Cheese—less than 3.5 miles
Beef and lamb—less than 7 miles
(Environmental Working Group—2010)

Carnitine. Question? What two supplements can literally make elderly rats "get up and do the Macarena?" According to Bruce Ames, a University of California biochemist, and his colleague, Tory Hagen, it's carnitine and a dash of alpha-lipoic acid. First, visualize elderly rats (roughly equal to 70 to 100-year-old humans) doing the Macarena. Seriously?

When fed the combination supplement of carnitine and alpha-lipoic acid the elderly rats actually doubled their activity levels compared to a second group of elderly rats who received only the placebo pellet. Carnitine pumps up the function of the energy producing mitochondria in the cells. Alpha lipoic acid functions as an antioxidant and the combination of the two works better than either supplement alone.

In fact, Ames and Hagen were so impressed with the combined supplements, they patented the combination and advertize it in health magazines as "Juvenon." Of course they swear by it, and both take it on a daily basis, as does health guru Dr. Andrew Weil.

Other studies have demonstrated that elderly rats also demonstrated brain benefits from the combination of carnitine and alpha-lipoic acid. They had less mitochondrial damage in their brains and better spatial and temporal memory than rats who consumed the placebo pellet. The doses were huge though, and studies haven't been performed on humans yet. By the way, Ames and Hagen also studied the combination in beagles and found that it improved beagle memory as well. That's a first—mice, rats, monkeys are the usual test subjects. What's up with the beagle studies?

CAROTENOIDS

Carotenoids. Carotenoids represent one of the most widespread groups of naturally occurring pigments. These compounds are largely responsible for the red, yellow, and orange color of fruits and vegetables, and are also found in many dark green vegetables. There are over 600 members of the carotenoid family. Give thanks that we're not going to discuss all of them. The most abundant carotenoids in the North American diet are beta-carotene, alpha-carotene, gamma-carotene, lycopene, lutein, beta-cryptoxanthin, zeaxanthin, and astaxanthin.

The carotenoids have many clinical benefits, and perhaps they are most well known for their "provitamin A" benefits. Approximately 50 carotenoids have "provitamin A" properties; the most well-known are "carotenes," especially beta-carotene. Carotenoids are also powerful antioxidants and immune boosters. Lutein and zeaxanthin are powerful carotenoids that protect the eyes from a degenerative process known as macular degeneration. These compounds will be discussed throughout the book—specifically for eye health and for the prevention of vitamin A deficiency.

Carotenoids and pink flamingos. Flamingos are grey when they hatch, but turn that luscious orange-pink from the carotenoid pigments in the algae and crustaceans they eat. Their liver metabolizes the food into orange and pink pigment molecules that are stored in their feathers. The more carotenoids consumed by the flamingo, the brighter their plumage.

CARROTS

Carrots. One raw carrot, about 7 inches long, has 2 grams of dietary fiber and 20,250 IU of vitamin A, approximately four times the recommended daily intake (RDI) for a man, and five times the RDI for a woman). Carrots are obviously an extraordinary source of vitamin A, derived from deep orange carotenoids (including beta carotene).

Large, naked raw carrots are acceptable as food only to those who live in hutches eagerly waiting for Easter. —Fran Leibowitz

Mel Blanc, the voice of Bugs Bunny, was actually allergic to carrots. B-deah, B-deah, B-deah, that's all folks...

Carrots as a rectal foreign object. Carrots have another claim to fame. They are tied with cucumbers as the number one popular food for rectal consumption. Let me explain. The September 1986 issue of Surgery published a fascinating review article entitled, "Rectal foreign bodies: Case reports and comprehensive literature review." The literature search found more than 700 identified items that had been removed from no less than 200 rectums, an average of 3.5 items per rectum. Note that those are just the items that could be identified. Who knows how many unidentified flying rectal objects (UFROs) there are out in the "anusphere."

Other foods were also popular, as you might imagine. In fact, the rectum was found to be a veritable fruit and vegetable cornucopia. Bananas, onions, and zucchini all came in a close second. A lemon and a jar of Pond's Cold Cream was removed from one gentleman's rectum. Upon questioning as to why those two items were conveniently located in the rectum, he answered: "I understand that it's a cure for hemorrhoids..." Interestingly, it must have worked as there was nary a hemorrhoid to be found. (Busch DB, Starling JR. Rectal foreign bodies: case reports and a comprehensive review of the world's literature. *Surgery* 1986 (September);100:512–59)

CAYENNE

Cayenne. Cayenne, a spice used for culinary and medicinal purposes, takes its name from its area of origin, the Cayenne region of French Guiana. The medicinal uses of cayenne reportedly go back at least 9,000 years ago, when Native Americans used the herb to treat a variety of diseases—from

HISTORICAL HIGHLIGHTS

Carrots were yellow until a gene mutation created an orange one in the 1700s. An observant farmer appreciated the beauty of the orange carrot and through the process of selective breeding continued the line of orange carrots.

indigestion to pain. The substance that confers the "spiciness" to cayenne is capsaicin.

Cayenne is also a rich source of nutrients and should be considered a nutritious addition to any meal. It contains carotenoids and vitamins C and E, lutein, quercetin, calcium, essential fatty acids, B vitamins, iron, magnesium, phosphorus and zinc. Now, if only you enjoyed spicy foods—some of us do, some of us don't.

Cayenne pepper as a remedy for cold extremities. Sprinkle one-eighth of a teaspoon of cayenne pepper into each shoe or glove to generate enough heat to keep the extremities warm. How does it work? The water-soluble components in the cayenne pepper are responsible for vasodilation of the superficial capillaries of the skin surface, resulting in an immediate sensation of heat. Within 15 minutes, oil-soluble compounds reach the deeper layers of the skin, generating warmth for hours. If you're planning to spend at least a few hours out in the frigid cold, perhaps a cayenne liniment is more suitable for keeping the digits warm and cozy. Mix one teaspoon of cayenne pepper with one pint of soy oil in a bottle made of dark glass or opaque plastic. Allow three weeks for the two ingredients to blend, giving the bottle a daily shake. Using a dropper, rub three drops on the soles of your feet, or the palms of your hands. Don't forget to keep your hands away from your eyes after applying the liniment to your hands. Use the liniment only on intact skin. If irritation or cracks occur, run cool water over the affected area and stop using the cayenne. (Rubman AL, ND, Director of the Southbury Clinic for Traditional Medicines in Southbury, CT.)

CELIAC DISEASE

Celiac disease. Celiac disease is an immune-mediated disease of the intestines caused by a chronic sensitivity to gluten. Gluten is a protein found in wheat, rye, oats*, and barley. (*Pure oats are not considered a problem; however, oats in the U.S. are usually milled with the other grains that contaminate the mixture with gluten and may trigger symptoms of celiac disease.)

The body's immune response to the gluten produces inflammation in the intestines that directly damages the absorptive surface. Malabsorption of nutrients such as iron, folate, calcium, fat-soluble vitamins A, D, E, and K, and protein can occur leading to nutritional deficiencies. Patients with celiac can present with iron deficiency anemic osteopenia and osteoporosis, as well as growth retardation in children.

Celiac disease is a common, inherited disorder estimated to affect as many as 1 in 100 persons in North America. Symptoms of celiac disease can present at any time—from the neonate to the nonagenarian. Approximately 20% of the cases are diagnosed over 60 years of age. The average age of diagnosis is between the ages of 30 and 50. In the Canadian Celiac Health survey of 2,681 adults with biopsy-proven celiac disease, the mean age at diagnosis was 46 years. Undiagnosed celiac disease has become more than four times as common in the past 50 years.

Celiac disease also presents in children. It should be considered in any child who has vomiting and diarrhea with failure to thrive, abdominal distention (swelling), short stature, delayed puberty, and persistent iron deficiency anemia. Children with celiac disease will rapidly improve when all gluten-containing foods are removed from their diet.

Celiac disease in adults presents with all grades of severity. Adult celiac disease does not always cause diarrhea and may present in mysterious ways. For example, adults may have recurrent aphthous stomatitis (painful ulcers of the gums and tongue), migraine headaches, weakness, anemia, and osteoporosis. Calcium deposition in the brain may manifest as seizures or the gradual development of dementia. These complications are the result of nutrient deficiencies such as iron, vitamins B12, vitamin D, folate, calcium, and amino acids.

Associated autoimmune symptoms include various "itises" such as dermatitis (skin inflammation), arthritis (joint inflammation), nephritis (kidney inflammation), and hepatitis (liver inflammation). If you are aware that certain foods always "upset your stomach," causing diarrhea and bloating for days, or that certain foods trigger headaches, consider testing for celiac disease. Blood tests for gluten antibodies (tissue transglutaminase autoantibodies) as well as a small bowel biopsy (taken from the duodenum, the first portion of the small intestine) will confirm the diagnosis. Once confirmed, call your friendly and knowledgeable registered dietician and read on for hints on changing your diet for a lifetime. (Ammoury RF, Croffie JM. Malabsorptive disorders of childhood, *Pediatrics in Review* 2010 (October);31(10): 407–416)

Celiac disease diet. How easy is it to obtain a "gluten-free" diet? It's about as easy as losing 20 pounds for your daughter's wedding by Saturday afternoon. And, it just so happens to be Friday afternoon when you decide to start your weight loss program. When advised to eliminate gluten from your diet, you will be surprised at the number of foods that have the glutens of wheat, rye, barley, and possibly, oats, in them. As mentioned earlier, oats are often contaminated by gluten during harvesting and processing in the U.S. At least one of the above glutens is present in all prepared foods including most breads, pasta, cookies, cereals, waffles, ice cream, ice milk, candies, chocolate, toffee, meat loaf, sausages, fried chicken, thick soups, sauces, many salad dressings, ketchup, soy sauce, mustard, horseradish sauce, bouillon cubes, curry powder, non-dairy creamer, vinegar, turkey (in its basting ingredients), the filler used in many pills (including over-the-counter drugs, so check with your pharmacist and/or go to www.glutenfreedrugs.com), beer, and some types of whiskey. Suffice it to say that reading labels is your safest bet for any unknown foods and especially foods that come in boxes, cans, tins, foils, bags, and bottles. Think of the positives—most of the foods you can eat are fresh—including fruits, plain meats, poultry, fish, eggs, soy, potatoes, corn, rice, broccoli and other fresh vegetables, nuts, seeds, legumes, cheese, yogurt, milk and a myriad of gluten-free products (available now at a grocery store in your neighborhood).

CEREAL

Cereal. William Keith Kellogg worked as an assistant to his brother, Dr. John Harvey Kellogg, who was a well-known nutritionist and the director of a hospital specializing in nutritional disorders. In 1884 he discovered a process of making flakes out of grains of maize (corn). By 1898 the process was industrialized. In 1906 the Kellogg brothers formed company to market cornflakes, and for over 100 years cornflakes have been regarded as an integral part of both the English and American breakfast.

Breakfast cereals that come in the same colors as polyester leisure suits make oversleeping a virtue. —Fran Leibowitz

---

Are all cereals created equal? The simple answer is no. When choosing a cereal, make an attempt to choose one that might be beneficial for your heart and your bowels. The key word for both systems is fiber. Cereals that contain whole oats reduce the risk of heart disease because of the soluble fiber provided by the whole oats. Cereals that contain *psyllium* can also make the claim that they good for you both above and below the belt. In other words, they are "heart healthy" and "bowel movers." Psyllium is the seed husk from the plantago plant. It is a concentrated source of soluble fiber, as well as a source of insoluble fiber. When you read soluble fiber on a product, think heart-and cholesterol-lowering effects; when you read insoluble fiber, think bowels and bowel movements. So, psyllium provides that double whammy effect on both ends of the body—top for the heart, bottom for the bowel.

Psyllium is the active ingredient of the over-the-counter laxative Metamucil, used by a myriad of average Americans for bowel-cleansing purposes. Unbeknownst to most average Americans that consume Metamucil for their daily constitutional, they are also providing a boost to their heart as well.

ASPARAGUS TIP

Consider the advice of a registered dietician—in fact, pick up the phone today and make the call. This advice can make all the difference in the world for a symptom-free existence.

Celiac organizations can also be great resources for understanding the gluten-free diet. In Canada you can call the Canadian Celiac Association (CCA) at 1-800-363-7296 or hop online to www.celiac.ca. In the United States you can call the Celiac Foundation at 1-818-990-2354 or go online to www.celiac.org.

ASPARAGUS TIP

If you increase your intake of psyllium, from any source or from multiple sources, you must increase your intake of fluids from all sources. If psyllium is taken by itself without extra fluids it has the exact opposite effect on the bowels. Instead of moving your bowels, it will stop them in midair.

Cereal selection. When selecting a cereal, try to find one with at least five grams of fiber and less than eight grams of sugar per serving (16 grams if it contains fruit). Keep an eye on those serving sizes—they can get out of hand when pouring from that big ol' cereal box. Add some fresh fruit (sliced peaches or sliced bananas, blueberries, strawberries) to give some added flavor and health benefits.

The following list contains a few of the top brands of cold cereal (and this list is not an all-inclusive list, by any means):

General Mills Fiber One Bran Cereal
Kellogg's All Bran Extra Fiber
Kashi GO LEAN
Lifestream Smart Bran
Health Valley Organic Apple Crunch Bran Cereal
Post's The Original Shredded Wheat
Lifestream 8 Grain Synergy
Kellogg's Complete Wheat Bran Flakes
Erewhon Fruit 'n Wheat

Not to be outdone, here are a few top brands for hot cereal:

Arrowhead Mills 4 Grain Plus Flax
Hodgson Mill Oat Bran Hot Cereal
John McCann's Irish Oatmeal
Roman Meal Cream of Rye
Wheatena
Instant Maypo Oatmeal (maple)

On April 17, 1998, a total of 13,797 people took part in a breakfast of cereal and milk at Dubai Creekside Park, Dubai, United Arab Emirates. The event was organized by Kellogg's, who provided all of the participants with miniature boxes of cereal. (Guinness Book of World Records, 1988)

CHAMPAGNE

Champagne. The bubbles in champagne are responsible for moving the alcohol into the bloodstream and straight to the brain faster than any other type of alcohol. It only takes five minutes for bubbly champagne drinkers to have a blood alcohol level of .054 mg per ml. The control group, drinking flat champagne, had blood alcohol levels of only .039 mg per ml after five minutes. After forty minutes the bubbly group had blood alcohol levels of 0.07 mg per ml, just 0.01 mg short of the legal limit for driving, whereas the flat champagne drinkers had only reached .058 milligrams. (University of Surrey in Guildford, U.K., 2009. *Alcohol and Alcoholism* 2010;(38):381)

Any ideas as to why? One thought is that the bubbles may loosen the pyloric sphincter (the sphincter between the stomach and the small intestine) and allow the alcohol to reach the small intestine and bloodstream more quickly. Another thought is that the fizz increases the rate of alcohol absorption in the stomach, allowing it to reach the bloodstream even quicker than waiting for it to arrive in the small intestine.

Come quickly; I am tasting stars!
Dom Pérignon exclaimed at the discovery of champagne.

Champagne, when to drink it.
I drink it when I am happy, and when I am sad.
Sometimes I drink it when I am alone.
When I have company, I consider it obligatory.
I trifle with it when I am not hungry, and drink it when I am.
Otherwise, I never touch it—unless I am thirsty.
—Madame Lilly Bollinger

Champagne cork. The carbon dioxide in champagne bottles creates 90 pounds of pressure per square inch, three times the pressure in automobile tires. Flying corks can cause retinal detachment, double vision, and blindness. Aim that cork away from anyone's face, eyes, head! Happy New Year! (Lee Aundra Keany. 20 Things You Didn't Know About Alcohol. *Discover Magazine* 2011)

HISTORICAL HIGHLIGHTS

The shallow champagne glass was made from wax molds of the breasts of Marie Antoinette. Hardly enough to make you giddy. Wax molds of Dolly Parton's famous breasts would be a better choice for a champagne glass for yours truly. Size matters.

CHEESE

Cheese. Did you know that the quality and flavor of cheese is inversely proportional to the thickness of the slice? So when that skinflint neighbor of yours serves you those wafer-thin slices of cheese and you mumble incoherently to no one in particular, "What a cheapskate, skimping on the cheese," he was actually enhancing your taste buds.

To keep the dentist away, eat a chunk of cheese after you finish a meal. It's been known for years that cheese, when eaten after a meal, slows down tooth decay. Tooth decay is caused by acid secretion from *Streptococcus mutans*, a bacterium that adheres to the teeth. It appears that when cheese is eaten at the end of a meal, when streptococcal acid secretion is on the rise, calcium and phosphate from the cheese diffuse into the bacterial colonies and blunt the acid rise. At least 12 different types of cheese, including cheddar, mozzarella, Edam, and Gouda, neutralize acids in saliva and help prevent tooth decay. Aged cheddar has also been shown to replenish enamel in decay-weakened tooth surfaces.

In 2009, the average American consumed approximately 32.9 pounds of cheese. The U.S. is number seven in the world in cheese consumption per person per year. France has always been number one on the list with the average person consuming 52.7 pounds of cheese ("fromage" to the average Frenchman) per year. Malta is second on the list with 50.4 pounds per person, Germany number three with 46.2 pounds per person, number four is Poland with 42.8 pounds per person, number five is Estonia with 41.7 per person, number six is Austria with 40.1 pounds consumed per Austrian per year.

This will come as absolutely no surprise to those of us who live in the Midwest—Wisconsin (the state with the most "cheeseheads") produces 25% of the cheese produced in the United States per year. California comes in a close second with 21.1%. Idaho, New York and New Mexico round out the top five cheese-producing states with 8.1%, 7.1%, and 7% respectively.

Over two thousand varieties of cheese are produced around the world. If you decided to try a new cheese once a week, it would take somewhere in the vicinity of 40 years to sample all the varieties.

There are cheese lovers, and then there are ***cheese love-love- lovers,*** and then there are cheese loathers. I don't fall into the cheese-loathing category, but I do fall into the category as finding the smell of cheese to be unpleasant. Apparently, I am not alone. In order to make cheese, milk has to be fermented—which is basically a controlled spoilage, hence the odor of decay. This particular smell has be compared to that of smelly feet by many famous and many not-so-famous individuals. The famous French poet, Leon-Paul Fargue (1876–1947), is said to have honored Camembert cheeses with the title l*es pieds de Dieu*—translated as "the feet of God."

With all of the different cheeses available and all of those pounds of cheese consumed per person, per year, does that mean that cheese is a health food? Well, not exactly. Thirty-two pounds of cheese per year is between a half pound and two-thirds of a pound of cheese per week, and most cheese is chock full of saturated fat, one of the bad fats if consumed in large amounts. Each ounce of full-fat cheese contains four to six grams of saturated fat. One yummy slice of a medium size pizza contains one ounce of cheese. If you are a cheese lover and you need to reduce your saturated fat intake, cut back to two ounces of cheese per week. Order your sandwiches, burgers, and salads without cheese and order your pizza with half the cheese. Look for "light" mozzarella, which has half the fat of regular cheese. The mozzarella that says "part-skim" cuts out only one gram of saturated fat per ounce. Not great, but better than the full-fat cheese.

So, what are the benefits of cheese? Cheese shares many of milk's nutritional advantages and disadvantages. The saturated fat component has been mentioned as more of a negative effect; however, cheese is a rich source of protein, calcium and energy. Eating cheese as a part of a well-balanced diet is fully compatible with good health. Cheese also contains a hefty amount of tryptophan, the precursor to serotonin. Serotonin can calm you down, make you sleepy, and make you happy. So a piece of cheese may be just what the doctor orders if you are anxious, tired, and depressed.

The 1964 World's Fair displayed a Wisconsin cheese made using 16,000 cows to produce 170,000 quarts of milk to make a 14.5 foot x 6.5 foot x 5.5 foot, 34,591 pound hunk of cheese.

If you want to clear your system out, sit on a piece of cheese and swallow a mouse. —Johnny Carson

---

The cheese stands alone, the cheese stands alone… After Mt. Vesuvius erupted in A.D. 79, 250 people ran to the beach conceivably to avoid the molten lava pouring down on the towns of Pompeii and Herculaneum. Unbeknownst to them at the time, this was not such a great idea. They were smothered in boiling mud that was running down the mountain to the ocean. Don't stop reading— there is actually an interesting end to this gruesome story.

The mud cooled rapidly and preserved their bones so well that scientists were able to do in-depth studies on the remains. They found that 20 percent of the people suffered from a disease known as brucellosis—a chronic flu-like disease caused by a bacteria from infected animals or animal products. How did the Romans acquire the brucellosis? Researchers could only scratch their heads until the discovery of a big ol' hunka cheese—in fact, a 2,000 year-old hunka cheese that was rife with *Brucella melitensis*, the bacteria responsible for brucellosis. Romans were known as avid "cheeseheads" (long before the "cheesehead" Wisconsin-ites), and the proof is in the mud-bone-pudding, so to speak. (Dr. Luigi Capasso, State University G d'Annunzio, Chieti, Italy; interview, Discover.com)

Cheese please.

Roquefort cheese. The name *Roquefort* is patented so that it only applies to cheeses aged in the caves on Mount Combalou near the French community of Roquefort-sur-Soulzon. Historically, the name *Roquefort* has been around for thousands of years. The famous Roman historian, Pliny the Elder, described a *Roquefort*-like cheese from that area in A.D. 79.

The romantic version of the story concerns a young shepherd watching his flock, gnawing on a piece of cheese with a loaf of bread at the mouth of a cave on Mount Combalou. As he gazed across the valley he spied a beautiful young shepherdess. Not surprisingly, he abandoned his meal to pursue the young maiden. If you're waiting for the ending where they fall in love and live happily ever after, it's not going to happen. So, the relationship didn't work out, and we'll fast forward to his return to the mouth of the cave several months later where he finds the abandoned piece of cheese. By that time, the cave's mold had transformed the cheese into something far tastier, and *Roquefort* cheese is presumably discovered.

Cheddar cheese. Unlike *Roquefort,* cheddar didn't patent its name, even though it is named after the English village, Cheddar, and the nearby Cheddar Gorge— an area teeming with caves where the climate is perfect for aging cheese. Throw a few farmers with excess milk in the mix and cheddar cheese began making its mark on the cheese world in the 12th century. Since the name cheddar isn't patent-protected, cheddar cheese today can come from anywhere around the world.

Monterey Jack. Part location and part person, the name of this cheese has its origins in Monterey, California where it was first produced by Franciscan Friars. The Jack part comes from a Scottish immigrant, David Jack, who started marketing his own version of the cheese.

Colby cheese. Colby cheese is named after a town in Wisconsin—you guessed it—Colby, Wisconsin.

Beware of queso fresco (fresh cheese) from "the old country." When families from the old country (Mexico) visit families living in the United States, they may bring products from the old country that do not pass the approval process in the United States. This can lead to some surprises in your clinical practice. A case in point: Thirteen Mexican immigrants were hospitalized with a foodborne illness known as listeriosis, caused by the bacteria *Listeria monocytogenes.*

The immigrants had all consumed noncommercial, unregulated *queso fresco* (fresh cheese) produced locally and sold by door-to-door vendors. All of the bacterial samples from the patients, samples from raw milk at the local dairy, and samples from the cheese sold door-to-door had the same

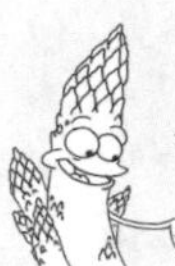

ASPARAGUS TIP

Wrap blue cheeses completely as mold spores spread readily not only to other cheeses but also to everything else in the immediate vicinity.

"signature" as the *Listeria monocytogenes* found in these patients. Listeriosis can be devastating to pregnant women and their fetuses. Unfortunately, of the 13 reported cases, there were five stillbirths, three premature births, and three neonatal infections. (Clin Infect Dis 2005 Mar 1;40:677–82; *MMWR* 2005 Mar 11;54:227–229)

The secret of staying young is to live honestly, eat slowly, and lie about your age. —Lucille Ball

---

Chew your food! Huh? Speaking of eating slowly, a recent study in the *American Journal of Clinical Nutrition,* found that if you chew your food 40 times instead of a typical 15 times, you would eat, on average, 12 percent fewer calories. In the study, obese patients had a higher ingestion rate and a lower number of chews per 1 gram of food compared with lean patients. Twelve percent fewer calories per meal equates to an approximate weight loss of 25 pounds per year. Blood tests taken 90 minutes after eating showed volunteers also had much lower levels of ghrelin (the hormone of hunger) when they had chewed each portion 40 times rather 15. Start chewing, chewing, chewing, chewing and chewing. I tried chewing scrambled eggs 40 times. Not pretty. Perhaps another food item would be a bit more amenable to 40+ chews—like pizza. (Li J. *Am J Clin Nutri* July 20, 2011)

A survey of 1,000 people in 2010 by the sandwich chain Subway, found that the average person in Britain chews their food just six times before swallowing it.

Chia seeds. Chia seeds come from the *Salvia hispanica* plant, a flowering plant in the mint family, native to central and southern Mexico and Guatemala. One tablespoon of chia seeds contains 1 gram of protein, 3 grams of fat (57% is ALA or alpha linolenic acid/omega 3), and 4 grams of dietary fiber. They also contain phosphorus (95 mg), manganese (0.2 mg), calcium (63 mg), potassium, and sodium in amounts comparable to flax seeds and sesame seeds.

Research is sparse and inconclusive as to health benefits of chia seeds as of this moment; however, will eating chia seeds cause a problem? Nope. Will they save you from the ravages of chronic disease? Maybe. One study published in a 2007 issue of *Diabetes Care* found that chia supplementation was superior to wheat bran supplementation for the reduction of cardiovascular risk factors in patients with type 2 diabetes. Of course, that was one study and only for 12 weeks. Stay tuned.

Any other claim to fame from the chia plant?

Yes…the CHIA PET. Chia sprouts are sometimes grown on porous terracotta figurines. An American, Joe Pedott, marketed the first CHIA PET in 1977 as *ChiaGuy.* Chia Pets became widely popular in the early 1980s with the chia ram, and the catchphrase, "Ch-ch-ch-chia," sung in the TV commercial as the chia sprouts shoot out of the head in a time lapsed sequence. This catchphrase originated at a marketing meeting when one of the brainstorming marketers pretended to stutter the name. As of 2007, 500,000 Chia pets have been sold annually, and remarkably, they are only sold during the holiday season. All sorts of Chia pets are sold today—turtles, pigs, puppies, frogs, kittens, hippos, and cartoon characters including Garfield, Homer Simpson, Shrek, and Sponge-Bob.

CHICKEN

Chicken. In 1975, the average American consumed 39 pounds of chicken annually; by 2006, the average American consumed 88 pounds of chicken (boneless, edible weight) per year. (U.S. Department of Agriculture, April 2007)

Chicken nuggets.

- Chickens have been used throughout history to foretell the future. Romans kept a chicken flock for their citizens to predict the affairs of the state. If roosters dropped a morsel food when they emerged from the coop in the morning, good things were going to happen that day for the Roman people.
- The Azande tribe in Sudan keeps chickens for the same reason but they do things a bit differently. They ask a question and then feed the chicken some poison. If the chicken dies, the answer is yes to that particular question, and remarkably if the chicken lives, the answer is no. I'm assuming there are no "maybes" for answers.
- Roosters can fertilize as many as 7 eggs with one episode of unprotected sex with a hen. Interestingly though, hens can lay eggs without being fertilized, and the majority of store-bought eggs in the U.S. and Canada today are unfertilized. Nutritional values are the same whether the egg has been fertilized or not.
- Chickens can run up to 9 mph; hence, catching a runaway chicken isn't so easy. And, they can actually fly—not far, but far enough and high enough to get into trees. The other hilarious fact about chickens trying to get away from a human is that when they run they zig-zag – making the human chasing them look like a complete idiot.
- What's a chicken gizzard? It's a small muscular organ located off the intestine that helps the chicken pulverize anything they might eat. When cage-free chickens peck at the ground they pick up small pebbles to store in the gizzard to use for grinding up the food they eat. If chickens are raised entirely in cages they are fed gravel in order for their gizzards to work. Chickens aren't fussy about what they will eat—chickens will

eat just about anything in addition to chicken feed. So, when they eat bones, twigs, cat food, and Styrofoam, the gizzard grinds them up into digestible morsels.

Chicken. Skin on or skin off? Should we eat our chicken skinless? When you remove the skin prior to consuming the chicken you remove two-thirds of the fat. So, if you're trying to cut back on fat and calories, cook it with the skin on, and then remove the skin prior to consumption, or take the skin off prior to cooking and save yourself the trouble of picking all of the fried skin off and the temptation to just "taste a little."

Chicken. White meat or dark meat? Leg, thigh, breast or wing? Did the chicken fly across the road or did the chicken walk across the road? Which came first, the chicken or the egg? Does a chicken have lips? How many questions are there about chickens? The muscles that get the most exercise contain large amounts of myoglobin for oxygen storage. This protein provides a darker color to the muscle (such as the leg), whereas a rarely used muscle will be much lighter in color (the breast for example). The majority of our domestic chickens spend little, if any, time in the air, as evidenced by the size of a chicken wing. When was the last time you saw a chicken fly across the road? Since chickens spend 99.9% of their time standing (caged) or walking (free range), it follows that the dark meat of leg and thigh are chock full of myoglobin and the white meat of breast and wing are pale in comparison. The next question? Is dark meat higher in calories?

A 2 oz. roasted chicken leg with the skin is 115 calories; without the skin it's 1½ ounces and 75 calories. A 3½ oz. roasted chicken breast with the skin is 195 calories and without the skin it's 3 oz. and 140 calories.

Chicken Soup. "The Jewish penicillin." Can chicken soup cure the symptoms of the common cold? Studies have found that the broth actually has anti-inflammatory properties (via the inhibition of neutrophils, the cells that trigger inflammation). Inhibiting inflammation reduces nasal congestion; however, "curing the symptoms" is not the appropriate term when it comes to chicken soup and the common cold. Perhaps "easing the symptoms" would be a better description.

The other benefit of chicken soup, or any soup for that matter, is the hot steam from the soup that helps to break up thick mucus in the airways and helps clear the nasal passages. (Rennard S, et al. Chicken soup inhibits neutrophil chemotaxis in vitro. *Chest* 2000 (October);118:1150–1157)

Chili peppers. Some of the more common food products made from the various types of chilies are curry powder, cayenne pepper, crushed red pepper, dried whole peppers, chili powder, paprika, pepper sauce, pickled and processed peppers, pimento, and salsa picante. In 1992, the monetary value of sales of salsa picante, also known as just salsa, a bottled sauce of Mexican origin made with chilies, onions, and tomatoes, overtook that of ketchup in the U.S.

What gives the chili pepper its heat-searing, eye-watering, nose-running, throat-burning wallop? Remember capsaicin? Zip back a few pages to refresh your memory. Capsaicin is produced by the "placenta" of the pepper, not the seeds. In fact there are a few different kinds of capsaicin, and they all have varying degrees of "burn." Three of them cause the "rapid burn" at the back of the palate and throat, and two others cause a long, low-intensity burn on the tongue and the middle palate. Differences in the proportions of these compounds account for the characteristic "burns" of the different types of peppers.

The degree of heat in peppers has actually been measured and documented. This scale is referred to as the Scoville Organoleptic Scale. Your basic mild pepper (the green bell pepper variety) gets a big fat zero on the Scoville Scale. Poblano peppers receive a score of 1,000–1,500; jalapeño peppers have a rating of 2,500–5,000; cayenne pepper rates 30,000 to 50,000; and the hellishly hot Red Savum Habanero scorches in at a walloping 350,000–570,000 Scoville Heat Units. (*Guinness Book of World* Records, 2001)

CHOCOLATE

Chocolate is the main by-product of cacao, also known as, "the drink of the gods." Cacao is derived from the seeds of a fleshy pod, the fruit of the cacao tree. Chocolate is a plant product and is cholesterol free. Americans are the leading consumers of ***all*** forms of chocolate. The Swiss eat the most chocolate per person per day and the Norwegians and Austrians lead the world as the drinkers of chocolate. When consumed in small amounts, chocolate can be considered part of a healthy diet, but before you run out and pop for a pound of chocolate, be advised that the American Cocoa Research Institute, an arm of the Chocolate Manufacturer's Association, published this morsel of information. The Center for Science in the Public Interest doesn't agree, but here are some chocolate facts for you to nibble on.

Chocolate contains saturated fat; however, the type of saturated fat is primarily stearic acid, which does not elevate blood cholesterol as much as other saturated fats do. One of those other saturated fats in chocolate is palmitic acid, which unfortunately ***does*** raise cholesterol.

One delicious ounce of chocolate contains 140–150 calories and 9–10 grams of saturated fat. If you add nuts to that ounce of delicious chocolate, add another 20 calories. So, even if chocolate only raises cholesterol slightly, it increases the size of your waist significantly.

On the other hand, chocolate is rich in antioxidants known as polyphenols (like tea and wine) which may help protect against coronary heart disease and cancer; one ounce has about as much as a half cup of brewed black tea. Warning—before you make the giant leap connecting a few pounds of Godiva with a reduction in your risk for heart disease, you might want to wait until additional data is available. It will most likely be a long wait, so don't hold your breath thinking that a box of chocolates is cardioprotective. The phenolics in chocolate have not yet been shown to act as antioxidants after absorption. In addition, the "other" ingredients found in chocolate, such as the saturated fats mentioned earlier, the sugar, and the calories, may negate any positive effect of the phenolic compounds. Oh well, it's worth dreaming about.

Chocolate and acne. Contrary to popular belief, chocolate is not the cause of acne. This myth has been floating around for over 100 years. Actually there are have been no definitive studies proving that various foods promote acne or protect you from acne. There is some evidence that food high in antioxidants such as blueberries, pomegranates, and green tea may contribute to less acne and positive skin health. Other studies have implicated dairy and carbohydrates as promoters of acne. None of the studies have been proven definitively. One thing we do know…hormones play a role. Testosterone is a major culprit, and you can't increase testosterone levels with a Hershey bar.

> **Jackie:** "Pity there's no such thing as Sugar Replacement Therapy."
> **Victoria:** "There is. It's called chocolate."
> —Victoria Wood (1953-:Mens Sana in Thingummy Doodah, 1990)

HISTORICAL HIGHLIGHT

The British firm Cadbury, the leading confectioner in nineteenth century England, first emphasized the connection between boxes of chocolate and romance. Chocolates and flowers became tokens of romantic love and were the typical presents given to women.

Henri Nestlé was a French chemist who first discovered powdered milk. He combined his talents with another Frenchman and they produced milk chocolate bars in the mid-nineteenth century.

Milton Hershey had the vision in the twentieth century to concentrate on the mass production of chocolate. His chocolate manufacturing plant, about 30 miles northwest of Lancaster, Pennsylvania was completed in 1905. Fast forward to World War II when the Army asked Hershey to supply the troops with chocolate bars. These bars were called Ration D Bars and Tropical Chocolate Bars. The Army mandated that the Ration D bars could only weigh 1 to 2 ounces, it couldn't melt when temperature reached 90 degrees, and the most unusual request—it had to have an unpleasant flavor so the troops wouldn't develop a craving for them. The chocolate bars were a hit and the Army asked Hershey to make a second bar that would not melt in tropical zones. He called it the Tropical Chocolate Bar. The combined production of both bars during World War II was 3 billion. The Hershey plant produced 24 million ration bars per week by the end of World War II.

Chocolate and cockroach allergies. Yes, that's the title of this section and yes, if you're allergic to chocolate, it's not the cocoa. It's the cockroach parts contained within the chocolate. The FDA has stated that 100 grams of chocolate can contain up to 60 insect parts and still be considered safe for consumption. The usual number of cockroach parts per 100 grams of chocolate is 8, but if you're allergic it doesn't matter if it's 8 legs or 60 legs. It's virtually impossible to avoid natural contamination in certain foods. Cockroach parts are also found in peanut butter, macaroni, fruit, cheese, popcorn, and flour. (Teich M, Allergist. Mt. Sinai School of Medicine, 2012).

Chocolate cravings and PMS. Fluctuating hormones in women may trigger chocolate cravings. Peak cravings often appear premenstrually, when estrogen is moderate and progesterone is high. The combination of PMS symptoms and a craving for chocolate may be responsible for a woman's capacity to commit homicide for a bag of M&Ms.

Chocolate, dark chocolate. Consumption of dark chocolate has been shown to have similar cardiovascular benefits to kicking back a glass or two of red wine. The dark chocolate (in moderation) reduces platelet aggregation or stickiness and may help prevent acute coronary syndromes (heart attacks) and strokes. Dark chocolate has also been shown to improve endothelial function and help lower blood pressure in overweight adults. Unfortunately, the sugar content may attenuate these effects. What is the healthiest way to have chocolate? Enjoy small amounts (one-half to one ounce) of dark chocolate as a treat. Make sure your chocolate pick has at least 70% cocoa, so you get the highest amount of the healthy polyphenols. (Corder R. Red wine, chocolate, and vascular health: developing the evidence base. B*r Med J.* (2008);94:821–23; Faridi Z et al. Acute dark chocolate and cocoa ingestion and endothelial function: a randomized controlled crossover trial. *The American Journal of Clin Nutr* (2008);88(1):58–63)

Chocolate and dental plaque. On another positive note—cocoa contains tannins, substances that may inhibit dental plaque formation and cavities.

Chocolate and dogs. Is chocolate really toxic to dogs? YES. Can chocolate actually kill a dog? YES. Should I panic if Fido eats 6 milk chocolate M&Ms? No. So what's the scoop? The scoop is that chocolate contains theobromine, a xanthine compound in the same family of caffeine. It takes a fairly large amount of theobromine to cause a fatal reaction in dogs. The amount, 100–150 mg/kg is dependent on the size of the dog, the individual reaction of the dog, and the concentration of theobromine in the type of chocolate ingested.

Although dogs should never have any type of chocolate, milk chocolate isn't nearly as dangerous as semi-sweet or unsweetened (baker's) chocolate. Unsweetened baker's chocolate contains 8 to 10 times the amount of theobromine as milk chocolate. Semi-sweet chocolate falls roughly in between the two for theobromine content. White chocolate is not a problem as it contains negligible amounts of theobromine. Another interesting source of theobromine is mulch made from cocoa beans. Yes, I said mulch—the stuff that your clueless neighbor might use for fertilizer.

The following provides approximate amounts of theobromine levels of different types of chocolate per ounce:

Dry cocoa powder = 800 mg/oz
Unsweetened (Baker's) chocolate = 390–450 mg/oz
Cocoa bean mulch = 255 mg/oz
Semisweet chocolate and sweet dark chocolate = 150–160 mg/oz
Milk chocolate = 44–64 mg/oz
White chocolate—fuggitabout it—insignificant amounts of theobromine
(Source: Merck Veterinary Manual 2012 online)

The toxic dose of theobromine is 100–200 mg/kilogram. To convert kilograms to pounds remember that 1 kilogram = 2.2 pounds, so a 10 kilogram dog is 22 pounds, a 20 kilogram dog is 44 pounds. Easy peasy. Now, that being said, the ASPCA poison control center states that problems can be seen at much lower doses—20 mg/kilogram. If this is translated into a "typical" scenario, a 50-pound dog would have to consume 9 ounces of milk chocolate to consume the 20 mg/kg amount of theobromine. Some dogs will not experience problems with this amount, but it's better to be safe than sorry when calculating the dose.

Dogs are especially at risk as they have a "sweet tooth" similar to that of most humans. The following signs and symptoms can be observed within 12 hours of ingesting a toxic dose of theobromine:

Excitement/ nervousness/ trembling
Vomiting/diarrhea
Excessive thirst/ excessive urination (with higher doses of theobromine)
High fever
Muscle spasms
Seizures
Coma (rare)
Death (rare)—but is usually due to heart irregularities (cardiac arrhythmias)

Is there an antidote for a chocolate overdose in dogs? Unfortunately, the answer is no. The half-life of chocolate is 17.5 hours in dogs. If you have no idea how much chocolate the dog has consumed, it would behoove you to induce vomiting as soon as possible—within one to two hours after the ingestion. Two tablespoons of hydrogen peroxide will do the trick. Activated charcoal may also inhibit the absorption of theobromine. Call your vet immediately. Try to have some idea of the amount of chocolate ingested so that the vet can treat appropriately.

Thankfully humans don't have the same toxicity to chocolate. Humans can metabolize and excrete theobromine much more efficiently than dogs.

Chocolate and Ex-Lax. Laxatives have a long history of mixing with various foods, including honey, sugar and citrus rinds. In 1905 a Hungarian pharmacist named Max Kiss had an epiphany. He knew that local wine merchants were adding the chemical phenolphthalein to wine—for what reason no one knows. However, one of the results of the added phenolphthalein was diarrhea on the morning after a night of heavy wine consumption. The phenolphthalein turned out to be a very effective laxative and he decided to try to appeal to the masses by adding chocolate. It was an explosive hit and he initially called it Bo-Bo, but decided to reconsider and name it an EX-cellent LAXative, hence, the name Ex-Lax. (Panati E. Extraordinary Origins of Everyday Things. Harper and Row Publishers, NY, 1989)

Today's ExLax contains the natural laxative, senna. Phenolpththalein was removed because it had the paradoxical effect of constipation if taken daily for long periods of time.

Coprastasophobia: Fear of constipation

Chocolate and feelin' groovy. Cocoa powder and chocolate also contain substances that might trigger a cluster of neurons in the limbic system of the brain and produce a feeling of well-being. Cocoa contains several stimulants, including theobromine, caffeine, and serotonin. All three stimulants can provide a little pep to your step—it doesn't last that long, but it might get you to where you're going if it's a short distance.

Chocolate. Hershey's Kiss or a human kiss? The verdict is in…a passionate human kiss cannot, in any way, compete with the pleasure of a milk chocolate treat when it comes to a long-lasting feeling of euphoria. Researcher David Lewis found that a chocolate treat gives a body buzz that lasts up to four times longer than the most passionate kiss. In laboratory experiments researchers monitored heart rates and brain metabolism during an encounter with a partner and during an encounter with a chocolate bar. The chocolate bar not only increased the heart rate over a longer period of time but it also had powerful effects on the brain as well. So forget the romantic smooch and dive straight into the bag of Hershey's Kisses. Bottom line: Everyday deserves a Hershey's Kiss.

P.S. One Hershey's kiss contains approximately 22 calories. Half of those calories are from fat. Who cares? The Original Hershey's Kisses Brand Milk Chocolates have been a favorite American treat since 1907.

Choking on foods. What are the five most common foods that cause kids to choke? Hot dogs, candy, peanuts, grapes, and cookies/biscuits.

Cholesterol. Despite the bad rap given to the lipid, cholesterol, over the years, the fatty, waxy cholesterol molecule is an irreplaceable component of many key parts of body physiology—from being a major structural component of cell membranes to a being a major component of hormones throughout the body, including cortisol, estrogen, progesterone, and testosterone.

In order for cholesterol to be transported through the blood it has to be coated with proteins called apoproteins. The combination of the lipid with the protein is cleverly called a lipoprotein. Lipoproteins come in three varieties based on their density when viewed under a special instrument in the lab called a spectrophotometer. The three varieties are high-density lipoprotein (HDL), low-density lipoprotein (LDL), and very low-density lipoprotein (VLDL). They have not yet discovered a "horribly low-density lipoprotein" (HLDL) as of this printing.

A brief digression is needed at this point. The VLDL number is a calculated number. The patient's triglyceride level is determined from a blood test and that number is divided by 5 to determine the VLDL number. For example, if the triglyceride level is 200 mg/dL (5.18 mmol/L), the VLDL will be calculated by dividing 200 by 5, which of course, is 40 mg/dL (1.03 mmol/L). So, 40 mg/dL (1.03 mmol/L) is the VLDL and that will be plugged into the formula for determining total cholesterol.

The sum of the three lipoproteins equals the total cholesterol (TC) number: HDL + LDL + VLDL = TC. In the clinical setting cholesterol is described in terms of LDL-cholesterol, HDL-cholesterol, and triglycerides. Little mention is ever made of a "VLDL level" as that level is only used to determine the total cholesterol.

So, just exactly what are the functions of each of these lipoproteins? LDL, the so-called "bad" cholesterol, is the most "atherogenic" of the bunch. When LDL is oxidized it scoots into the major arteries and forms large lipid plaques called atheromas. The higher the LDL levels the greater the risk for atherosclerosis throughout the cardiovascular system.

HDL, the "good" cholesterol, has three properties that help protect the cardiovascular system. It helps remove LDL from the blood and transports it to the liver, where it is turned into bile and excreted. HDL also has anti-inflammatory and anti-oxidant properties. Oxidation is the process by which LDL is deposited into the arterial walls. The anti-oxidant effects prevent LDL from being deposited into the arterial walls to form "fatty plaques." The anti-inflammatory effects prevent the rupture of any fatty plaques that have already formed in the arterial walls. If HDL-cholesterol levels are too low, LDL continues to pack into artery walls and form fatty plaques. Protection from cardiovascular disease is best accomplished by not only increasing HDLs, but also by decreasing LDLs.

What about triglycerides? Triglycerides are also implicated in cardiovascular disease. Underlying causes of high triglycerides include diabetes, metabolic syndrome (insulin resistance), obesity, hypothyroidism, excessive alcohol consumption, and the nephrotic syndrome.

So what are the numbers? Total cholesterol? Is that number even important? Not really. As health care practitioners, we are more interested in knowing what "type" of cholesterol "makes up" the total (known as the lipid profile or lipid panel), but for the sake of being thorough, here are the numbers for total cholesterol: Less than 200 mg/dL (5.18 mmol/L) is desirable, 200–239 mg/dL (5.18–6.19 mmol/L) is considered borderline-high risk, and greater than 240 mg/dL (6.21 mmol/L) is considered high risk for cardiovascular disease.

The GOOD—HDL levels should be greater than 40–50 mg/dL (1.03–1.29 mmol/L) for the average American man and greater than 50–60 mg/dL (1.29–1.55 mmol/L) for the average American woman. An average HDL level of less than 40 mg/dL (1.03 mmol/L) for men and less than 50 mg/dL (1.29 mmol/L) for women is considered to be a risk factor for heart disease; optimal levels are greater than 60 mg/dL. In fact, levels above 60 mg/dL (1.55 mmol/L) are considered to be cardioprotective.

The BAD—VLDL levels should be less than 30 mg/dL (0.77 mmol/L) (remember that this number is calculated by dividing the total triglycerides number by 5; if your triglycerides are 150 mg/dL (3.88 mmol/L), the VLDL is 30 mg/dL, or 150 divided by 5 = 30…got it?) And, as an FYI, the optimal triglyceride level is less than 150 mg/dL (less than 1.7 mmol/L). Remember this: If the triglycerides are high, the HDLs are low. You don't want your HDLs to be low as low HDLs increase the risk of heart disease.

The UGLY—Optimal LDL levels should be less than 100 mg/dL (2.59 mmol/L). If you have no risk factors for heart disease, or only one risk factor, an LDL of 101 mg/dL(2.60 mmol/L) to 129 mg/dL (3.34 mmol/L) is near optimal. Levels of 130 (3.36 mmol/L) to 159 mg/dL (4.11 mmol/L) are considered borderline high, 160 (4.14 mmol/L) to 189 mg/dL (4.89 mmol/L) high, and above 190 mg/dL (4.92 mmol/L) is considered to be over the top. (*American Heart Association,* What your cholesterol levels mean. March 2010)

Cholesterol lowering via the dietary approach. What dietary changes give you the biggest bang for your buck when it comes to lowering LDL-cholesterol? Phytosterols, soluble fiber, lowering saturated fats, and lowering carbohydrates are your best bets. So, how can you change your dietary preferences to lower your risk of cardiovascular disease?

Let's start with phytosterols. Phytosterols, which encompass plant sterols and stanols, are similar in structure to cholesterol (sharing the same last name, "sterol"). Their mechanism of action is to block food-based cholesterol from being absorbed from the GI tract back into the bloodstream. They were originally introduced into spreads, after finding that stanols could be mixed in with margarine. Especially high sterol levels are also found in rice bran, wheat germ, corn oils, and soybeans. Many juices have added plant sterols. Some products that work in synergy with plant sterols include red yeast rice, garlic, and Co-Q10. The National Cholesterol Education Program

(NCEP) states that 2–3 grams of plant sterols or stanols daily will reduce LDL-cholesterol by 6%–15%, and recommends daily consumption of 2 grams of phytosterols as part of its Therapeutic Lifestyle Changes (TLCs). To sustain LDL reductions, individuals need to consume sterols or stanols daily.

Now, what about soluble fiber? Whole grains, fruits (apples, oranges, mangoes, and prunes), vegetables (root vegetables such as sweet potatoes, carrots, and onions), legumes (beans, peas, soybeans, and peanuts), and nuts (almonds and pecans) are particularly high in soluble fiber.

Replacing saturated fats and trans fats with unsaturated fats—such as polyunsaturated fats and monounsaturated fats—also helps to lower cholesterol. So, replace butter with polyunsaturated oils like soybean, corn, and sunflower or with high monounsaturated fats such as canola, olive, and safflower oils.

If you are going to decrease the trans and saturated fats you don't want to substitute copious amounts of carbohydrates, because they can raise triglycerides. When triglycerides go up, HDL typically goes down. Some people are more carbohydrate sensitive than others. People who are overweight tend to be more "carb-sensitive."

Let's look at the lowering carbohydrates just a bit more. A month-long study published in the June 8, 2009 *Archives of Internal Medicine*, found that a high-protein/low-carb diet trumped a low-fat/high carb diet for reducing LDL-cholesterol and total cholesterol. Weight loss was similar, but the LDL was significantly reduced.

Cholesterol found naturally in foods. Cholesterol found naturally in food, such as shrimp and shellfish and eggs, is not "the bad guy." The major dietary factors that raise LDL-cholesterol are trans fats and saturated fats. Although a three-ounce serving of shrimp has 166 mg of cholesterol—more than half of the 300 mg that are recommended as a daily intake—it has almost zero saturated fat and absolutely zero trans fats. So shrimp and shellfish are good substitutes for entrees containing meat and dairy fat, both of which are high in saturated fats. And, a three-ounce serving of shrimp is only 84 calories. Just don't coat it in batter and fry it in Mazola oil and then dip it in butter.

Choline and the rat brain. Rat brains and human brains have similar hippocampuses, the medial area of the temporal lobe responsible for memory. Researchers at Duke University have found that feeding choline to pregnant rats during a critical period of fetal development (the equivalent to the human third trimester when the pathways are being formed in the brain) would significantly improve memory in infant rats. The offspring of rats deprived of choline during this critical period of development showed a marked decrease in their ability to learn and remember information. Since the areas of learning are so similar in the rat and human, researchers are speculating that the same process might occur in human fetal development. Choline appears to enhance pathway formation, essential for neuronal transmission in both the brain and spinal cord. Subsequent rat studies found that the benefits of choline were both prenatal and postnatal. Both periods of choline exposure corresponded to neurogenesis and synaptogenesis (new neurons and new connections). Converted to "human years," the effect of choline would occur up to the age of four years. (Zeisel SH. The fetal origins of memory: The role of dietary choline in optimal brain development. *The Journal of Pediatrics* 2006;149:131–136)

Bring on the human studies! It's always nice to hear that we have smart rats in the lab, but let's see if these studies can be reproduced in human developing brains.

The average human consumes 8.4 mg/kg per day for males and 6.7 mg/kg per day for females. The average pregnant woman should boost her choline intake in order to provide adequate amounts of the nutrient for the developing fetus. Choline, an amino acid and the building block for acetylcholine, the neurotransmitter of cognition, is found in egg yolks, milk, nuts, liver, and wheat germ. Choline is also abundant in breast milk and in some infant formulas. Soy-derived infant formulas have less total choline than human and bovine milk formulas. An extra egg or two or a handful of nuts just might be the difference between high school and Harvard. Moms-to-be, say yes to liver and eggs!! (Shaw SL, et al. Periconceptional dietary intake of choline and betaine and neural tube defects in offspring. *Am J Epidemiol* 2004;160:102–109. Fischer JA et al. Ad libitum choline intake in healthy individuals meets or exceeds the proposed adequate intake level. *J Nutr* 2005;135:826–829)

CHROMIUM

Chromium picolinate and diabetes. The Institute of Medicine recommends 20 to 30 μg per day for women and 30 to 35 μg for men. Many multivitamins have closer to 120 μg which is considered safe. For our bodies to properly use insulin to keep blood sugar levels under control, we need chromium, an essential trace element, which we mostly get from food. New research suggests certain supplemental minerals may help control diabetes or may even help to avert the development of type 2 diabetes—and one of those minerals is chromium picolinate. It appears as if some individuals who develop type 2 diabetes are deficient in chromium. Chromium assists insulin in moving glucose into the cells and may help overcome the insulin resistance seen in type 2 diabetes. One of the major causes of insulin resistance

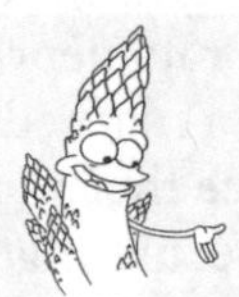

ASPARAGUS TIP

Do ***not*** use chromium in diabetic patients with impaired renal function.

in type 2 diabetes is an increase in the hormone, angiotensin II. Chromium supplements have been shown to reduce circulating angiotensin II.

The recommended safe and adequate intake of chromium is 50–200 µg per day. Most of us in the U.S. get about 50 µg from our diet. Whole grains are an excellent source of chromium. A study comparing 1,000 µg of chromium per day with the 200 µg dose showed minimal, if any, positive benefit from the 200 µg dose. Chromium is considered a safe mineral and side effects are rare; however, it is not advisable to start taking chromium on your own without discussing it with a health professional. (Anderson RA, et al. Elevated intakes of supplemental chromium improve glucose and insulin variables in individuals with type 2 diabetes. *Diabetes* 1997 (November);46: 1786; Preuss HG, *Science News* 2008 (January 15);173:13; Austin RP, *Diabetes Forecast*, July 2011)

Chromium and memory. A small study, but one you might want to remember, found that chromium picolinate may be an effective memory booster. Twenty-six adults with mild memory loss took a 1,000 µg chromium picolinate supplement or a placebo daily for 12 weeks. The supplement group performed better on memory tests while the placebo group showed no change from baseline.

Why might chromium picolinate help? This essential trace mineral reduces insulin resistance, a condition in which the body's cells don't use insulin properly. Too little insulin in the brain may contribute to memory loss. What's the dose? Even though the study used a 1,000 µg dose, it appears as if a 400 µg dose taken daily is beneficial for memory. Drugs that reduce blood sugar may need to be adjusted if chromium is used in a diabetic. (Robert Krikorian, PhD, Associate Professor of Clinical Psychiatry, University of Cincinnati, Ohio, December 2010)

Cinnamon, diabetes and weight loss. Studies show conflicting evidence as to whether or not cinnamon lowers blood glucose and contributes to weight loss. The natural food gurus tout it as a nutraceutical that lowers serum glucose and speeds up metabolism. The American Diabetic Association doesn't recommend it. Most stores in the U.S. sell cassia cinnamon, the type most commonly used for baking and cooking. This is the type that most researchers have used to determine cinnamon's effectiveness in lowering blood sugar. Interestingly, it appears as if the type that gives you the most health benefits has not been the type that has been researched. Presumably the best health benefits come from Ceylon cinnamon, the cinnamon from Sri Lanka. What to do? Cinnamon is safe…why not give it a whirl. It won't interact with the drugs for diabetes, it's tasty, it's cheap, so a teaspoon or two a day might give you benefits—or it might not. If you do plan on buying a cinnamon supplement, choose a brand label with a quality seal. These include the NSF International, The USP label, or Consumer lab seal. This helps assure that the supplement contains the ingredients stated on the label. It also helps guarantee that the product does not contain any harmful contaminants or ingredients. (American Diabetic Association, 2012)

Studies are mixed as to the benefits of lowering blood sugar. Richard Anderson of the U.S. Department of Agriculture's Diet, Genomics, and Immunology Lab gave 1 gram, 3 grams, or 6 grams of ground cinnamon or a placebo to 60 Pakistanis with diabetes. After 40 days, fasting blood sugar hadn't changed in the placebo group, but had dropped by approximately 25% in those who got 1 gram of cinnamon, 18% in those who took 3 grams, and by 29% in those who received the 6 grams. (*Diabetes Care.* 2003;26:3215) Unfortunately, subsequent studies in various countries failed to obtain the same results. (*Diabetes Care.* 2007;30:813)

Some researchers, including Anderson, continue to be believers. The active ingredient in cinnamon appears to be polyphenol type-A polymer, which activates insulin receptors on cell membranes, much like insulin does. If you decided to try cinnamon for its glucose-lowering effects, use a supplement made from a water extract of the spice. It has the active ingredient, but not some of the other things that you don't want—like coumarins which can interact with coagulation factors and increase the risk of bleeding.

Citrus fruits. Citrus fruits have been around for 4,000 years where they first originated in Southeast Asia. Citrus fruits are well known for their amazingly high vitamin C content—a medium-sized orange has 163% of the Daily Value based on a 2,000 calorie diet. Vitamin C has numerous effects on body functions as you will read in Chapter V. However, vitamin C isn't the only nutrient packed in citrus fruits. The fruits are rich in essential vitamins and minerals such as potassium, folate, calcium, thiamine, niacin, vitamin B6, phosphorus, magnesium, copper, riboflavin, and pantothenic acid, as well as fibers including pectin and lignin. More than 170, yes, I said 170 phytochemicals have been found in citrus fruits including limonoids, flavonoids, and carotenoids—all of which have documented antioxidant, anti-inflammatory, immune-boosting, and anti-cancer effects. So, add citrus to your daily consumption of delicious foods. Include oranges, grapefruit, kumquats, lemons, and limes in salads, cocktails, and snacks.

Claviceps purpurea is the natural form of LSD (lysergic acid diethylamide), perhaps the most famous hallucinogen of all. It grows as a fungus on rye, and can cause hallucinations and bizarre behavior after eating infected rye. Mary Kilbourne Mattosian, a researcher and author on the effects of disease on history, observed that many of the seventeenth-century witch hunts (including, Salem, Massachusetts) occurred in places where rye was widely cultivated, and after weather that favored the growth of this fungus.

Clostridium perfringens. Poorly prepared meat and poultry are the main culprits in harboring *C. perfringens.* Poorly prepared, in this instance, means not heated properly or the meat may be well prepared, but too far in advance of consumption. So, as the meat sits, waiting to be consumed, germination of the *C. perfringens* spores occurs and infective bacterial colonies develop.

Symptoms typically include abdominal cramping and diarrhea. Vomiting and fever are unusual. The course of the disease is usually less than 24 hours. Very rare, fatal cases can occur with a specific strain of *C. perfringens.*

Many cases of *C. perfringens* food poisoning remain subclinical, as antibodies to the toxin are common among the population. This has led to the conclusion that most of the population has experienced food poisoning to *C. perfringens.*

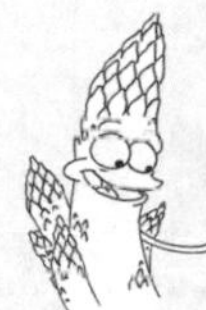

ASPARAGUS TIP

C. perfringens is the main leavening agent in salt-rising bread. The baking process is thought to reduce bacterial contamination.

Coca-Cola Classic and the absorption of antifungal drugs. The antifungal drugs all have the last name "conazole." For example, itraconazole is Sporanox, ketoconazole is Nizoral, and fluconazole is Diflucan. The "con-

HISTORICAL HIGHLIGHT

In 1886, a pharmacist named John Pemberton was working on his newest concoction in Atlanta, Georgia. He was working on a remedy to relieve exhaustion, aid the nervous tremors, and soothe the headache of a hangover. He mixed his new elixir with a boat oar in a large brass kettle heated over an open fire in his backyard. He took his new elixir to the Jacobs Pharmacy in Atlanta and instructed his assistant to mix the syrup with water and chill it with ice. His assistant accidentally added carbonated water instead of plain water.

They both agreed that the mixture would be a huge success, but not as a hangover remedy. He would advertise it as a fountain drink and an alternative to root beer and ginger ale, the only other two fountain drinks available at that time. He had to come up with a name, so he combined the name of two of the ingredients, coca leaves and cola nuts.

In 1891 another pharmacist, Asa B. Chandler, who had taken Pemberton's elixir for headaches, acquired the rights to Pemberton's formula for a walloping $2,000. Eight years later he set up the franchising system that is the basis of the company's success today, and bottled the drink Coca-Cola.

azoles" absolutely must have an acid environment in the stomach in order to be absorbed. The condition known as achlorhydria, also known as "the lack of stomach acid," makes it impossible to absorb drugs that require an acid environment. Enter Coca-Cola Classic—taking an ounce of this brand of soft drink will enhance the absorption of this important class of drugs. Why, you might ask?

The acid content (pH) of Coca-Cola Classic is similar to that of the gastric acid in the stomach, or battery acid in your car for that matter.

FACTS: When Coca-Cola was first sold as a fountain drink in 1886, sales averaged 9 drinks per day. Today Coca-Cola is consumed in 155 countries with 393 million sold per day.

In 1902 the average American drank 12 sodas per year. Today that number is 600 per year.

One 12-ounce can of Coca-Cola = 10 teaspoons of sugar (40 grams of sugar)

The Coca Cola bottling company is the world's largest consumer of sugar.

Cockroaches and catnip. Researchers from Iowa State University have found that as attractive as catnip is to cats, it's just as repulsive to roaches. Toss a little catnip into a roach-infested cabinet and they scatter as if a nuclear bomb has been dropped in their midst. The only problem is, it doesn't decimate the pesky critters, it only scatters them…but hopefully into the apartment next door. (Peterson C, Coats J. Insect repellents—past, present and future! *The Royal Society of Chemistry,* Pesticide Outlook – August 2001)

A digression on the dreaded cockroach: "The cockroach's reputation as a filthy creature is undeserved," says Michael Bohdan, professional exterminator and proprietor of The Cockroach Hall of Fame, in West Plano, Texas. He goes on to state: "They are clean and cautious creatures. They're more careful of where they step with their padded feet than the average person. When I watch them I can see how they react with each other and how they use their antennae to test an area before they walk over it. They groom themselves continually." Has this changed anyone's mind about cockroaches?

Cockroaches and socialites are the only things that can stay up all night and eat anything. —Herb Cohen

---

Cochineal. Cochineal is a red dye made from the dried and pulverized bodies of beetles and is used as an artificial coloring for candy, ice cream, yogurt, and beverages…and you wondered why some drinks, such as Fruitopia, that are colored *red* made *you* red, itchy, wheezy, and sneezy. Cochineal has caused severe allergic reactions in individuals with known allergies—from hives to life-threatening anaphylactic shock. After reading this tidbit you may have another type of severe reaction, centered in the organ of nausea, as you drink your Fruitopia colored with dried and pulverized insect bodies. (*Nutrition Action Newsletter,* May 2008.)

*NEWS FLASH…*March 30, 2012. Starbucks is in hot, hot water right now. The company recently began using ground up cochineal beetles from Mexico and South America to color their Strawberry Frappuccinos. Their rationale was/is to steer clear of artificial ingredients and substitute the artificial for natural. How much more natural can you get? Beetle juice? Going green means going beetle juice.

The vegans are enraged. Strawberry Frappuccinos are no longer vegan.

Cocktail. The term "cocktail" was invented in Elmsford, New York. A barmaid named Betsy Flanagan decorated her bar with the tail feathers of cocks. One day a patron asked for "one of those cock tails." She served him a drink with a feather in it and the name was coined.

Coconut oil and Alzheimer's disease. Fact or fiction? As of this very moment (July, 2012), there is no evidence-based medicine that coconut oil is beneficial as a preventative therapy or cure for Alzheimer's disease. The theory that it may be beneficial is based on the fact that the damage caused by amyloid plaques and neurofibrillary tangles in the brain of a patient with Alzheimer's results in the inability to use glucose as an energy source. Coconut oil contains medium chain triglycerides that can be converted to ketones. The brain can use ketones as an alternative source for energy.

Remember the medical axiom—"Do no harm." So, the risks of trying coconut oil are few and the cost isn't outrageous. Yes, it can cause GI disturbances (diarrhea is the primary problem), if you give too much, too soon. So, start low (1 tablespoon) with meals, and go slow, increasing by ½ tablespoon as tolerated, up to 3 tablespoons per meal. Each tablespoon contains 12 grams of fat so patients should reduce the other sources of fat in their diet. Some older patients may have to start with even less, so keep an eye on those ever-present bowels.

Stay tuned to the Alzheimer's Organization for continued information on the topic. Who knows? This just might be helpful once further studies are evaluated. (www.alz.org)

Coconut oil and other health benefits? Is this a super-dooper food as some websites claim? Can it increase metabolism, boost the immune system, and aid in the prevention of viral and bacterial infections? Not so fast…so far little evidence from scientifically rigorous studies have proven any of the claims made by the purveyors of coconut oil. And, virgin coconut oil has a very high concentration of saturated fats, primarily lauric acid that experts consider neutral to beneficial. One tablespoon of coconut oil contains 117 calories, 13.6 grams of total fat, 11.7 grams of saturated fat, and less than one gram each of mono- and polyunsaturated fats. Until more research has proven the claims, stick with the canola and olive oils—vegetable oils higher in mono- and polyunsaturated fats and lower in saturated fats. (*Food and Fitness Advisor,* July 2010)

COFFEE

Coffee. Coffee was first introduced as a beverage in Arabia around 1,000 A.D. It was called *bunc* and it was believed to be useful as a medicinal tonic. It was finally accepted as a social beverage in the sixteenth century. Napoleon called coffee the "intellectual's drink." Voltaire reportedly drank approximately four gallons of coffee per day, and Bach wrote a sonata, *Coffee Cantata,* as an ode to the drink. Saudi Arabia and Turkey had laws in the past stating that a woman could divorce her husband if he failed to provide her with coffee.

It is estimated that 5,537,000 tons of coffee are produced each year. The average American coffee drinker downs 1.87 cups of coffee per day, whereas the average Swedish coffee drinker averages 5.7 cups of coffee per day.

Coffee and blood pressure. It takes at least four to five cups of coffee to increase blood pressure, not one cup. The rise in blood pressure is not sustained; therefore it's a nonissue in people who regularly consume caffeine. It's important to realize that the effects of caffeine vary greatly from individual to individual, so blood pressure should be monitored if there is any evidence of a chronic elevation.

Coffee as a treatment for asthma. *The Edinburgh Journal* of 1859 promoted strong coffee as the treatment for asthma. The caffeine in coffee is a potent bronchodilator. Italian researchers found that the caffeine in three cups of coffee had the same bronchodilating effect as a standard dose of theophylline. They also found asthma to be less prevalent among coffee drinkers than non-coffee drinkers. (Welsch EJ et al. Caffeine for asthma. *Cochrane Database Syst* Rev 2010 (January 20).

Coffee in the science lab. Oh, those mad scientists are soooo funny. Just a hoot. Here is a perfect example of humor found in the science lab—a description of a lab partner drinking coffee would go something like this: "Approximately 100-kg bilaterally asymmetrical male hominid currently imbibing 100–200 ml of aqueous 1,3,7-trimethylxanthine solution." A knee-slapper, eh? (Courtesy of Kevin J. Hricko, Sr., Pfizer)

HISTORICAL HIGHLIGHT

One day when Winston Churchill was delivering a speech on the floor of the House of Commons, Nancy Astor, the first woman elected to the House of Commons, stood up and angrily interrupted him. "Winston," she shouted, "if you were my husband, I would flavor your coffee with poison!" Churchill, ever the quick wit with perfect timing replied, "Madam, if I were your husband, I should drink it!"

Coffee and cholesterol. The good news: caffeine in coffee is not linked to increased blood cholesterol or to LDL-cholesterol oxidation and fat deposition in the arteries. The bad news: the culprit called terpenes in coffee is responsible for these unwanted health effects. The good news: using paper or gold filters when you make coffee helps trap the terpenes and keeps them out of the cup. The bad news: coffee made with the French plunger or French press, or espresso coffees, including cappuccinos and lattés contain terpenes.

Coffee and headaches. The headache experienced postoperatively by many patients may have absolutely nothing to do with anesthesia or the surgery—it may simply be due to caffeine withdrawal in patients who have been coffee-deprived 12 hours or more prior to surgery. (Weber JG, Ereth MD, Danielson DR. Perioperative ingestion of caffeine and postoperative headache. *Mayo Clinic Proceedings* (1993);68:842–845)

Coffee and Parkinson's disease. Researchers have found that the consumption of coffee is associated with a lower risk of Parkinson's disease, as compared with matched controls. In one Japanese study, the risk for developing Parkinson's disease among those who did not drink coffee was double that of those drinking just one to two (4-ounce) cups of coffee per day, and was five times greater than the heaviest coffee drinkers (who drank more than seven cups per day).

The molecular basis for this relationship is not known and the findings provide no reason to recommend increased coffee consumption in order to prevent Parkinson's disease. However, those with a strong family history may consider this as an option. As an extra bonus, the risk for Parkinson's disease is reduced with increased caffeine consumption from any source, including soft drinks and tea. (Hu G, et al. Coffee and tea consumption and the risk of Parkinson's disease. *Movement Disorders* (2007); 22(15):2242– 2248; Webster RG, et al. Association of coffee and caffeine intake with the risk of Parkinson disease. *JAMA* (2000);283:2674–2679)

Coffee and suicide in women. A study in the *Archives of Internal Medicine* concluded that there was a strong inverse relationship between coffee consumption and suicide as well as deaths from all external causes of injury, including motor vehicle accidents. The higher the coffee intake, the lower the risk of suicide. What's that all about? Hmmmm…could it be that depressed individuals consume caffeine to elevate their mood which in turn increases energy and their sense of well-being. Non-coffee drinkers may not benefit from this effect. (Kawachi I, et al. A prospective study of coffee drinking and suicide in women. *Archives of Internal Medicine* 1996;156(5):521–525)

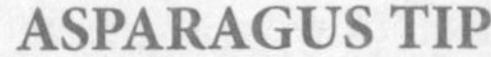

ASPARAGUS TIP

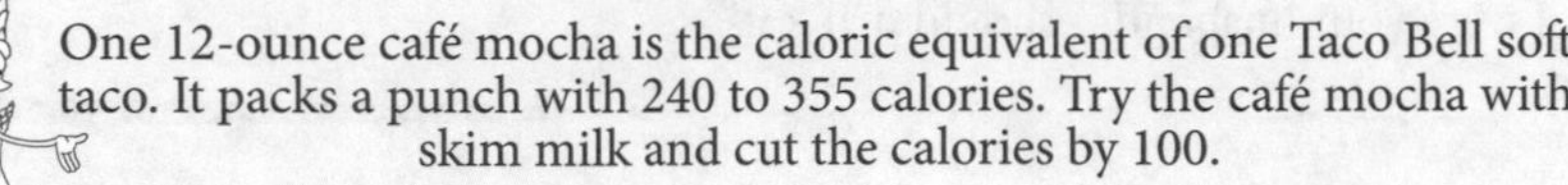

One 12-ounce café mocha is the caloric equivalent of one Taco Bell soft taco. It packs a punch with 240 to 355 calories. Try the café mocha with skim milk and cut the calories by 100.

Coffee enemas for detoxification. Doin' it the old-fashioned way. Nursing textbooks from the 1920s through the 1950s touted the beneficial effects of detoxification via coffee enemas for a variety of conditions ranging from arthritis to schizophrenia. The *Merck Manual* included coffee enemas as recommended therapy for detoxification until 1977. Coffee enemas were dropped from the *Manual* in 1977 because they had fallen out of fashion with the changing technological advances. Today however, with the re-emergence of complementary and alternative therapies, twice daily coffee enemas have resumed their place as detoxifying agents in an alternative cancer therapy program known as the Gonzalez/Kelley treatment regimen for advanced pancreatic cancer. In addition, various alternative practitioners favor coffee enemas as a means of enhancing liver function and removing metabolic toxins and waste. (National Cancer Institutes, www.cancer.gov/cancertopics. 2/10/12)

The mechanism of action is presumed to be smooth muscle relaxation of the hepatic ducts resulting in increased secretion of toxins from the liver into the GI tract and out of the body. This only occurs when the caffeine is administered rectally—drinking coffee does not have the same effect on the biliary system.

Coffee mugs and disease-causing bugs. Don't assume that your office coffee mug is as clean and tidy as you may think, even though you give it a quick rinse after using it every day. A food safety specialist at the University of Arizona rounded up 53 cups from office kitchens throughout the campus. Of the 53 cups, 22 were coated with significant numbers of coliform bacteria. To put it bluntly—coliform bacteria are bacteria that reside in your rectum.

Lest one forget, looks can be deceiving. Even the coffee mugs that looked squeaky clean harbored gazillions of the coliform critters. As the investigators continued their search they uncovered the common denominator causing the cup contamination—the dreaded office sponge or dishcloth used to clean all of the cups.

Mugs cleaned with communal sponges or dishcloths were commonly contaminated with coliform bacteria. Simply running the sponge or dishcloth through the dishwasher or zapping either of them for a moment or two in the microwave kills all the bacteria Two other options are to replace the sponge or dishcloth weekly, or clean your own mug with a sudsy, disposable paper towel.

Coffee myths. Coffee has been blamed for a variety of ailments—from heart disease to fibrocystic breasts to pancreatic cancer. However, very little, if any research substantiates the claims. There is no link between heart disease or pancreatic cancer and coffee. Coffee has no connection with fibrocystic changes observed in women's breasts. The risk for osteoporosis is questionable, but coffee does not appear to increase the risk, especially when milk is added to the coffee. Coffee has been suspected to increase the risk of miscarriage and birth defects; however, studies haven't substantiated these claims either. Still, it is recommended that pregnant women drink no more than two cups of coffee per day. So, if you like coffee, drink it. If you're pregnant drink only two cups a day. Coffee seems to have more positives than negatives when it comes to health.

Coffee. The most hazardous food spilled while driving. And more… (from worst to not-so-bad).

- Coffee
- Hot soup
- Tacos
- Chili-covered foods
- Juicy hamburgers
- Barbecue
- Fried chicken
- Jelly- and cream-filled doughnuts
- Soft drinks
- Chocolate

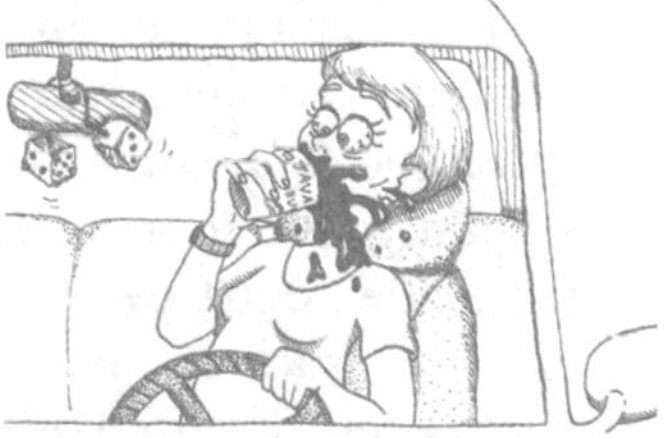

Whoa…it's obvious why coffee might be the top hazard but why would chocolate be hazardous when driving? Think about it for a millisecond. You have just dropped a chunk of a Hershey's chocolate bar down the front of your freshly ironed shirt or blouse. As you try to pick it up it smears all over everything that you touch. You are so busy trying to remove the chunk of chocolate that your attention is on everything but the road. Thus it has made the top 10 list as one of the most dangerous foods consumed while behind the wheel. (National Highway Traffic Safety Administration and the Network of Employers for Traffic Safety—2002)

Color-coded cuisine. Here's a quick test to see if your diet is diverse enough: Count the colors on your plate. If there are four or more, your diet is "as good as it gets."

Comfort food. Can't get enough of that comfort food? Apparently you're not the only one. According to information collected from Information Resources, Inc, (IRI), a company that monitors spending at more than 30,000 grocery stores throughout the U.S., the sales of comfort foods skyrocketed after the terrorist attacks of September 11, 2001.

In the month after the terrorist attacks, sales of frozen appetizers such as frozen pizza puffs, egg rolls, and other bite-sized morsels were up 35% from the same time in the previous year. The sale of Oreo cookies jumped 18%. Instant mashed potatoes and Cheerio sales were up 11%, frozen pizza sales up 8%, macaroni and cheese up 7% and peanut butter up 6%. Ice cream sales rose by 8% and pastries, doughnuts, potato chips and tortilla chips were all up by 4%.

Of course the bottom line to the increase in comfort foods is an increase in the bottom size. Packing on the calories in the form of salts and sweets relieves tension and, as an unwanted side effect, sends the scale soaring to heights previously thought unreachable.

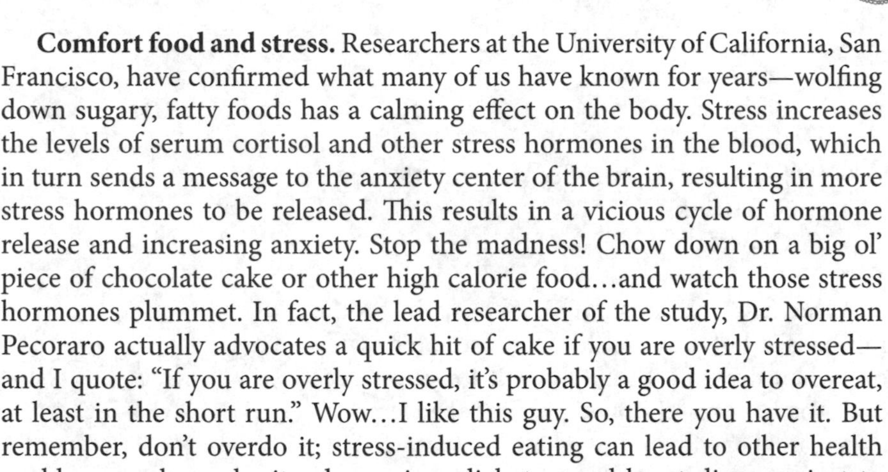

Comfort food and stress. Researchers at the University of California, San Francisco, have confirmed what many of us have known for years—wolfing down sugary, fatty foods has a calming effect on the body. Stress increases the levels of serum cortisol and other stress hormones in the blood, which in turn sends a message to the anxiety center of the brain, resulting in more stress hormones to be released. This results in a vicious cycle of hormone release and increasing anxiety. Stop the madness! Chow down on a big ol' piece of chocolate cake or other high calorie food…and watch those stress hormones plummet. In fact, the lead researcher of the study, Dr. Norman Pecoraro actually advocates a quick hit of cake if you are overly stressed—and I quote: "If you are overly stressed, it's probably a good idea to overeat, at least in the short run." Wow…I like this guy. So, there you have it. But remember, don't overdo it; stress-induced eating can lead to other health problems such as obesity, depression, diabetes, and heart disease…just to name a few. Sugar buzz kill.

Can it be a mistake that STRESSED is DESSERTS spelled backward?

Competitive eating. The 2003 International Federation of Competitive Eating champion, Sonya Thomas, won the Thanksgiving meal Invitational contest in New York by eating seven and three-quarters pounds of Thanksgiving dinner in 12 minutes. She won several other eating contests in 2003—one by eating 23 barbeque sandwiches in 12 minutes, and another snarfing down 43 tacos in 11 minutes. She also holds two women's worlds records—24 hotdogs in 12 minutes and 68 hard-boiled eggs in 8 minutes. Sonya, by the way, is 36-years old and weighs only 100 pounds.

COOKIES

Cookies, chocolate-chip. Ruth Wakefield invented the chocolate-chip cookie by mistake in 1930. Mrs. Wakefield was the proprietor of the Toll House Inn, a restaurant located on the toll road between Boston and New Bedford, Massachusetts. One day, while mixing a batch of chocolate cookies, she ran out of baker's chocolate and substituted pieces of semisweet chocolate in the dough. She thought that the semisweet chocolates would melt in the dough, but much to her dismay, they didn't. And the rest is history—the chocolate-chip cookie made its debut at the Toll House Inn— hence, the original name, Toll House cookies. Fifty percent of all cookies baked in American homes are chocolate-chip cookies.

If you cheat on your husband or commit murder, that's bad. A cookie is just a cookie. —Emme Aronson, plus-size model, on a saner approach to diet.

Cookies. Chocolate-chip cookies and willpower. How much willpower do you have when it comes to resisting a freshly baked plate of chocolate-chip cookies? One study from researchers at Case Western Reserve suggested not much. Sixty-seven college students were asked to work alone tracing geometric figures for as long as they could while a plate of freshly baked chocolate chip cookies sat nearby. The students who were allowed to taste the cookies prior to starting the project worked an average of 19 minutes, while the students asked to ignore the cookies gave up after only 8 minutes of toiling away at tracing geometric designs. Apparently the will to resist completely drained the students' self-discipline to continue working.

Overwhelming stress can be drastically reduced through simple meditation… as long as it is followed by two martinis, very dry, and a 10-pound bag of chocolate chip cookies. —Anonymous

---

Cookie dunkin'. Yes, there has actually been a study on how long a cookie should be dunked into a glass of milk before it breaks apart. Dr. Len Fisher, a professor of physics at the University of Bristol, England, used a fancy mathematical formula (the Washburn equation, if you're interested) that provided the definitive answer—you should only dunk a cookie in a glass of milk for 3.5 to 5 seconds. That's enough time for the cookie to absorb the liquid through its pores, but not enough time for the cookie to turn to mush. He also found how you dunk makes a difference. If you dunk the cookie fairly flat so that only one side gets wet, it will last four times as long—14–20 seconds—as a vertically dunked cookie. Fisher also found that the more milk a cookie held, the better its "flavor release." To determine this last piece of information he ate milk and cookies with a plastic tube shoved up his nose to analyze the gases wafting up from his palate. Seriously?

Cookies, Girl Scout. Girl Scout cookies have been sold since 1934. A Philadelphia Girl Scout Leader came up with the idea of selling a vanilla cookie in the shape of the Girl Scout seal. One day she heard that reporters would be interviewing actresses at a local flower show. She sent a group of Girl Scouts to the flower show with the cookies and the rest is history.

So after all these years of personally consuming hundreds, if not thousands of thin mint Girl Scout cookies—what is my favorite Girl Scout cookie? Sales data from 2010 confirm that my favorite thin mints are the biggest sellers.

- Thin mints top the list with 25% of total sales
- Samoas and Carmel Delights comprise 19% of the sales
- Peanut Butter Patties and Tagalongs—13%
- Peanut Butter Sandwich/Do-Si-Dos—11%
- Shortbread and Trefoils—9%
- Other varieties including Lemon Chalet Cremes, Shout Outs!, Thank U Berry Munch, Ducle de Leche, et al.—23%

Cookies, Oreo. The Oreo cookie is the world's top selling cookie. Over 491 billion Oreo cookies have been sold since they were first introduced, making them the best selling cookie of the 20th century. Thirty-five billion Oreo cookies were sold in 2011. March 6, 2012 was the 100th birthday of the Oreo cookie. (Toops, Diane: Top 10 power brands, Retrieved on June 7, 2007; Oreo Cookie facts, 2012)

ASPARAGUS TIP

Don't forget that the consumption of Oreo cookies can cause stools to be dark, as in black, and can be confused with melena (definition: black, tarry, "pasty" stools resulting from the breakdown of blood in the gastrointestinal tract over 14 hours). I'm sure you could have lived another 56 years without knowing what melena means—and that Oreo cookies are even mentioned in the same sentence.

Copper. Copper is an essential mineral with an established RDA of 900 micrograms (0.9 milligrams) per day for adults and a Tolerable Upper Intake Level or UL of 10,000 micrograms per day. Copper plays a role in cardiovascular health. Adding copper-rich foods may also be particularly beneficial in women since dietary surveys show that women have copper intakes that are 10–25% lower than the RDA. Foods high in copper content include shrimp, lobster, crab, whole grains, nuts, seeds, beans, lentils and mushrooms. It's virtually impossible to overdose on copper from food sources. A three-ounce serving of shrimp contains 163 micrograms of copper. High levels of zinc interfere with copper absorption.

CoQ10

CoQ10. CoQ10, also known as Coenzyme Q10, is a vitamin-like substance that plays a key role in the production of energy in every cell in the body. Its major function is to act as a cofactor the conversion of sugar into energy and to boost energy in skeletal and cardiac muscle cells. Because it is found in every cell in the body, in other words it is ubiquitous, it has been given the name ubiquinone.

CoQ10 is also a potent antioxidant that helps to reduce free radical formation when food is oxidized. Numerous health claims have been made as to its benefits on "making old hearts healthy," preventing the myalgias (muscle aches and pains) from the "statin" drugs, slowing down the progressive degenerative diseases including Parkinson's, Huntington's disease, and Lou Gehrig's disease, boosting athletic performance, and preventing periodontal disease. Wow. Too good to be true? Yes, and no.

We get about half of our CoQ10 from eating fatty foods (beef, sardines, peanuts) and the other half we make in our cells. CoQ10 is found muscles that require a great deal of energy—the heart and skeletal muscles come to mind. In fact, CoQ10 is involved in creating 90% of cellular energy in the heart. CoQ10 levels decline as we age—what else is new? It appears as if CoQ10 levels are particularly low in hearts that have failed, leading to speculation that supplementation would be beneficial. A study in the journal *Biofactors* (December 2010) showed that the ejection fraction in heart failure patients who took CoQ10 supplements rose from an average of 22% to an average of 39% after six to 12 months. The research is not definitive; however, it certainly wouldn't hurt a patient with heart failure to take this supplement (side effects are non-existent)—it would only hurt the pocketbook. It's an added expense to your daily meds but if you have heart failure and money to burn, pick up a bottle at WalMart, K-Mart or Target. Try Healthy Origins, or Jarrow Formulas, available through www.provitaminas.com for 99.9% pure natural CoQ10. (Peter H. Langsjoen, MD, founding member of the International Coenzyme Q10 Association, www.icqa.org)

A small study in 2002 from UCSD (University of California at San Diego) demonstrated milder symptoms in Parkinson's patients taking CoQ10 for 16 months vs. the placebo group. Larger clinical trials in the U.S. and Canada are currently following Parkinson's patients to determine whether or not CoQ10 slows the progress of the disease.

In a 2007 study in the *American Journal of Cardiology* (99:140), patients on statin drugs were randomized to take 100 mg of CoQ10 per day vs. patients taking 400 IU/day of vitamin E. After 30 days, patients taking CoQ10 reported a 40% decrease in muscle pain severity and a 38% decrease in the interference of pain in their activities of daily living. The vitamin E group reported absolutely no difference in their symptoms. There were no negative side effects in either group. This study suggests that CoQ10 may be of benefit in patients on statin drugs that report muscle aches and pain. On the flip side, a study from New Zealand showed no difference in patients with muscle aches and pains taking a placebo or 200 mg of CoQ10. There's no convincing evidence on statins and preventing muscle aches and pains with CoQ10, but it wouldn't hurt to try it as there are no known risks or side effects of taking a 200 mg per day dose.

Should healthy patients take CoQ10 just for the health of it? At this point there is no evidence that this supplement will benefit healthy humans.

Is CoQ10 present naturally in foods? Yes, primarily in organ meats including liver, and in smaller amounts in beef, sardines, mackerel, and peanuts.

CoQ 10 for the prevention of migraines. Preliminary evidence suggests that 150 mg/day of CoQ10 may be an effective preventative supplement for migraine headaches. CoQ10 is a cofactor in several metabolic pathways and it boosts mitochondrial function in muscle cells. It may take about three months to work, but it's worth a try if you suffer from repeated migraines. (*Prescriber's Letter,* June 2002)

Cosmeceuticals. All sorts of dietary products are found in cosmetics today. Read some labels and you'll be surprised to see that cucumber, chamomile, grape seed, pineapple extract, papaya, vitamins C and E, beta carotene, and green tea are just some of the wide variety of nutrients that have been added to cosmetics. Are these nutrients beneficial in the overall scheme of skin care? Evidence for some of the claims made by the companies is just about as scarce as hens' teeth, so don't believe everything you read. Vitamin C may help protect the skin from the sun, but sunscreen does it even better. Vitamin E is rather oily so it may help as a moisturizer, but mineral oil and petrolatum are just as effective at half the cost. Alpha-hydroxy acids (AHAs) are derived from milk and fruits such as papaya, pineapple, jojoba, and grapefruit. AHAs have been proven to help with wrinkles and aging spots since they remove the top layer of skin. It's the acid that does the abrasive work, and this removal of the top layer of skin can help improve the appearance of the skin. Remember that once the top layer is removed the skin is more vulnerable to the sun, so burning might be an unwanted side effect. And of course, burning results in skin damage, which was probably the reason you were using AHAs in the first place. The vicious cycle continues.

Cows. Did you know that a little less than 50% of the cow is used for beef that is consumed by the average American? However, 99% of the cow is used for various and sundry purposes. Some wack-a-doodle even thought of using the fine hair from a cow's ear as the tip for high-quality paintbrushes for artwork. Beef tallow provides glycerin for cosmetics and toothpaste (vegans beware), soaps, cleaners, shampoos, and detergents. Some of the inedible fats from cattle are used for candles, automobile tires, chalk, crayons, fabric softeners, explosives, ink, and matches. The bones, horns, and hooves have been used for buttons, bone china, glues, animal feeds, piano keys, and fertilizer. The intestines are perfect casings for sausages. It takes the intestines from two cows to provide sufficient "cat" gut to make one tennis racket. Huh?

> Catgut is a misnomer that took hold over 200 years ago. At that time, sheep intestines were used to make violin strings. As the tale goes, the instrument sounded like a cat screeching (most likely during violin lessons), and this became the generic term for natural animal gut.

Back to the cow: Some of the edible by-products from the cow find their way into some margarines and shortenings and have been used for making chewing gums and candies. Beef by-products have also been used to make drugs, such as beef (bovine) insulin (used by diabetics in the past), glucagon for hypoglycemia, and thrombin to promote blood coagulation during surgical procedures.

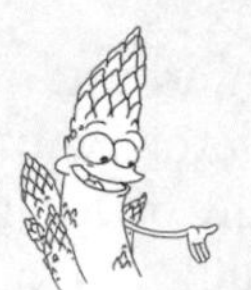

ASPARAGUS TIP

A cow needs three pounds of water to make one gallon of milk

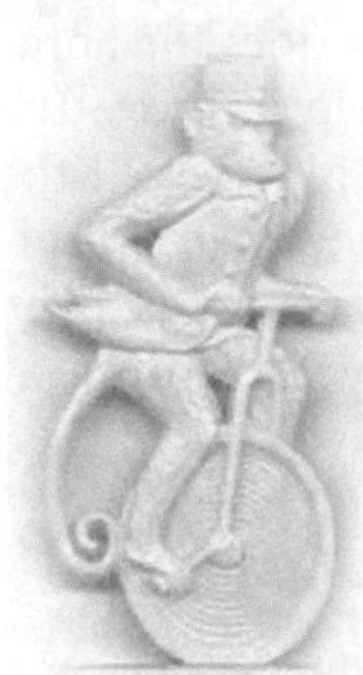

Cracker Jack. The most important part of a box of Cracker Jack is obviously the toy. The toy was added to each box of Cracker Jack in 1912. Since that time, 17 billion toys have been added to those boxes. In fact, those toys are so important to the image of Cracker Jack that each packing machine has three electronic eyes aimed at each box to make sure there is a toy contained within. Collectors of all things "Cracker Jack" have valued some of those toys at over $7,000.

Cracker Jack has been around since 1871, when two Chicago brothers, F.W. and Louis Rueckheim, were making and selling popcorn. They had a pretty good business and decided to add a bit of a twist to the run-of-the-mill popcorn. They added molasses and peanuts to the popcorn and sold it at the 1892 Chicago World's Fair.

It was a huge hit but didn't have a name. However, in 1896 a salesman was munching on the popular popcorn, molasses, and peanut combination and exclaimed, "That's a cracker jack!" And there you have it…the box of Cracker Jack became one of the most popular snack foods ever invented. If you stacked all of the Cracker Jack boxes that have been sold on end, they would reach around the Earth 63 times. And one last tidbit: there are nine peanuts per ounce of Cracker Jack.

Wellington's Law of Command: The cream rises to the top. So does the scum.

Croissants. The bakers in Vienna, Austria created the crescent-shaped pastry in 1683 to commemorate the city's successful stand against the army of Ottoman Turks in that year. The shape of the croissant is derived from the crescent emblem on the Turkish flag, and when the Viennese devoured the pastry, it symbolized Austria "swallowing up" the invading Ottoman army. Croissants made their way to France and became a major part of their *petite déjeuner* (breakfast). Croissants arrived in the United States during the 1920s, much to the delight of the average American.

Devouring croissants should not become a daily breakfast item. The nutritive value of a croissant is minimal, to say the least. A small croissant is 100 calories, and 50% of those calories are from saturated fats.

Cruciferous vegetables. This family of vegetables has been around for somewhere in the neighborhood of 2,000 years. The name cruciferous comes from the petals that form the shape of a cross. This healthy family of vegetables contains bok choy, broccoli, Brussels sprouts, cabbage, cauliflower, collards, kale, kohlrabi, mustard greens, radishes, rutabagas, and turnips. They are considered to be big guns when it comes to disease-fighting properties.

Broccoli and cabbage have been studied the most. They contain various phytochemicals (phyto = plant) including indoles and isothiocyanates. The isothiocyanates stimulate liver enzymes that detoxify carcinogens (cancer-causing substances), and they suppress tumor development in cells that have already taken certain steps toward developing a malignant tumor. Indoles detoxify carcinogens as well, but they also alter estrogen metabolism. The indoles convert the most potent of all endogenous estrogens, estradiol, into the least potent forms, including estrone. The least potent forms do not have breast growth stimulating properties that estradiol has.

Cruciferous vegetables and cervical intraepithelial neoplasia. A small study presented at the March 1999 meeting of the Society of Gynecologic Oncologists suggests that the indoles, the phytochemicals found in cruciferous vegetables, may play a role in *reversing* cervical dysplasia, also referred to as cervical intraepithelial neoplasia or CIN. Twenty-seven women with CIN were given either a supplement of indole-3-carbinol (I3C) at a dosage of 200–400 mg/day or a placebo. By the end of the three-month study, half of the women taking the I3C supplements experienced *complete* regression of the condition, while none of the women in the placebo group did. One third of a head of cabbage contains 400 mg of I3C; however, this supplement is also available in pill form in health food stores in the U.S.

Cauliflower is nothing but a cabbage with a college education.
—Mark Twain (1835 - 1910)

Cucumbers. Cleopatra used the juice of the cucumber to maintain her historically beautiful skin. Her beauty secret has been passed through generations. Cucumber juice continues to be used today in a myriad of facial creams, lotions, and potions to maintain the health and beauty of the skin

Cucumbers also have another claim to fame. They are tied with carrots as the most favorite vegetable for rectal consumption. In fact, the entire cucumber is used for this purpose and, on many occasions, has had to be removed surgically as voluntary expulsion was not an option.

For reasons unbeknownst to clinicians some patients have a tendency to insert all manner of foreign objects into their orifices. The children go for the orifices in the upper body—ears, nose, mouth, and trachea. Adults go for those in the lower body—vagina, anus, and urethra.
—Clifton K. Meador, MD. A Little Book of Doctor's Rules. 1992

Curcumin. Curcumin is a chemical contained in the plant turmeric, which has been used throughout India for thousands of years. It's the chemical that gives curry its spicy nature.

Curcumin and non-alcoholic steatohepatitis (NASH). Research from the department of pathology at St. Louis University has provided preliminary evidence that curcumin may be an effective therapy to treat and prevent the progression of this inflammatory type of fatty liver disease. More research is needed, of course, but if you are at high risk with obesity and diabetes, you may want to add a bit of curcumin/curry to your diet. (http://www.sciencedaily.com/releases November 10, 2010)

Curry. This popular Indian spice was named after a British general, Sir George Curry (1826–1890), who was stationed in India and became extremely fond of highly spiced foods.

Cutting boards—wood or plastic? Plastic. Plastic boards are dishwasher safe and easy to clean. They don't need the oiling that wood boards need, and they come in numerous sizes, shapes, weights, and colors to fit your kitchen needs. It is recommended that you have at least two cutting boards, one for meats and chicken, and the other one for everything else. Cook's Illustrated magazine actually suggests having three cutting boards available at all times, with the third one for garlic and onions. Soft plastic and wood cutting boards can retain the smell of garlic and onions, hence the suggestion to have a third board for the odiferous members of the onion family.

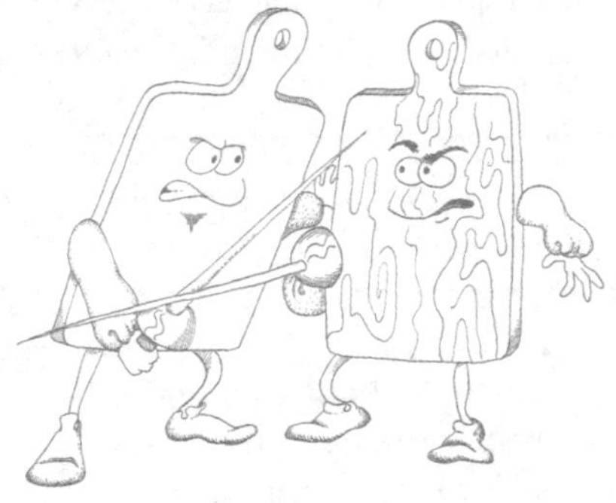

CHAPTER D

I never worry about diets. The only carrots that interest me are the number you get in a diamond.
— Mae West

Daily values (DV). This number is provided on the Nutrition Facts label as a percentage of the total amount of a specific nutrient recommended per day. The percent daily values (% DV) are meant to be used as a guideline to help the consumer understand whether a product is high or low in a given nutrient. The % DVs are based on the Reference Daily Intakes (RDIs) and the Daily Reference Values—obviously all the same words just changed around to confuse the consumer. The % DV is based on a 2000-calorie-day diet; however, it does not take into account the variations in nutrient needs due to age or gender. For example—the recommended daily intake of calcium for a 20-year old is 1000 mg and the recommended daily intake of calcium for a 50-year-old is 1200 mg. If you read the nutrition label on a carton of milk it will state that one cup contains 30% of the daily value of calcium. Hmmmm. Let's do the math. Thirty percent of 1000 mg is 300 mg for the 20-year-old. However, thirty percent of 1200 mg for the 50-year-old would only be 25% of the daily value. So, let's not get too picky. Bottom line: A Daily Value of 5% or less is low and a Daily Value of 20% or more is high. So, check out the DV of the nutrients you are specifically interested in to determine which products are best for your particular needs.

DASH

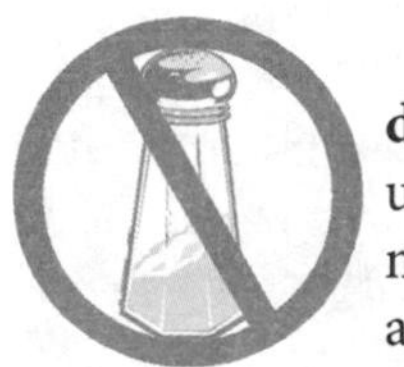

DASH (Dietary Approaches to Stop Hypertension) diet. Chalk up another plus in the fruit and vegetable column. In the original 1997 DASH study, scientists at six medical centers across the U.S. studied 459 hypertensive adults for eight weeks. The participants were divided into three groups. The control group ate the typical all-American diet—high in total fats and saturated fats, low in fruits, vegetables, legumes, and whole grains. A second group ate a similar high-fat diet, but rich in fruits and vegetables (9–10 servings per day). A third group ate an overall healthful diet—low in fat and high in fruits, vegetables, low-fat dairy foods (3 servings per day), and other low-fat protein sources. The two groups eating lots of fruits and vegetables demonstrated significant reductions in blood pressure within two weeks. The overall healthful diet (group #3) demonstrated dramatic reduction in blood pressure over the entire study. Blood pressure in this group dropped an average of 11.4 systolic points and 5.5 diastolic points. In fact, the blood pressure reductions observed in this group were equal to those observed with antihypertensive drug therapy. The findings were attributed to the abundance of magnesium, potassium, calcium and fiber found in the healthful diet. The bottom line: dietary changes that focus on whole foods rather than individual nutrients can lower blood pressure quickly and effectively without the numerous side effects of drugs. The DASH diet is defined as: 26 percent of total calories from fat (with less than 10% saturated fat), an increase in low-fat dairy products, 10–11 servings of fruits and veggies per day, and less than 3,000 mg salt per day.

Update on the DASH diet: As a follow-up to the 1997 DASH diet, researchers have examined the role of sodium restriction and the control of hypertension. All participants in the study received the DASH diet; however, subgroups received different amounts of sodium with the DASH diet. One group received 3.5 grams daily (high sodium), the second group received 2.3 grams daily (intermediate sodium), and the third group received 1.5 grams daily (low sodium). Mean systolic pressures ranged from 133 mm Hg in the high-sodium group to 124 mm Hg in the low-sodium group.

These results are basically the icing on the cake as far as sodium and hypertension are concerned. Dietary sodium restriction does lower blood pressure significantly and should be a part of the diet in hypertensive patients. (Sacks FM et al. Effects on blood pressure of reduced dietary sodium and the dietary approaches to stop hypertension *New England Journal of Medicine*, 2001 Jan 4;344:3–10; U.S. Department of Health and Human Services, National Heart Lung and Blood Institute, National Institutes of Health. *Your Guide to Lowering Your Blood Pressure with DASH.*)

DASH DIET. Daily Nutrient Goals Used in DASH Studies for a 2100-calorie eating plan.

Total fat	27% of calories
Saturated fats	6% of calories
Protein	18% of calories
Carbohydrate	55% of calories
Cholesterol	150 mg
Sodium	2300 mg*
Potassium	4700 mg
Calcium	1250 mg
Magnesium	500 mg
Fiber	30 g (grams)

*1,500 mg sodium was a lower goal tested and found to be even more effective for lowering blood pressure. It was particularly effective for middle-aged and older individuals, African-Americans, and individuals with pre-existing high blood pressure. (U.S. Department of Health and Human Services, National Heart Lung and Blood Institute, National Institutes of Health. *Your Guide to Lowering Your Blood Pressure with DASH.* NIH Publication No. 06-4082, Revised April 2006)

DEHYDRATION

Dehydration. What are some of the usual causes of dehydration? Exercise, high altitudes, alcohol, and hot weather can all cause dehydration. Even mild dehydration, defined as a 2% loss of body weight, can adversely affect health and exercise performance. How do you know if you are dehydrated? The point at which most people begin to feel thirsty is when 1–2 percent of their body water has been lost due to dehydration. So the key is to drink before you're thirsty—don't wait until you feel thirsty. (Food and Fitness Advisor 1999;2 (5):5)

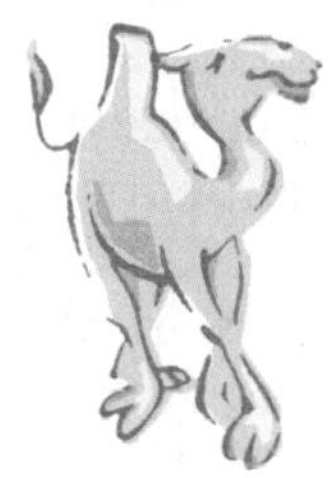

Question: How can you tell when a camel is dehydrated?

Answer: Contrary to popular folklore, it's not about the humps! The state of hydration in camels can be determined by the shape of the hollow in their sides behind the ribs. Diagnosis by this hollow area is so accurate that nomads can tell how dehydrated a camel is within 10 liters.

A well-hydrated camel usually drinks 10–20 liters or more per minute, with a maximum speed of 27 liters per minute. The camel gulps only 3–4 times when drinking one liter of water. The camel can drink as much as 100 liters after going several days without water. When a large quantity of water reaches the blood and tissues of camels, it is diluted to an extent that could not be tolerated by other mammals such as the human. That quantity of hypotonic solution would result in a drastic change in osmotic pressure causing our red blood cells to rupture. The red blood cells of camels can swell to 240 percent of their initial size without bursting. The turnover of water in a camel is also low—82 ml/kg per 24 hours for camels grazing in the summer. This is about half the rate of cattle grazing in the summer. The winter turnover of water in the camel is half that of the summer rate. (Gauthier-Pilters H, Dagg AI. The Camel: Its Evolution, Ecology, Behavior and Relationship to Man. 1981. The University of Chicago Press, Chicago IL.)

Dehydration and fatigue. Fatigue is one of the early signs of mild dehydration, according to Dr. Susan Kleiner, (*Journal of the American Dietetic Association,* February 1999) Dr. Kleiner recommends drinking 9–12 cups of fluids per day. Notice she didn't say 9–12 cups of water…any fluids will do.

Diabetes ("to siphon") Mellitus ("honey-sweet") (Latin) circa 1830).

Taste thy patient's urine; if it be sweet like honey, he will waste away, grow weak, fall into sleep and die. —Dr. Thomas Willis (1659)

Fortunately, Dr. Thomas Willis' prognosis has changed dramatically over the past 350+ years. There are more diabetics today than ever, but with a carefully controlled diet, exercise, and drug regimen, most of these patients can live happily ever after, and not "waste away, grow weak, fall asleep and die."

One million nine hundred thousand new cases of diabetes were diagnosed in Americans aged 20 years or older in 2010. (CDC National Diabetes Fact Sheet, 2011) Wow. The diabetes epidemic is here to stay unless we figure out a way to slow it down or to stop it altogether. Like that's really going to happen unless we make some significant lifestyle changes. Two ***significant*** lifestyle changes come to mind immediately—get up off the couch and portion control. But let's not get ahead of ourselves.

The pathophysiology of type 2 diabetes mellitus is characterized by two underlying problems. The first underlying abnormality is the body's inability to utilize insulin (known as insulin resistance), the hormone that transports glucose, fat, and protein into the cells to be used for metabolism. The second underlying abnormality is pancreatic beta cell dysfunction. In other words, there is an inappropriate release of insulin from the pancreatic beta cells in response to a glucose challenge.

One of the major reasons for the first mechanism, or insulin resistance, is the presence of excessive fat tissue in the body—especially fat tissue located centrally, also known as abdominal, or visceral, fat.

The maintenance of a healthy weight as well as the distribution of that weight is absolutely critical when treating and/or preventing type 2 diabetes. Of course, the simple solution would be to lose weight. Very funny, easier said than done; however, losing as little as 5–10% of the total body weight can reduce insulin resistance and can often avert the need for pills or insulin injections to control the blood sugars. (See Chapter W for weight loss pearls)

Diabetic Diet—circa 1917

Forty-eight hours after admission to the hospital the patient is kept on ordinary diet to determine the severity of his diabetes. Then he is starved, and no food allowed save whiskey and black coffee. Whiskey is given in the coffee: one ounce of whiskey every two hours, from 7 a.m. until 7 p.m. This furnishes roughly about 800 calories. The whiskey is not an essential part of the treatment: it merely furnishes a few calories and keeps the patient more comfortable while he is being starved. (Starvation Treatment for Diabetes—1917) Yikes, I love the whiskey for the comfort part, but I can't imagine the dearth of nutrients given the fact that coffee is the only other component of this starvation diet.

Diabetic diet—the evolution. Fortunately for all involved, the diabetic diet has drastically changed since 1917. From the early starvation diet of whiskey and coffee, to high-fat, low-fat, low-carb to high-carb, low carb, no carb, good carbs, bad carbs, no sugar, some sugar, various types of sugar, to low-calories or low-low calories, to high glycemic index foods and low glycemic index foods. Whew! What's a diabetic to do?

Between 1921 and 1950, diabetic diets were short on carbohydrates and high on fats. This was a complicated diet and compliance was lousy. Throughout the 1950s the percentage of calories from carbohydrates was increased and the "exchange" system was developed by not only the ADA but also the ADA. Huh? Yes, both the American Diabetes Association and the American Dietetic Association used the acronym ADA at that time. Names have changed but the groups remain the same. (The American Dietetic Association is now known as the Academy of Nutrition and Dietetics as of January 2012). The exchange diet offered lists of foods with their carbohydrate amounts, protein amounts, fats, and calories. Complex carbohydrates were encouraged and simple sugars were discouraged. The best news is that it was, and still is, patient friendly.

During the 1980s dieticians started discussing the "glycemic index" of various types of carbohydrates. The University of Toronto developed this index to compare how quickly carbohydrates in food are broken down in the body, converted to glucose, and released into the bloodstream. One of the most surprising findings was that a packet of pure sugar had less of a glycemic effect than refined carbohydrates such as white bread, white potatoes, and white rice. In other words, pure sugar didn't raise the blood sugar as rapidly and as high as a bowl of white rice or a slice of white bread. All of a sudden, it didn't seem that pure sugar was so bad after all. Comparisons of various foods were made—pears had a lower glycemic index than bananas. Heck, even a bag of M&Ms was better for you than a banana. Woohoo…how fabulous is that, as I devour a small package of peanut M&Ms while writing this section. Well, not so fast. Toss those M&Ms and zip over the Chapter G for more on the glycemic index.

HISTORICAL HIGHLIGHT...

...and a "honey" smell. H.G. Wells, a short, dumpy, bald diabetic author with a large head and a high-pitched squeaky voice was well known as a "ladies man." After that description, one might wonder why? According to one of his lovers his body "smelled of honey," which may have been the reason the old rascal had affairs into his seventies with women up to 40 years younger than he was. Obviously erectile dysfunction was not one of the side effects of his long-standing diabetes.

The concept of counting carbohydrates became popular in the '80s and the percentage of carbohydrates in the diet was increased to 50 to 60% of the total calories. At this time fat became the criminal as it was associated with atherosclerosis and cardiovascular complications. The total amount of fat in the diet was reduced to 30% of the total calories. And, of course, the types of fat became the talk of the town. Trans fats and saturated fats were taboo, whereas polyunsaturated fats and monounsaturated fats were encouraged.

So, what is the bottom line about nutrition and diabetes today? There is no specific "diabetic diet." The diet for every diabetic should be individualized and based on healthy eating concepts. Animal protein should be limited, especially if the kidneys are at risk. The DASH diet is a superb diet to follow—lowering sodium, increasing potassium, and increasing calcium. The Mediterranean diet also has numerous benefits with an abundance of fresh vegetables, fish, and olive oil— and wine. An appointment with a registered dietician is the best bet for all persons with diabetes. He/she can individualize a patient's dietary needs and can come up with a meal plan containing an amount of carbohydrates, fats, and protein best suited for each diabetic patient. (Diabetes Forecast, August 2008)

Diabetes and sugar intake. Sugar, per se, is no longer considered an absolute no-no for individuals with diabetes; however, there is new evidence that sugar may play a role in the *development* of diabetes. Researchers from the Harvard Medical School found that women who ate diets high in refined carbohydrates and low in fiber were 2.5 times more likely to develop type 2 diabetes, regardless of age, weight, or family history. Remember that refined carbohydrates, such as white bread, white potatoes, and white rice increase blood sugar much faster than just a packet of sugar. Yikes. Pump up that fiber! Fiber slows down the glucose rise and the subsequent bolus of insulin released from the pancreas. You may want to dump the "white foods" and consume whole grains, bran cereals, beans, and more beans, and also nix the ice cream, cake, and cookies, all of which contain trans fats. (Liu S, et al. A prospective study of whole-grain intake and risk of type 2 diabetes mellitus in US women. *Am J Public Health* (2000);90:1409–1415)

DIET

Dietary supplements. On any given day approximately 160 million Americans will take a dietary supplement. Americans spent $26.9 billion on dietary supplements of all types in 2009, up from $20.4 billion in 2004. In 2009, vitamins accounted for 34% of total supplement sales, totaling $1.9 billion.

Approximately one in four persons taking a prescription medication also takes a dietary supplement. Asthma, insomnia, depression, chronic GI disorders, pain, memory problems, and menopausal symptoms are the medical conditions for which supplements are most commonly used. Patients at high risk for interactions, such as those with seizure disorders, cardiac arrhythmia, hypertension, and heart failure, often report supplement use. (Gardiner P, Phillips R, Shaughnessy AF. Herbal and dietary supplement-drug interactions in patients with chronic illnesses. *Am Fam Phys* 2008 Jan 1;77(1): 73–78)

There are more than 54,000 dietary supplements listed in the Natural Medicines Comprehensive Data base with only 33% showing some degree of scientific backing for their effectiveness. Approximately 12% have been flagged for safety issues. Do ***not*** use the following: Aconite, bitter orange, chaparral, colloidal silver, coltsfoot, comfrey, country mellow, germanium greater celandine, kava, lobelia, and yohimbine*. (Michele Erskine, UCLA, Division of Geriatrics, 2011)

*Yohimbine is the supplement added to most of the over-the-counter erectile dysfunction drugs sold on late night TV between midnight and six a.m. It has only been proven to boost erectile function in rats—in fact, male rats copulated with female rats 45 times in 15 minutes when given yohimbine. The female rats were not amused. The problem with yohimbine in humans is that it sends your blood pressure into orbit…you will by-pass the bedroom for the emergency room with a hypertensive crisis. Steer clear of those late night commercials touting performance enhancement, guys.

Probably nothing in the world arouses more false hopes than the first four hours of a diet. —Dan Bennett

---

Diets and high school wrestlers. A survey of 2,532 Michigan high school wrestlers uncovered the most common methods for quick weight loss used by these young athletes. Sixteen percent tried to spit the weight away every day, while 22% did so 1–4 days a week. Brilliant. Who said wrestlers were Rhodes Scholars? Other wrestlers wore plastic or rubber suits, fasted for more than one day, restricted fluids, took diuretics, laxatives and/or diet pills, and purged after eating a huge meal. (Kiningham RB, Gorenflo DW. Weight loss methods of high school wrestlers. *Medicine and Science in Sports and Exercise* (2001);33:810–813)

Diets. Wikipedia lists over 100 different types of diets…from the alkaline diet to the Zone diet. How can we *not* lose weight? Look at all of the choices we have. High protein, low carbs, low fat, no carbs, no protein, vegetables only, fruits high in water content only, grapefruit with every meal, protein at breakfast only, veggies only…Surely there's a diet for all of us. Here are a few of the popular diets today and how they are supposed to be the "end all and be all to one and all."

Alkaline diet: The alkaline diet is based on a scientifically unsupported theory that certain foods help to maintain the balance of the slight alkalinity of blood. Clinical benefits are unknown.

Atkins diet: A very low carbohydrate diet, high in protein, protein, and protein—any protein—red meat, white meat, all meat, a few vegetables, and very little fruit (especially in the induction phase). The Dr. Atkins Diet Revolution was first published in 1972. In his second book, he modified parts of the diet but didn't alter the original concepts of low carbs and high protein. He also added exercise on the second go-around.

Cardiologist's Diet: "If it tastes good, spit it out."

Jenny Craig. Jenny Craig and her husband, Sidney, founded this diet, also known as "Jenny," in 1983. Jenny's "clients" are provided with individual, private counseling sessions with program consultants. Clients are required to join a plan and purchase prepackaged foods or order for home delivery. Plans are directed toward specific groups—men, women, teens, diabetics, and the elderly. Jenny Craig's diet menus are based on the glycemic index of foods. (See chapter G for the Glycemic Index)

Dukan diet. One of the most popular current diet programs in France is designed by the French nutritionist, Pierre Dukan. The protein-based diet plan is based on over 100 allowed foods and is divided into four phases: attack, cruise, consolidation, and stabilization. This is the current diet used by "the stars" to shed a few pounds rapidly. (Dukan P. The Dukan Diet. Random House, NY. 2011)

Eat This, Not That. This guide is aimed squarely at male readers who eat mainly at fast-food restaurants. Zinczenko and Goulding's idea of a "diet" is to substitute one bad meal for another bad meal with fewer calories—in other words, eat a Big Mac (540 calories) instead of a Whopper with cheese (760 calories). Actually its not a bad book—if you're going to make lousy choices to begin with, make better lousy choices by taking this book with you to McDonald's, KFC, and Burger King. (David Zinczenko, with Matt Goulding. Eat This, Not That! Rodale)

Genotype diet. Naturopathic physician, Dr. Peter J. D'Adamo has identified six genotypes and gives food dos and don'ts for each. And if you believe this one, I have a bridge to sell you. (Dr. Peter J. D'Adamo and Catherine Whitney. Eat Right For Your Blood Type. Broadway Press)

Old Country Buffet Diet: "I'm gonna have the buffet, do you have another one for my husband?"

PALEO diet. Eat like a caveman. Walk like an Egyptian. Speaking of cavemen, The Otzi caveman, whose frozen remains were found after 5,300 years, had his stomach contents analyzed and the following foods were found: wild cereals, wild goat called ibex, some flowering plants, and red deer. His last meal was a wild goat eaten within one hour of his demise. So, even tho' everyone discusses the PALEO diet as all natural fruits and vegetables, it appears as if cavemen also dined quite a bit on wild meat. So, with this caveman diet, what did his health show? Scans and other studies revealed arteriosclerosis (hardening of the arteries), gallstones, arthritic knees (perhaps related to Lyme disease), and intestinal whipworms (parasites) and fleas. So much for the epitome of caveman health.

Skinny Bitch in the Kitch. No sugar, no dairy, no white flour, no coffee, no diet drinks and no artificial sweeteners. Probably the "b" word is appropriate if you have to cut all of the above out of your diet. And it's all vegan. And it's hysterical. (Rory Freedman and Kim Barnouin, Running Press)

South Beach Diet. A diet plan designed by a cardiologist, Dr. Robert Agatston and dietician Marie Almon as an alternative to low-fat approaches touted by Dr. Dean Ornish and the Pritkin diet. It's based on "good carbs" vs. "bad carbs" and "good fats" vs. "bad fats." The carbs were "good carbs" if they have a low glycemic index. (www.southbeachdiet.com/)

TV ad diet. If you based your entire diet on foods seen in TV ads, you would eat 25 times the recommended servings of sugars and 20 times the recommended servings of fat. You would also eat an overabundance of salt, but an undersupply of vitamins A, D, and E. (*Journal of the American Dietetic Association,* June 2010)

Weight Watchers: Jean Nidetch, the founder of Weight Watchers, weighed 214 pounds when she had the brainstorm to start her business in 1963. One of the best approaches compared to other diets, Weight Watchers uses the combination of teaching helpful habits, eating smarter, pumping up the exercise, and providing intensive support, the so-called "power of the group." Weight Watchers is the only commercial weight loss program whose efficacy has been demonstrated in a large, multisite, randomized, controlled trial. It produces a mean loss of approximately 5% of initial weight, which in most cases is sufficient to prevent or ameliorate weight-related health complications. (Tsai AB, Wadden TA. Systematic review: An evaluation of major commercial weigh loss programs in the United States. *Annals of Internal Medicine.* 2005;142(1):56)

Weight Watchers has substantially changed its weight loss program. Their *POINTS* program has been updated to *Points Plus,* which takes into account research on protein, fiber, and satiety, and shifts away from processed foods to more whole, natural foods. One big change is that most unsweetened fruits and vegetables—except starchy vegetables like corn and potatoes—will be counted as zero in the *Points Plus* program. (www.WeightWatchers.com)

Zone diet. This diet is the 40:30:30 ratio of calories—40% carbohydrates, 30% proteins, and 30% fats, respectively. (www.zonediet.com)

The biggest seller is cookbooks, and the second is diet books….how not to eat what you have just learned to cook. —Andy Rooney

---

Dioxin and other closely related dreaded chemicals. This toxic chemical group consists of dioxin, furans, and PCBs (polychlorinated biphenyls). All three contain nasty benzene rings, and can enter into the nucleus of cells to wreak havoc with the genetic material. Chemical damage to DNA can result in birth defects such as neural tube defects (spina bifida syndromes) and uncontrolled cellular proliferation leading to cancer. In fact, the Environmental Protection Agency estimates that the cancer risk increases by one in 100 for the most dioxin-sensitive individuals.

Another known toxic effect includes developmental delays in children. Reproductive changes in males have been observed and include a reduction in testicular size, lower testosterone levels, and reduced sperm counts. In women, dioxin has been linked to an increased risk of endometriosis and infertility. Immune dysfunction may also occur in dioxin-exposed individuals. Children may be less responsive to vaccines, and allergy symptoms may be aggravated in individuals with allergic disorders. There is also some evidence that these chemicals may increase the risk of autoimmune diseases.

Dioxins, furans, and PCBs are released into the air via municipal waste incinerators, hospital incinerators, electrical transformers, chemical and pesticide manufacturing, and pulp and paper bleaching. Inhalation of particles may occur; however, this is not the major route of entry. The toxins settle on grazing land, in lakes, ponds, rivers, and streams, and in other bodies of water. Cattle eat the dioxin-laden grass, and fish and shellfish ingest small particles of dioxin-laced sediment. Dioxin-tainted grain is also fed to hogs and cattle where it concentrates in fat tissue.

Dioxin works its way up the food chain as humans consume fish, shellfish, beef, and pork. In fact, the "fattier" the fish, beef, or pork, the greater the concentration of dioxin. Vegans, who eat no animal products, obviously ingest the lowest levels of dioxin. In contrast, the followers of various high animal protein diets, i.e. the Atkins diet, ingest the most.

More than 90 percent of human exposure comes from fish and shellfish, meat, poultry, and non-skim dairy products. If you are a lobster eater, note that the dioxin is concentrated in the "green stuff" that is pulled out of the body of the lobster. (By the way, that "green stuff" is actually the liver and pancreas of the lobster, combined in one green, gooey mass—ick.) Pregnant women dining on lobster should be especially aware of the dangers to the developing fetus, and make sure that none of that gooey green stuff is ingested.

Freshwater fish contain the highest amounts of dioxin, furans, and PCBs, with an average of 274 picograms per 4 ounces of fish. Farm-raised shellfish and fish are next at 95 and 70 picograms per 4 ounces, respectively. Beef measures in at 33 picograms, 4 ounces of pork at 26 picograms, two eggs at 13 picograms and one cup of whole milk at 11 picograms. Choose your foods wisely. Be careful about freshwater seafood, especially if you are in the mood or the mode to get pregnant.

Most of the seafood consumed in the U.S. is farm-raised fish, and therefore has lower levels of dioxin than wild freshwater fish. Two of the most commonly eaten fish are pollock—the white fish that ends up in most fish sticks and fried fish sandwiches—and tuna. If you are a catfish and trout lover you are in luck. Most catfish and trout are farm-raised and fed largely on plant meal, therefore their dioxin levels are miniscule compared to the catfish and trout swimming in streams and in the mighty Mississippi. (*Nutrition Action Newsletter,* October 2000.)

Disliked foods. The most disliked foods of the average Americai tofu, liver, yogurt, Brussels sprouts, lamb, and prunes.

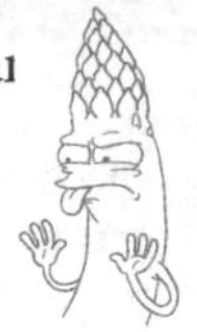

Q: What is the difference between Brussels sprouts and boogers?

A: Children will eat their boogers…

Gross. But true.

Diuretics. Diuretics (thiazide and "loop" diuretics—hydrochlorothiazide/HCTZ, furosemide/Lasix, bumetanide/Bumex) are not only one of the oldest classes of drugs used for hypertension, but they are also considered first-line therapy for many patients with hypertension. By lowering blood pressure, diuretics lower the risk for heart attacks, strokes and all other causes of death from cardiovascular diseases. Diuretics increase the excretion of water from the kidneys and subsequently reduce the blood volume. When blood volume is lowered, the blood pressure falls. One of the side effects of diuretics is directly related to their ability to increase the excretion of water via the kidneys. The problem is that electrolytes (particularly sodium and potassium) are excreted right along with the water. Patients taking diuretics generally need to increase their intake of potassium-containing foods if their serum potassium levels become too low.

Interestingly, one of the presumed effects of the low potassium associated with diuretics is an *increased* risk of type 2 diabetes. Potassium plays a role in the regulation and secretion of insulin—not enough potassium? Insulin secretion decreases and blood sugar levels rise. Easy fix—increase the amount of foods that contain potassium! *Really?* Does that work? Yes, actually it does. So flip over to the P chapter and look at all of the delicious foods that contain large amounts of potassium. Recommend these potassium-containing foods to your patients who are taking diuretics for blood pressure control.

Diverticulitis, diverticulosis, diverticular disease. The terms diverticulosis and diverticular disease usually refer simply to the presence of ***un***inflamed diverticula. The term diverticulitis is an inflammation of the diverticula.

What are diverticula? And how do they become "itised" or inflamed? Diverticula are defined as herniations (pouches) of the lining of the large bowel or colon. They occur at the weakest areas of the bowel wall right next to blood vessels that penetrate the wall of the colon. Diminished stool bulk from insufficient dietary fiber leads to a reduction in gastrointestinal transit time (a fancy way of saying that stool sits in the large bowel for way too long), which subsequently elevates pressure within the colon and causes the bowel lining to herniate. Once diverticula are present, particles of undigested food become lodged within the pouch. The opening of the diverticula becomes blocked or obstructed, setting the stage for inflammation and the overgrowth of normal colonic bacteria. It is estimated that symptomatic inflammation of the diverticula, referred to as diverticul***itis,*** will develop in

It was a long held assumption that patients with diverticulosis should refrain from eating nuts and foods containing seeds. This erroneous piece of advice has no scientific basis and eliminates many nutritious and high-fiber foods. (McNally PR. GI/Liver Secrets Plus. 2010 4th edition. Mosby)

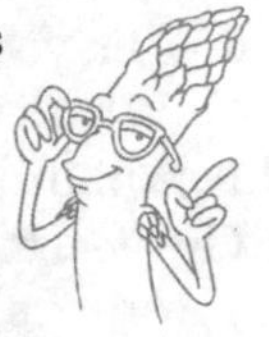

only 20 percent of the patients with diverticula. Diverticulosis is extremely common in Western society, affecting approximately five to 10 percent of the population over 45 years of age and almost 80 percent of the population over 85 years of age.

The treatment for acute diverticulitis is oral hydration consisting of a liquid diet and 7–10 days of a broad-spectrum antibiotic such as ciprofloxacin (Cipro) or metronidazole (Flagyl). Once the acute attack has resolved, the patient should be instructed to maintain a high-fiber diet to keep things moving through the colon. In other words, "eat like a vegetarian" and eat lots of high-fiber fruits and vegetables. You want to "get the food in" and "get the food out." You don't want food to hang around in the colon for long periods of time.

A recent 12-year study of 47,000 people found that the 33 percent who were vegetarians were 31 percent less likely to develop diverticulitis, be admitted to the hospital for the disease, or to die of the condition. Vegans were at an even lower risk. Participants who ate the most fiber had a 42 percent lower risk; meat-eaters with the highest fiber intake had a 26 percent lower risk than meat-eaters who ate the least fiber. Fibers speeds the passage of foods through the digestive system, which can reduce internal pressure in the intestines, and reduce the risk of developing diverticula in the first place.

Doctrine of Signatures. Translations from medical texts from 700 B.C. describe an interesting concept called the Doctrine of Signatures. This doctrine is based on the concept that for every part of the human body there is a corresponding part in the world of nature. The ancient physician-priests used this doctrine as the basis for their medical therapies.

For example, if you had jaundice (a medical condition with yellowing of the skin or whites of the eyes, arising from excess bilirubin in the blood), you might be treated with a mixture based on an eviscerated yellow frog. Liverwort plant, with leaves shaped like the liver, would be the correct treatment for diseases of the liver. So a dash of eviscerated yellow frog wrapped in the leaves of the liverwort plant may be just the remedy for the "yellow" jaundice caused by liver disease.

The whole ginseng root, resembling a human body, became known as the "whole-body tonic." And, interestingly, if you read the indications for ginseng, most state that ginseng is good for "whatever ails ya'"—from a bunion to a brain tumor.

Carrots have always been used for "eye-health" due to the large amounts of vitamin A (carotenoids such as beta carotene, a precursor to vitamin A). A carrot that has been cut horizontally has the appearance of the iris of the eye.

Walnuts closely resemble the two halves of the human brain, the cerebral hemispheres. Walnuts have one of the highest contents of alpha linoleic acid, the precursor to omega-3 fatty acids. And, we all know that omega-3s are "brain food." (See chapter O for Omega-3 fatty acids)

Eggplant, avocado, and pears target the health of the uterus and cervix. Interestingly it takes an avocado exactly nine months to grow from the blossom to the ripened fruit.

Kidney beans? Look like??

Sweet potatoes have a similar shape to the pancreas. Sweet potatoes help to balance the glycemic index. The pancreas is instrumental in producing insulin and glucagon in order to control blood sugars.

Oysters and the testicles? The oyster and the testicle not only resemble one another, but the testicle also benefits from the highly concentrated amount of zinc contained in the oyster. Males with zinc deficiencies fail to produce enough testosterone and sperm, resulting in erectile dysfunction and infertility.

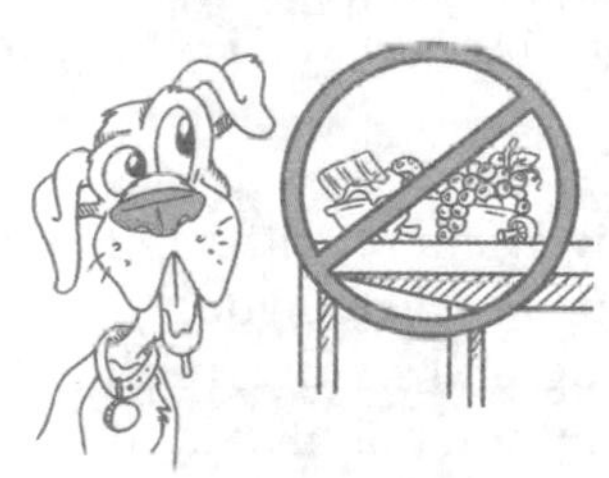

Doggie don'ts. Chocolate, avocado, any fruit pit, raisins or grapes, mushrooms, potato peelings, sugarless chewing gum with Xylitol…

As pet owners we often like to share with our pets all of the things we love and enjoy in life, including food. However, there are a couple of reasons that you should always be very careful when considering introducing human treats to your pet. The first and most obvious reason is that the food you want to share may not be a particularly healthy food item, and therefore you should think twice about allowing your pet to acquire a taste for something they shouldn't have. Secondly and most importantly, although you may very well enjoy a particular food yourself, it might actually be very poisonous for your pet. The following is a list of foods that your pet should avoid, as they are all poisonous to some degree.

Alcoholic Beverages: Any type of alcohol can be poisonous to your pet and aside from intoxication, can cause coma or even death. Hops (as in beer) may cause panting, elevated temperature, increased heart rate, seizures and possibly death.

Apricot pits, cherry pits, and peach pits: All of the listed pits may cause respiratory difficulties such as breathing, coughing and sneezing in pets.

Chocolate and Coffee: The theobromine in chocolate and coffee may result in rapid respirations, an increased heart rate, restlessness and agitation.

Grapes: Large amounts of grapes can be poisonous to pets and can cause vomiting, diarrhea, lethargy, abdominal pain, lack of appetite and kidney damage.

Macadamia Nuts: Macadamia nuts may cause vomiting, lethargy, high fever, abdominal pain, stiff joints, lameness and tremors.

Moldy Foods: Moldy foods can have varied effects on pets, including vomiting and diarrhea.

Mushrooms: Various types of mushrooms can have varied effects on pets including depression, diarrhea, nausea and vomiting, abdominal pain, tearing, hallucinations, defecation, liver failure, seizures, drooling, urination, kidney failure, heart damage, hyperactivity and in some cases, death.

Onions and Onion Powder: Onions and onion powder can cause gastrointestinal problems such as vomiting and diarrhea.

Raisins: Large amounts of raisins can be poisonous to pets and result in vomiting, diarrhea, lethargy, abdominal pain, lack of appetite and kidney damage.

Salt: Salt in large quantities can cause electrolyte imbalances.

Walnuts: Walnuts can cause gastrointestinal problems such as vomiting and diarrhea, as well as respiratory issues such as sneezing, breathing and coughing.

Xylitol: Xylitol is a popular sugar substitute used in sugarless chewing gum and candy. It's found in a variety of other products as well, including baked goods, chewable vitamins, throat lozenges, and over-the-counter medications. It is totally safe for human consumption…but, it is *LETHAL* for dogs.

The ASPCA Animal Poison Control Center has received reports of dogs ingesting large amounts xylitol that have developed liver failure within 72 hours. In dogs, xylitol promotes insulin release resulting in severe hypoglycemia, with loss of muscle control in standing or walking, and seizures. Call your veterinarian immediately if your dog consumes any amount of xylitol-containing products. The ASPCA Animal Poison Control Center also offers around-the-clock consultations. Call (888) 426-4435 for a fee of $65.00. (Cummings School of Veterinary Medicine at Tufts University, *Your Dog*, May 2011)

Yeast Dough: Yeast dough can be dangerous as it will expand and result in gas, pain and possible rupture of the stomach or intestines in your dogs.

Dr Pepper. Why did Dr Pepper bottles have the numbers 10, 2, and 4 written on the sides? These are the times that a person's blood sugars are lowest and can therefore be "revived" by a sugary drink such as Dr Pepper. P.S. There is no period after Dr in Dr Pepper. This is not a typing error. (The Book of Answers. New York Public Library, 1998)

Drug interactions with dietary supplements and foods. The Food and Drug Administration (FDA) has recently teamed up with the National Consumers League to publish a list of foods people should avoid when taking

HISTORICAL HIGHLIGHT

In 1885, a pharmacist named Charles Alderton created a 23-flavor beverage. He gave the recipe to his boss, Wade Morrison, the pharmacists who owned the drug store. Morrison thought it was pretty tasty and served it in the soda fountain of his Old Corner Drug Store in Waco, Texas. Customers came from far and wide to taste the new delicious drink from the soda fountain. Morrison named the drink Dr Pepper. Why? Some say it was named after Dr. Charles T. Pepper, the pharmacist who gave Morrison his first job. Others say it isn't so. Rumor has it that Morrison had a crush on Dr. Pepper's daughter, another doctor, Minerva Pepper.

common medications. The following are a few examples of food and drug interactions. For a comprehensive list of "Food and Drug Interactions," call 1-800-639-8140.

Anticonvulsants such as carbamazepine (Tegretol, Epitol) and phenytoin (Dilantin) increase folic acid metabolism and decrease intestinal absorption of folic acid, resulting in decreased folic acid levels. Anticonvulsants also increase the rate of vitamin D, metabolism leading to decreased levels of vitamin D. Give supplements of folic acid and vitamin D if clinical judgment warrants it.

The caffeine in chocolate can interact with stimulant drugs, such as Ritalin, and increase their effect. Monoamine oxidase inhibitors, used to treat depression, and chocolate interact to create a sharp rise in blood pressure.

Taking Cipro (ciprofloxacin) with calcium-fortified orange juice results in a 40 percent decrease in serum levels of the antibiotic. Cipro should be taken with water to ensure the best absorption and bioavailability. (*Journal of Clinical Pharmacology,* April 2002)

Digoxin (Lanoxicaps, Lanoxin). The pectins in apples may bind to digoxin and reduce the effectiveness of the drug. Advise patients to avoid apples while taking digoxin. Licorice causes potassium loss and may also increase the risk of digoxin toxitiy.

Glucocorticoids such as cortisone, Prednisone, and dexamethasone prescribed for long-term administration result in calcium and vitamin D depletion with steroid-induced osteoporosis. Supplementation with calcium and vitamin D as well as a bisphosphonate (such as Fosamax) is necessary.

Isoniazid (INH, Laniazid) interferes with vitamin B6 metabolism. Patients receiving greater than 10 mg/kg/day of INH should be supplemented with 50–100 mg of pyridoxine (B6) per day.

Ginseng—this herb can interfere with the anti-coagulant effects of warfarin/Coumadin. Ginseng can enhance the antiplatelet effects of anti-inflammatory drugs such as aspirin and non-steroidal anti-inflammatory drugs, including Naprosyn and ibuprofen.

Grapefruit juice. The drug interactions with grapefruit juice are so numerous that a large section of Chapter G has been devoted to this topic.

Green tea and simvastatin.Green tea increases the bioavailability of simvastatin (Zocor). Increased bioavailability means a higher risk of drug toxicity and side effects including muscle aches and pains.

Vitamin E interacts with blood thinning medications such as warfarin/Coumadin and contributes to an increased risk of bleeding.

(U.S. Food and Drug Administration, U.S. Department of Health & Human Services. "Avoiding Drug Interactions." Last updated 6/10/2010)

Dry scalp and brittle, damaged hair? Try the following recipes:

Do you have problems with dry scalp?

½ of a cucumber,

½ of an avocado,

1/3 cup of sour cream and

one large cube of a eggplant

Blend the cucumber, avocado, and sour cream together in a blender and scoop onto your dry scalp. Massage the concoction into your hair and scalp with the eggplant cube. Cover your hair with a shower cap or saran wrap for 30 minutes finishing with a rinse that will leave your hair follicles moisturized and scalp soothed.

OR:

Is your problem brittle, damaged hair?

1 packet of Knox Gelatin (unflavored) melted in ½ cup of water

3 egg yolks,

4 tablespoons of grape seed oil or olive oil

3 capsules of primrose oil

Go with the grape seed oil if you want a less "oily" feel. Mix everything together, puncturing the primrose capsules for their oil only. Toss the remainder of the capsule. Saturate hair and scalp with the mixture and cover with a shower cap or saran wrap. Leave on for 45 minutes to an hour. You can kick it up a notch by running a hair dryer over your wrapped head. You might want to even take a hot bath while this is on your head as the heat will open up the scalp pores and penetrate the mixture into the root of the hair shaft. (Marina Valmy, director of Marina Valmy Skincare).

Whenever I feel like exercise,
I lie down until the feeling passes.

—Robert Maynard Hutchins (1899–1977), former president and chancellor of the University of Chicago, dean of the Yale Law School, and chairman of the board for the Encyclopedia Britannica.

Edamame. Fresh soybeans, known as edamame (Japan) and maodou (China), are soybeans that are picked before they are fully mature. Harvested at 80 percent maturity, fresh soybeans are sweeter, crisp, and more palatable than fully mature soybeans. Toss them in a pot of boiling water for a few minutes, add a pinch of salt, and spray with a few squirts of olive oil and enjoy!

EGGS

Eggs. Sometimes called "nature's perfect food," the egg is known as a high nutrient-density food. High nutrient-density foods provide a wide range of nutrients in proportion to their calorie count. Eggs are a great source of protein, the B vitamins, B12 and riboflavin (B2), choline for brain function, lutein and zeaxanthin for eye health, phosphorus, and vitamin D (41 IU)—and, only about 72 calories per large egg. The nutrients in an egg actually depend on what the hen eats. Corn's yellow pigments—lutein and zeaxanthin—are what make the egg yolks so yellow. In areas where hen feed is wheat-based, yolks are lighter in color. Egg producers may supplement the feeds with marigold petals and other additives to deepen the color. In addition, egg producers boost nutrients like omega-3s and lutein in eggs simply by adding them to the hens' feed. The only major downside, but not much of one for most people—the egg yolk contains an average of 185 mg of dietary cholesterol. The following is the comparison of a whole egg vs. the egg white:

Whole egg | Egg white
Calories 72 | 17
Cholesterol 185 mg | 0
Protein 6.3 g | 3.6 g

Total fat 5.0 g | 0.6 g
Saturated fat 1.5 g | 0 g
Vitamin D 41.0 IU | 0 IU

How many eggs can you eat per week? If your cholesterol levels are normal, one full egg a day is fine. If your total cholesterol is high and/or your LDL-cholesterol is high, you should limit your whole egg consumption to three or four per week. To cut back on cholesterol and saturated fat substitute two egg whites for one whole egg. Eat plant proteins instead of meat at one meal if you choose to have an egg every day. (USDA, February 2011)

A study reported in the April 2008 issue of *The American Journal of Clinical Nutrition,* found absolutely no link between men who ate up to six eggs a week and the risk of dying (from any cause) or having a heart attack or stroke. What they did find, however, is that this does not apply to men with Type 2 diabetes. As the egg intake increased in this group, the risk of dying or having a heart attack or stroke increased as well. The diabetic men who ate just one egg a week were 30% more likely to die than those eating less than one a week; those who averaged an egg a day were twice as likely to die. One of the big flaws of the study just so happened to be that the men who ate the most eggs also had the highest risk factors for heart attacks, strokes, and death. In other words, they were older, smoked more, were less physically active and had hypertension—all of which can increase mortality rate.

The research also didn't control for trans fat and saturated fat intake. So, it's a study that is fairly difficult to interpret. It's best to use caution with egg intake if you are a diabetic male or female. If you're not a diabetic, scramble, poach, or boil up an egg a day.

Eggs—the numbers. Americans consume 80 billion eggs per year. The average American, as of 2009, consumes 246.1 eggs per year. (United Egg Producers, A National Egg Producer Organization, June 10, 2010. http://www.unitedegg.org/useggindustry_generalstats.aspx)

U.S. hens lay enough eggs per year to circle the equator 100 times.

Egg laying. Did you know that a hen's "reproductive effort," defined as the "fraction of body weight that an animal deposits daily in her potential offspring," is 100 times greater than a human's? Each egg is about 3% of the hen's weight, so in a year of laying eggs, the hen converts about eight times her body weight into eggs. One-fourth of her daily energy expenditure goes toward egg-making. Heck, that's only half of what a duck puts forth—one-half of the female duck's daily energy expenditure goes into egg-making. Count your blessings, ladies of the human race.

Today's typical industrialized hen, (also known as a "layer"), is born in an incubator, eats a diet that originates largely in the laboratory, lives and lays on a wired floor under the lights for about a year, and produces between 250 and 290 eggs. These cages, called battery cages, have five to eight hens per cage, and are not only crowded, but inhumanely so. Each hen has 67 inches of floor space, less than a sheet of 8 x 11 typing paper. It's a horrible way to live and a filthy way to produce eggs.

The term "free-range" can be misleading. It sometimes means that the chickens live in a slightly larger cage or that the chicken has a five-minute access to the outdoors in a 24-hour period. Other terms can be trusted to provide more information about how the hens are treated:

.....USDA Organic means that the hens are uncaged inside barns or warehouses and must have outdoor access. Hens are fed an organic, all vegetarian diet that is free of antibiotics and pesticides. Hens cannot have received any antibiotics after they were 3 days old.

.....American Humane Certified: Hens can be confined in cages or can be cage-free.

.....Animal Welfare Approved: Hens are raised by independent farmers in flocks of no more than 500 birds that spend their adult lives outside. The animals aren't fed any animal byproducts.

.....Certified Humane: Hens must be uncaged inside barns or warehouses, but may be kept indoors at all times.

.....United Egg Producers Certified: Meets minimum voluntary industry standards, which according to the Humane Society, "permit routine cruel and inhuman factory farm practices."

Eggs—the incredible edible egg—more facts:

- The yolk accounts for one-third of the weight of the egg but provides three-fourths of the calories and most of the iron, thiamin (B1) and vitamin A. Each egg yolk contains approximately 185 mg of dietary cholesterol, which is 62% of the recommended daily value of dietary cholesterol.
- Eggs are graded by the size of their yolks and the thickness of the white, qualities that affect appearance but not nutritional values. The higher the grade, the thicker the yolk and the thicker the white will be when you cook the egg. So, buy Grade AA eggs if you want to cook them sunny side up. Grade B eggs will look rather puny and anemic on the breakfast platter. Nearly all eggs are sold as grade A.
- Egg yolks also contain choline, an essential B vitamin for optimal liver and brain function. Choline may also help protect against cardiovascular disease and play a role in cancer prevention. Here's the bad news: choline intake decreases with age, so eat more eggs! Choline is also found in wheat germ and liver.
- The typical egg yolk naturally contains about 25 mg of DHA and 25 mg of ALA. DHA (docosahexanoic acid) is the most potent omega-3 fatty acid, and levels can increase to about 100 mg per egg if the company making the eggs feeds the chickens fishmeal or algae. ALA (alpha linolenic acid) is much less potent. Egg yolks can also contain omega-3 fatty acids if the hen has been fed flaxseed or canola oil. The omega-3 from flaxseed or canola oil is alpha-linolenic acid, which is much less potent even though the label

will read 350 mg per egg yolk. If you just eat egg whites you'll miss out on the omega-3s. (*Environmental Nutrition,* April 2008) P.S. The FDA has banned all omega-3 claims on eggs, but that hasn't stopped producers from making the claims on the carton.

- The regular egg sizes (Jumbo, Extra Large, Large, Medium, Small) are determined by how much the eggs weigh per dozen. Large eggs are the standard for cake mixes and in other recipes. Using any other size may change the outcome—and not in a good way.
- One ostrich egg will make 11½ omelets.
- A cup of eggnog has 343 calories, 19 grams of fat, 34 grams of carbohydrate, and 150 mg of cholesterol.
- Most hard-boiled eggs end up with off-center yolks. This is why deviled eggs have defied automation for all these years.
- Two proteins found in the egg white, lysozyme and ovotransferrin, are responsible for inhibiting bacterial growth in the raw egg. When the eggshell is intact, the chick embryo is protected from nasty pathogens. However, if the shell is cracked, the enzymes become ineffective, and the egg is highly susceptible to bacterial growth. Once the shell is removed, raw eggs should be consumed within two days. Two other ways to keep eggs safe from pathogens include storing eggs with the small end down and not washing the eggs prior to storing them in the refrigerator. When the eggs are stored with the small end down the yolk is completely submerged in the egg white. The egg white contains the natural antibacterial proteins that protect the yolk of a developing chick embryo in a fertilized egg. If you wash the eggs before storing them, the water will make the eggshell more porous, allowing pathogens a perfect portal of entry.
- *Salmonella* loves eggs. In fact, *Salmonella* can slip through the pores of an intact shell, without providing a clue to the unsuspecting consumer that they have a contaminated egg. So, as a general rule of thumb, never eat a dish or beverage (such as eggnog) made with raw fresh eggs, especially if you are immunocompromised. Cooking eggs to an internal temperature of 145° F destroys the *Salmonella.* Egg-milk dishes such as custards must be cooked to an internal temperature of 160° F.
- Speaking of pores…the eggshell has between 7,000 and 17,000 pores that help it breathe. Odors can permeate the egg through the pores, allowing the egg to absorb the odors of the surrounding foods in the 'fridge. Keeping the eggs in their original carton prevents the evening leftover Chinese takeout moo goo gai pan from permeating your freshly scrambled breakfast eggs. So, when purchasing your new refrigerator, don't pay extra for an "egg tray." It's a waste of money because you don't want to remove the eggs from their original carton for storage.
- Brown eggs or white eggs? The color of the egg's shell depends on the breed of the hen and has nothing at all to do with the nutritive value or the taste of the egg. For most color-egged chickens the pigment is added to the outer layer of the shell as the egg passes through the oviduct on its way to being laid. The brown or mottled-brown eggs come from a class of pigments called the porphyrins that are produced by the breakdown of red blood cells.

- So, what about the "Martha Stewart" blue and green eggs? These multicolored eggs come from the Araucana chicken breed that hails from Chile. This breed produces a pigment called oocyanin ("oo" is the prefix for egg, and cyanin comes from the term cyano, or blue) Oocyanin is actually a byproduct of bile production and it penetrates the entire shell as the pigment is added early in the formation of the egg. False claims stating that the Araucana chicken eggs have less cholesterol have hit the talk show circuits and the Internet. Actually, the Araucana chicken egg has a higher cholesterol content than the White Leghorn, the breed that dominates the commercial U.S. egg market. (Document PS19 Animal Science Department, Florida Cooperative Extension Service, Institute of Food and Agricultural Sciences, University of Florida; original publication date, June 1997. Reviewed March 2009. http://edis.ifas.ufl.edu)
- Beaten egg whites can be used as a facial mask to make your skin temporarily look smoother. The mask works because the egg proteins constrict as they dry on your face, pulling at the dried layer of cells on top of your skin. When you wash off the egg white, you wash off some of these loose cells. You can also use egg whites as a rinse or shampoo. The protein in a beaten raw egg can temporarily make your hair look smoother and shinier by filling in the chinks and notches in the hair shaft.
- Eggs are one of the top 8 foods that trigger 90% of food allergies.
- Eggs refrigerated at an optimal 27 degrees are safe for up to four to five weeks past their expiration dates.
- Vaccines grown in egg cultures or in chick embryos include the live-virus measles vaccine, live-virus mumps vaccine, and flu vaccines. These may trigger allergic reactions in people with a history of anaphylactic reactions to eggs.
- It takes 100 million fertilized chicken eggs to supply the U.S. with the flu vaccine. This method of vaccine preparation was developed more than 50 years ago—a bit outdated, labor intensive obviously. It's time to move the flu preparation process into the 21st century.

Can patients who are allergic to eggs get the flu vaccine? Perhaps. People who can tolerate a small amount of egg in baked goods may actually have no problems with the tiny amount of egg protein that is used in vaccines. The 2010 flu vaccines, *Agriflu* and *Fluarix* had less than 1.2 μg/mL of egg protein. If vaccines contain egg proteins, give one-tenth of the dose and wait 30 minutes. If the patient has no difficulties with breathing or a falling blood pressure during those 30 minutes, the rest of the dose can be given. Stay tuned—it won't be long before making vaccines with eggs will be a thing of the past. www.cdc.gov/vaccines/recs/vac-admin/default; *Pediatrics* 2010;125:e1024.

Eggs and eye injuries. Microwave ovens and hard-boiled eggs may be hazardous to your eye health. A case study in the *British Medical Journal* (2004;328:1075) reported extensive eye injuries in a 9-year-old girl who had microwaved a previously boiled egg. She microwaved the egg, in its shell, for

ASPARAGUS TIP

The French are the most serious when it comes to food. Who else would codify 295 ways to prepare eggs—not counting omelets! In fact, the 100 pleats in a French chef's tall white hate, la toque blanch, traditionally signifies the number of ways he/she must know how to prepare eggs in order to qualify as a member of the profession.

40 seconds, and as she was carrying the egg to the breakfast table it exploded like a hand grenade, sending shell fragments into her eye and face. Her right eye sustained extensive injuries, including corneal perforation and a ruptured lens due to imbedded shell fragments. NOTE: Even without the shell, a ruptured egg yolk can explode if its membranous yolk sac is intact. Moral of the story: Do not microwave your eggs in a shell or with the yolks intact. Puncture the egg yolk if you must, but to be completely on the safe side, only microwave previously scrambled eggs.

Egg salad sandwich—a clinical use to diagnose gastroparesis. The condition known as gastroparesis is defined as a "chronic symptomatic disorder of the stomach characterized by delayed gastric emptying in the absence of mechanical obstruction (a blockage)." In other words, food sits in the stomach for too long a period of time causing early satiety (feeling full), nausea, vomiting, bloating, upper abdominal discomfort, and weight loss. Gastroparesis is a miserable condition and not one that you would wish on your worst enemy.

The top three causes are diabetes, surgery and medication-induced gastroparesis. Other conditions include pregnancy, collagen vascular disease such as scleroderma, Parkinson's disease, thyroid and liver disease, and chronic renal insufficiency.

In order to determine the emptying time of the stomach, the researcher needs to test for how fast it takes a meal to get out of the stomach, i.e., gastric emptying. Gastric-emptying scintography of a solid-phase meal is considered the gold standard for the diagnosis of gastroparesis. Most centers use 99MTc sulfur colloid-labeled (radioactive) egg salad sandwich as a test meal. Yum. (Ali T, Hasan M, Harty RF. Gastroparesis. *Southern Medical Journal* 2007 March;100(3):281–286)

Empty stomach and drugs. Many drugs are best taken on an empty stomach. The bisphosphonates, prescribed for the treatment of osteoporo-

ASPARAGUS TIP

In a healthy young adult, the usual time that it takes to empty the stomach from any meal is 90 to 120 minutes. Of course, liquids empty the fastest, followed by solids that have been reduced in size (by the chewing process) to particles of 1 to 2 mm.

sis, include alendronate (Fosamax) and risedronate (Actonel), ibandronate (Boniva). This class of drugs should be taken with absolutely *no* food, only an 8- ounce glass water. Complete non-absorption occurs with any amount of food resulting in the failed management of osteoporosis. The antibiotic azithromycin (Zithromax) should be taken on an empty stomach for the best absorption whereas an antibiotic in the same class of antibiotics, clarithromycin (Biaxin), should be taken with food for better absorption. This confuses one and all so please read the following tip.

ASPARAGUS TIP

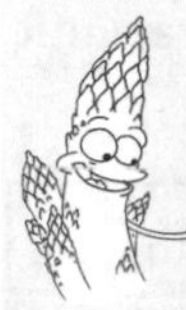

Follow the instructions on the prescription bottle! If the Pharmacist has slapped a sticker on it that says Take with food, then do it!! If the sticker says Take on an empty stomach, then do it! There's a method to their madness—and it all has to do with increasing the effectiveness of the drugs that you are spending your monthly paycheck on.

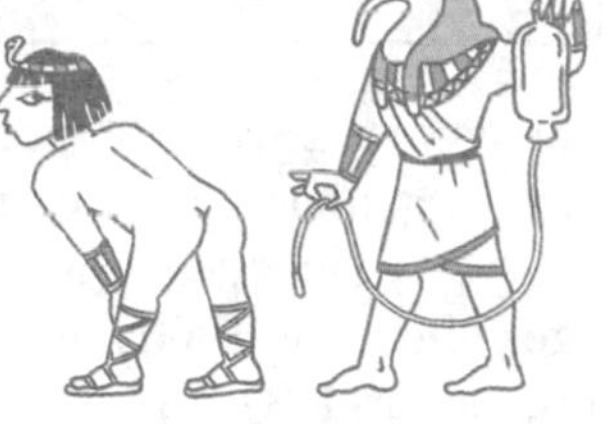

Enemas to cleanse the bowel from "rotting food." Ancient Egyptians were deathly afraid of rotting food in their gastrointestinal tract; hence, their adamant belief in enemas three days a month. They believed that enemas were invented by the god Thoth. Royalty were especially cognizant of the importance of the bowel—one mighty Pharaoh had his own "Keeper of the Royal Rectum." And, of course, we all have heard the stories about Louis XIII, the King of France from 1610–1643. He had an average of 212 enemas per year. Individuals who were not lucky enough to be a Pharaoh or a King had their enemas administered by pharmacists who were dubbed *limonadiers du posterior* (or to put it more eloquently, "lemonade-makers of the rear-end."

Energy drinks. Red Bull was first introduced as an energy beverage in Austria in 1987 and hit the ground running a decade after that in the U.S. Since that time hundreds of energy drinks have been marketed, with caffeine as the major ingredient. Some energy beverages have a meager 50 mg of caffeine per can or bottle, whereas others pack a walloping 505 mg per container. The top four best selling energy drinks include Red Bull, Rockstar, Monster, and Full Throttle. Each energy beverage has a list of ingredients from B vitamins to ginseng, ginkgo and guarana* extract. This list of ingredients is referred to as an "energy blend." Combining all of the ingredients with caffeine makes it difficult to predict the effects of each of the energy drinks.

*Guarana is actually just another source of caffeine…similar to coffee beans, cola nuts, and tea or mate leaves. Note that guarana is usually not counted as caffeine on labels.

For example, Red Bull has 160 mg of caffeine per 16-ounce can vs. Full Throttle with 141 mg per 16 ounce can. Another major component of energy drinks is sugar (glucose/sucrose). Each 16-ounce can contains approximately 13 teaspoons of sugar (just a bit more than ¼ cup of sugar). Rockstar contains the highest amount of sugar with 62 grams compared to Red Bull and Monster with 54 grams. Rockstar has the most calories per 16-ounce can as well—280 calories vs. 200 for Monster and 220 for both Red Bull and Full Throttle. Most of the other ingredients contained in energy drinks (taurine, B vitamins, gingko, ginseng) have little therapeutic effect because the amounts of each are far below the amounts expected to deliver therapeutic benefits.

Red Bull has a 65% share of the $650 million energy drink market in the U.S. (2005) The U.S. is the world's largest consumer of energy beverages with 290 million gallons, averaging 3.8 quarts per person per year in 2007. However, this number is a bit misleading. The major group consuming energy drinks are between the ages of 11 and 35 years of age.

What are the short-term effects of energy beverages? Physiologic effects occur immediately after drinking the first can. In one study of healthy volunteers between ages 18 and 40, drinking 2 cans (500 mL) of an energy beverage containing 1000 mg of taurine and 100 mg of caffeine, as well as vitamins B5, B6, and B12, glucuronolactone, and niacinamide, daily for one week found the following effects:

1) Within 4 hours of energy beverage consumption, the maximum systolic blood pressure increased by 8% on day 1 and 10% on day 7.
2) Within 2 hours of energy beverage consumption, the maximum diastolic blood pressure increased by 7% on day 1 and 8% on day 7.
3) Heart rate increased by 8% on day 1 and 11% on day 7.
4) Throughout the study, heart rates increased between 5 and 7 beats/min, and systolic blood pressure increased by 10 mm Hg after energy beverage consumption.
5) Throughout the study, heart rates increased between 5 and 7 beats/min, and systolic blood pressure increased by 10 mm Hg after energy beverage consumption.
6) No clinically important ECG changes were observed.

BOTTOM LINE: Energy beverages should NOT be consumed if you have blood pressure problems.

A few more studies have been published with case reports on the immediate effects of energy beverage consumption. These are summarized as follows:

1) Four documented cases of caffeine-associated death have been reported, as well as 5 separate cases of seizures associated with energy beverage consumption.

2) An otherwise healthy 28-year-old man had cardiac arrest after a day of motocross racing and continued consumption of energy beverages.
3) A healthy 18-year-old man died playing basketball after drinking 2 cans of Red Bull.

(Higgins JP, et al. Energy Beverages: Content and Safety. *Mayo Clin Proc* 2010;85(11):1033–1041; Steinke L, et al. Effect of "energy drink" consumption on hemodynamic and electrocardiographic parameters in healthy young adults. *Ann Pharmacother.* 2009;43(4):596–602; Ballard SL, et al. Effects of commercial energy drink consumption on athletic performance and body composition. *Phys Sportsmed.* 2010;38(1):107–117; Clauson KA, et al. Safety issues associated with commercially available energy drinks. *J Am Pharm Assoc.* 2003;49(3):e55–e63)

Enteral feedings after gastrointestinal surgery. The time-honored NPO (nothing by mouth) sign over the bed for days after elective gastrointestinal surgery has "gone the way of the dinosaur." A new meta-analysis examined 11 studies comparing any form of gastric stimulation (either oral feedings with a sip or two of clear liquids or a tube inserted into the small bowel with fluids) with absolutely "nothing per os" or NPO—"os" by the way, means 'mouth' in the Roman vernacular). Once the verdict was in from the studies, the results definitely favored the early enteral feedings over NPO to reduce complications from elective gastrointestinal surgeries. In addition to reducing post-operative infections, the early bowel stimulation also reduced the mean length of stay by one entire hospital day. You might not think that this is a big deal…one day, hrumpffff, you say. However, the average cost of just the room for one hospital day in 2008 was $1993.48! (Noblett HD. Bowel management after surgery. *ADVANCE for Nurse Practitioners.* February 2010;45–51)

E. COLI 0157:H7

Escherichia coli *(E. Coli O157:H7).* This bacteria is a combination of two bacteria— the usual run-of-the-mill E. coli that inhabits the usual run-of-the-mill colon of humans, and a very nasty bacteria that produces a nasty toxin known as *Shigella.* So how did the two bacteria get together and combine to make one big nasty bug? No one knows exactly how the *Shigella* toxin Shigatoxin gene jumped to the unsuspecting run-of-the-mill E. coli. But what they do know is that when the *Shigella* gene inserted itself into E. coli, the gene was slightly altered in a way that made the new *E. Coli O157:H7* produce a toxin even deadlier than the original toxin made by *Shigella.* Most likely this transfer of genes occurred in a cow's bowel in Venezuela in the mid-1970s. The very first confirmed case in the U.S. was in a Naval Officer in San Diego in 1975, but this wasn't discovered as the cause until after a few outbreaks occurred in the 1980s.

The first known outbreak of *E. Coli O157:H7* in the U.S. was in White City, Oregon, in December 1981 when a dozen people arrived at the Emergency Room complaining of diarrhea and abdominal cramping. Their stools were watery at first but within hours the diarrhea turned into pure, bright red blood. Cultures were negative for any known organism at that time, but all of the patients had one thing in common— they had all dined at the local McDonald's.

The second outbreak was in Traverse City, Michigan in 1982, and all of the patients had also eaten at a McDonald's restaurant. A microbiologist at the Center for Disease Control in Atlanta was working on the stools obtained from the group in White City, Oregon, and found a new strain of bacteria called *E. Coli O157:H7*. No one believed at the time that this was a toxic strain, but when the same strain showed up in the Michigan group, eyebrows were raised. In July 1982 the investigators found what they were looking for. A plant in Ohio that had supplied the lot of hamburger meat to the McDonald's in Traverse City was the culprit. The plant, as part of its quality control program, just happened to have saved ground beef from the suspected lot of hamburger. And it just so happened that *E. Coli O157:H7* was also found in that lot of hamburger.

At the same time a mysterious illness was being investigated in children in Toronto. In the space of 10 days, 14 children were admitted to the Hospital for Sick Children in Toronto, all with the same symptoms beginning with watery diarrhea progressing to bloody diarrhea. About a week later the children developed acute kidney failure. Two children died and others were left with severe, permanent damage to their kidneys.

The researchers in Toronto found a toxin produced by the bacteria, and named it *Shigatoxin*.

One of the most notorious outbreaks of this foodborne illness involved the Jack-in-the-Box restaurants in Seattle-Tacoma in 1993 where four children died and hundreds of people became ill.

The bacteria surfaced again in 1996 in cases traced to contaminated apple juice and lettuce. In August, 1997, when 17 people in Colorado got sick after eating hamburgers from beef processed by a Hudson Foods plant in Nebraska. Hudson Foods, based in Rogers, Arkansas, recalled 25 million pounds of its ground beef, the largest meat recall in history. The plant in Nebraska closed its doors after the outbreak.

E. Coli O157:H7 can cause diseases from standard diarrhea that resolves by itself within 5 to 20 days to severe anemia, kidney failure and death. The symptoms of *E. Coli O157:H7* infection typically appear within 3 to 8 days after exposure. However, the usual time is 3 to 4 days following exposure. In adults, *E. Coli O157:H7* infections generally resolve within one week. About one third of children will carry and shed the organism in their stool for up to three weeks.

Another outbreak occurred in 2006 with spinach. What started out as a limited number of contaminated plants from a small farm in San Benito, California turned into a public health nightmare. According to the plant records, 41,760 bags of spinach were packaged that day for the U.S. market, and 720 bags were shipped to Canada. Three weeks later the Wisconsin Health Department reported that four people had been diagnosed with hemolytic uremic syndrome (HUS), a kidney disease resulting in acute renal failure and anemia. By the end of the outbreak, 205 people in the U.S. and Canada were diagnosed with the *E. Coli O157:H7* infection, 103 were hospitalized, 31 developed HUS, and 3 died. Sales of spinach and leafy greens took a nose-dive, costing California producers and processors $100 million. No one has any idea as to how the spinach became contaminated. Finger pointing was rampant…the blame game started with wild pigs pooping on the spinach leaves. The next finger pointed to rainwater draining from a nearby cattle pasture and splashing cow manure on plants. The answer has never been found, so the wild pigs and next door cattle have continued to shoulder the responsibility for this outbreak.

Notes on this nasty bug:

…..*E. Coli O157:H7* is infectious in low doses. Comparing an infectious dose with cholera emphasizes the difference. Whereas cholera requires the presence of 1,000,000 to 10,000,000 organisms before clinical illness occurs, *E. Coli O157:H7* can produce clinical symptoms with as few as 10–100 organisms.

…..*E. Coli O157:H7* is referred to as acid-tolerant. This means the normally protective, high-acid pH of the stomach will not destroy the bacteria as it passes through the first line of defense known as the stomach.

…..*E. Coli O157:H7* is unaffected by freezing. However, it cannot survive for long at temperatures warmer than 120° F (49° C).

…..Most slab meat is safe, because the *E. Coli O157:H7* organisms are only found on the exterior of the meat and are easily killed during the cooking process.

…..Hamburger meat, not steak, is the real culprit because of the method by which it is processed. Ground meat, with *ground* being the operative word, is produced from the "trimmings" or remnants of higher-grade cuts of meat. These remnants are ground together in a big vat with the scraps of other animals parts. This grinding process is a highly efficient way of distributing *E. Coli O157:H7* throughout the meat. As a result, each hamburger patty may be chock-full of the bacteria. If the burger patty is not thoroughly cooked at temps above 160° F, the organisms at the center of the patty can remain viable and cause significant disease. (USDA Mean and Poultry Hotline 1-800-535-4555) By the way, this is what happened at the Jack-in-the-Box outbreak in Seattle-Tacoma. The new grills at the restaurant chain were not cooking the burgers to the recommended 160˚F. The burgers on the peripheral part of the grill were only being cooked to 140˚F and the epidemiologists traced the outbreak to the consumers who ate the burgers from the peripheral portion of the grill.

…..Forming contaminated ground beef into hamburger patties can leave a residue of about 10 million *E. Coli O157:H7* on your hands. In fact, this form of *E. coli* can survive on a stainless steel counter top for up to 60 days. Clean the counter tops and cutting boards with soap and water and don't prepare other foods in the same area as raw hamburger. And don't forget to wash your hands after handling raw hamburger.

…..Estimates of the percentage of burgers sold that now contain detectable levels of *E. coli* range between 0.1–10% .

.....Hamburger meat is the major culprit in the majority of outbreaks. However, alfalfa sprouts, bean sprouts, lettuce, and unpasteurized apple ciders have all been responsible. Other animals can carry *E. coli* as well. Eleven family members in Oregon got sick after eating contaminated venison jerky. The deer had been infected, and the *E. Coli O157:H7* survived the brining process for curing the meat. Other reports have involved kids who have gone to petting zoos and acquired the illness after petting goats. The Department of Public Health reported a 1996 outbreak that sickened scores of children at a Twin Cities day-care center after eating meat from a cow carcass that one child's family had in their freezer.

.....The use of antibiotics during the infection is discouraged. Antibiotics kill the bacteria in the bowel and cause the release of more toxins. The use of antibiotics has been associated with an increase in the incidence of hemolytic uremic syndrome and acute kidney (renal) failure in kids.

.....Since the organism is passed in the feces, infected persons with diarrhea and those who are unable to control their bowel habits (particularly children in day care centers and older adults in nursing homes) should be isolated until symptoms have resolved. Specific guidelines regarding return to work or school may vary depending on individual parameters; consultations with the local or state health department is recommended. (Qadri SM, Kayalis S. *Enterohemorrhagic E. Coli.* Postgraduate Medicine 1998;103(2):179–187. Buchanan RL, et al. The rising tide of foodborne and waterborne infections. *Patient Care* 1997;May 15:31–72; Wisconsin Department of Health Services, accessed February 15, 2012)

Esophagus. It takes 4–8 seconds for a bolus of food to move through the 10-inch esophagus to the stomach.

Exercise. "With the possible exception of diet modification, we know of no single intervention with greater promise than physical exercise to reduce the risk of virtually all chronic diseases simultaneously." (Booth FW, Gordon SE, Carlson CJ, Hamilton MT. Waging war on modern chronic diseases: primary prevention through exercise biology. *Journal of Applied Physiology.*2000;88:774–787)

Exercise before you eat? Eat before you exercise? Should you exercise before or after a meal to lose weight? It depends on whether you are skinny or fat. Lean individuals burn more calories when they exercise after a meal; however, obese individuals burn more calories when they exercise before a meal. The difference in the number of calories burned isn't astounding. Lean individuals burn 7 more calories after eating and obese individuals burn 19 more calories when they exercise before eating.

The only reason I would take up jogging is so that
I could hear heavy breathing again. — Erma Bombeck

CHAPTER F

A fruit is a vegetable with looks and money. Plus, if you let fruit rot, it turns into wine, something that Brussels sprouts never do.

—PJ O'Rourke

FAST-FOOD FACTS

Fast-food facts. Since the 1970s, the number of fast-food restaurants has grown at a rate of 7% per year. The percentage of every American food dollar used for eating out has nearly doubled since that time, from 20% to 38%. Portion sizes of restaurant meals, take-out foods, and snacks have also increased, in some cases by more than 100%. The majority of fast-food restaurants offer entrees with more than one portion size, e.g., "small-size," "regular-size," "queen-size," "king-size," "super-size," "mega-size," "monster-size," "double-double," and "triple-size." A typical bagel, once a skinny 2–3 ounces, has ballooned to twice that size, from 4–6 ounces. The following are just some of the items taken from various menus and their nutritional "values."

- Stuffed baked potato skins: 79 grams of fat, 40 grams of which are saturated. Eight stuffed potato skins is equivalent to bombarding your heart with 2.5 pounds of Tater Tots. If I'm going to kill myself, I would rather do it with Tater Tots.
- Boneless buffalo wings with a blue cheese dipping sauce: 1060 calories, 81 grams of fat, 14 grams of saturated fat, 3330 mg sodium.
- Chicken Caesar salad garnished with croutons and tossed with Caesar salad dressing: 46 grams of fat, 11 of which are saturated. The full-fat dressing is the culprit here. The croutons add only a few grams of fat.
- Bacon and cheese grilled chicken sandwich with mayonnaise: 30 grams of fat, 12 of which are saturated. The bacon, cheese, and mayonnaise turn a heart-healthy grilled chicken sandwich into a heart attack between two buns.
- Oriental chicken salad with dressing: 49 grams of fat, 12 of which are saturated. Like the Caesar salad, this salad has some semblance of health under all that gooey, fatty dressing. The skinless chicken breast

sliced over lettuce, cabbage, and carrots is perfectly healthy. But keep the lid on that dressing. Also steer clear of the crunchy fried noodles piled on top.

- Fried chicken fingers: 34 grams of fat, 13 of which are saturated. A typical five-finger order is as bad for your left main coronary artery as a Big Mac followed by a hot fudge sundae. How about if you add French fries to those chicken fingers? Don't even think about it.
- Baby-back ribs: 54 grams of saturated fat, 21 of which are saturated. Add the French fries and coleslaw and you can turn your dinner into a double bypass surgery. The combination adds up to over 1,500 calories to fill those extra stretchy sweat pants with the elastic waistband.

Fast food expenditures. In 1970, Americans spent 6 billion dollars on fast food. In 2008, Americans spent 110 billion dollars on fast food. Another way to look at it? The average American spends 5.6% of their salary on fast food. A 25-year-old with a $32,000 per year salary spends $1,820 per year on fast food.

Fast foods and liver enzymes. Many practitioners are perplexed by intermittent elevations of liver enzymes in their patients. McDonald's, Kentucky Fried Chicken (KFC), and Burger King may just be the answer. Researchers assigned 18 healthy volunteers to fast-food-based diets for 4 weeks. During the study period, mean ALT levels (a liver enzyme), increased significantly. Fourteen of the 18 patients developed elevated ALT levels within the first week, but only two participants developed fatty livers. All participants' ALT levels returned to normal within several weeks after stopping the diet. Fat intake was unrelated to ALT levels; however, sugar and carbohydrate intake correlated with rising ALT levels. (Kechagias S, et al. Fast-food based hyperalimentation can induce rapid and profound elevation of serum ALT in healthy subjects. *GUT* 2008 Feb 14)

FATS

Fats. Contrary to popular belief, fats are an essential component of the diet. Fats are necessary for proper growth and development of the brain and central nervous system. Fat provides essential fatty acids for cell membrane structure and prostaglandin formation. Fat also acts as a carrier for fat-soluble vitamins. Fat storage is important for energy production. So who said fat wasn't good for us?

An interesting paradox has occurred in the diets of the American public over the past two decades. Past U.S. Department of Agriculture's Dietary Guidelines stressed eating ***less*** fat and ***more*** carbohydrates. So the average American actually listened and started to reduce their intake of *fats*. Paradoxically, we started getting even fatter and consuming more calories than ever, all the while, reducing fat intake. So what was happening here? Instead of eating high-fiber carbohydrates, Americans decided to eat sweet, calorie-dense (translation: lots of calories in a small amount of food), low-fiber carbohydrates, so that the low-fat diet became a high-calorie, processed carbohydrate diet. The pounds started piling up. To quote a friend of mine: "Every time I go to Hilary's house to eat she only has low-fat food—low fat this, low-fat that. Everything in Hilary's house is low-fat except Hilary."

Of course, the realization finally hit the officials that make the U.S. dietary guidelines. Mon dieu! *Calories do count.* Surprise, surprise. We also now realize that the type of fat is more important than the amount of fat. Fats known as monounsaturated fats and polyunsaturated fats such as omega-3 fatty acids provide numerous health benefits. Saturated fats should be consumed in small amounts and trans fats should be consumed in minuscule amounts, if at all. So, the average American diet can contain anywhere from 18% fat to 40% fat, depending on the type of fat, the number of calories and the individual. The American Heart Association recommends that total fat intake should be less than 25% to 35% of your total calories per day. Saturated fats should be approximately 7% of the total daily calories and trans fat intake should be less than 1% of your total calories per day. The remaining fat should come from sources of monounsaturated fats and polyunsaturated fats such as nuts, seeds, fish, and olive oil.

So, let's just say you are a sedentary 31–50 year-old female sitting here reading this fun, fact-filled book. You will need approximately 2,000 calories a day to maintain your lifestyle of sitting on the couch. Of the total 2000 calories, you should consume less than 16 grams of saturated fat, less than 2 grams of trans fat and between 50 and 70 grams of total fat daily. So, up you go…off the couch, walk to the grocery store and stock up on fish, almonds, and pumpkin sees. See below for more on the specific types of fats.

Patience is one of the missing nutrients in most people's diets.
— Keith Ayoub, Ed.D., R.D. American Dietetic Association

Fat types. Here fat, there fat, everywhere fat-fat—low fat, high fat, some fat, no fat, mono fat, trans fat, poly fat, sat fat, fish fat. So where do we start? How about from the really bad fats to the really good fats?

Trans fats. "When you're bad you're really, really bad." Trans fats are formed when vegetable oils have hydrogen molecules chemically *added* in the lab. Hydrogen molecules are added for three reasons:

1) To make the fats solid at room temperature
2) To make the product able to withstand frying temperatures
3) To extend the shelf-life of products

Even though the reasons seem reasonable, the problem with trans fats is the increased risk of cardiovascular disease. Trans fats increase total cholesterol and the bad LDL-cholesterol even more than saturated fats do, the other bad guys. In very high amounts they lower the good HDL-cholesterol levels. Any slight decrease in HDLs equals a big increase in heart disease. In fact, a 1-mg/dl decrease in HDL equates to a 2–3% increase in heart disease. In terms of heart disease, trans fats may be slightly worse than saturated fats, but suffice it to say, they are both bad for you when consumed in significant amounts.

Trans fats are abundant in stick margarines, shortening, pastries, packaged cookies and crackers, French fries, and other deep-fried fast foods. Recommendation: minimal intake of trans fats, or as mentioned above—less than 1% of your total daily caloric intake. Just looking at a buttery croissant will supply you with all the trans fats you need for the day. The current trans fats intake of the average American should be as low as possible per day.

The good news about trans fat is that there has been a 58% drop in trans fat intake between 2000 and 2009. In recent years, many food companies have taken trans fats out of their products and many big chain restaurants have switched to healthier oils. A government regulation now requires food manufacturers to list the amount of trans fats on the nutrition facts panel of food labels. And it appears as if consumers are reading the labels since the consumption of trans fats has dropped considerably. (CDC report, 2012; *JAMA*, February 8, 2012)

A food can contain up to 0.5 grams of trans fat in one serving, but the manufacturer may list 0 grams of trans fat on the Nutrition Facts label or on the front of the package. This is a labeling loophole permitted by the U.S. Food and Drug Administration. Look on the ingredient list…if it says partially hydrogenated oil then the food contains trans fat. If it says fully hydrogenated oil, then it contains saturated fats.

Saturated fats—the bad. Saturated fats are the other bad guys, but they are one rung above the trans fats on "the bad fats" ladder. Saturated means that their chemical structures are chains of fatty acids "saturated" with hydrogen molecules. That means that damaging oxygen molecules do not have a place to attach, making these fats less likely to be "oxidized" and become rancid. Saturated fats are abundant in animal foods such as red meat, poultry (especially dark meat), butter, cheese, milk, and cream. They are also abundant in certain oils including coconut, palm, and palm kernel oils. There is *no doubt* in anyone's mind today that saturated fats, in abundance, contribute to cardiovascular disease.

Polyunsaturated fatty acids (PUFAs)—climbing up the ladder. The polyunsaturated fats have chains of fatty acid with hydrogen bonds; however, there are two or more free areas for oxygen molecules to attach to. There are two types of polyunsaturated fats: the omega-6 fatty acids and the omega-3 fatty acids. The ratio of omega-6 fatty acids to omega-3 fatty acids in our diet should be less than 10:1.

The primary omega-6 fatty acid is linoleic acid, an essential fatty acid that the body cannot make on its own. Omega-6 fats are heart-friendly because they lower LDL and total cholesterol levels. The problem is that too many omega-6s upset the balance between the omega 3s and the omega 6s. Omega-6 fatty acids currently make up over 90% of the polyunsaturated fats in the average American diet, mostly in the form of vegetable oils also known as seed oils. Soybean, corn, sunflower, and safflower oils are packed with omega-6 fatty acids. Corn oil, for example, has a ratio of about 74 omega-6s to one omega-3. Yikes, that's quite a bit more than the recommended ratio of "less than 10:1."

There are three omega-3 fatty acids—eicosapentaenoic acid (EPA), docosahexanoic acid (DHA), found primarily in certain types of fish, and alpha-linolenic acid (ALA), the primary plant-based omega-3. Do not confuse the omega-6 alpha linoleic acid with the omega-3 alpha linolenic acid. Easily done—the only difference is the additional "n." Annoying.

What do the omega-3s do for you? Actually the better question is: What don't they do for you? Chapter O will delve into the plethora of benefits of the omega-3 fatty acids but here's a brief preview:

Omega-3 fatty acids reduce clotting, prevent cardiac arrhythmias, boost immune function, have anti-inflammatory properties, promote eye and brain development, improve cognitive function and dampen mood swings, and the list goes on. Fish oils are the richest source of omega-3 fats, especially fatty fish. Flaxseed oil is a front runner as a plant-based omega-3 fatty acid. Most average Americans do not consume enough omega-3s, hence the recommendation to bump up the weekly fish intake to at least twice, if not thrice, weekly.

Monounsaturated fatty acids (MUFAs)—the really good, top of the ladder fats. Monounsaturated fatty acids are the clear winner in the fat category. A monounsaturated fatty acid has one free spot (hence, the term "mono" or "one") on its chain to which oxygen molecules bind. Two of the best sources are olive oil and canola oil; peanut oil and peanuts are high in monounsaturated fats as well. Avocados, olives, hazelnuts, macadamia nuts, almonds and almond oil are other foods with high levels of MUFAs.

When monounsaturated fats are substituted for saturated fats in the diet, cholesterol levels will improve. Monounsaturated fats may also offer some protection against breast cancer. Notice the word *may.* More research is needed to make a definitive statement, but until that time it wouldn't hurt to increase the monounsaturated fat intake while decreasing trans and saturated fats.

If you live in the Mediterranean countries your diet is traditionally composed of 40% fat. However, the majority of that fat comes from olive oil. Mediterraneans who follow the Mediterranean diet have a much lower incidence of heart disease, stroke, and other chronic conditions because of their intake of the heart healthy monounsaturated fats. Unfortunately today there are too many fast food restaurants infiltrating the Mediterranean countries and the true Mediterranean diet has become somewhat of a thing of the past. (Knoops KT et al. Mediterranean diet, lifestyle factors, and 10-year mortality in elderly European men and women: the HALE project. *JAMA*. 2004 Sep 22;292 (12):1433–1439)

Fat content food—the blot test. Just how high is the fat content of that piece of chicken, slice of pizza, or helping of Cheeseburger Hamburger Helper? Place the item on a paper napkin or paper towel and observe the grease mark. If it leaves an obvious grease mark, the item contains at least 3 grams of fat. The greasier the spot, the greater the amount of fat. So when you bring home that bag of French fries and the entire bottom third of the bag is covered with grease, you know the fat content is waaay up there. Here's the good news…toss the fries on a paper towel and blot, blot, blot before you eat them. Blotting will help remove lots of those extra fat calories.

Can you imagine a world without men? No crime and lots of happy fat women." —Nicole Hollander

---

Fat cells and gender differences. The average American has 40 billion fat cells. A person who is born overweight or who develops extreme obesity may have upwards of 250 billion fat cells in her body. The fat cells of a 120-pound female can store an extra 74,000 calories; those from a 160-pound man can store an extra 95,000 calories. A healthy range of body fat for men

ASPARAGUS TIP

Fat facts:

…. It takes 1,000,000 fat cells to store the calories in a Life Saver.

….When calorie intake exceeds calorie expenditures, fat cells can expand to as much as six times their minimum size and begin to multiply, from 40 billion in an average adult to up to 250 billion in the extremely obese adult.

….Losing weight causes fat cells to shrink in size and become less metabolically active, but it's tough to lose the number of fat cells you have. The irony—gaining fat cells is easier than losing them. Sound like a familiar refrain?

….Excess abdominal (visceral) fat triggers immune system cells known as macrophages to enter the fat tissue. The macrophages and the fat cells release inflammatory mediators—presumably to fight the foreign substance which may be an infection to the macrophage but it's actually just fat. Presumably, this is part of fat's intended function; inflammation fights infection, which for the most of history was more pressing than a large bag of Nacho chips. Scientists have found that in an obese person's visceral fat tissue, macrophages compromise up to 40% of the cells.

HISTORICAL HIGHLIGHT

If you have ever "chewed the fat," credit the crews of the old days of "wooden ships and iron men" who talked and grumbled while chewing their daily ration of brine-toughened salt pork.

is 10–15%, and a healthy range for women is 20–25%. A body fat percentage over 20% for men or 30% for women is considered an indication of obesity. (Vella CA, Kravitz L. Gender differences in fat metabolism. *IDEA Health and Fitness Source* 2002;20(10):36–46)

Fat intake and migraine headaches. Reducing total daily fat intake to less than 20% of the total daily calories has been shown to reduce the frequency of migraine headaches by 70%, the intensity of the migraine by 68%, and the duration of the attack by 74%. (American Association for the Study of Headaches, Scientific Assembly, May 31–June 2, 1996, San Diego, CA.)

No diet will remove all the fat from your body because the brain is entirely fat. Without a brain you might look good, but all you could do is run for public office. —Covert Bailey

---

Fava beans. The fava bean, also known as the broad bean, is the largest of the commonly eaten legumes. Fava is the Italian word for broad bean; however, China, not Italy, is the world's largest producer of the fava bean.

Favism. Favism is a disorder characterized by a hemolytic reaction (destruction of red blood cells) to the consumption of fava beans. It is closely linked to an inherited enzyme deficiency found in over 400 million people worldwide. Normally, the enzyme, G6PD (glucose-6-phosphate dehydrogenase), protects red blood cells from free radicals. Free radicals can kill red blood cells easily if G6PD is not present, resulting in a severe hemolytic anemia. Why fava beans and not black beans, white beans, red beans, or green beans? Fava beans contain high levels of oxidants known as vicine, divicine, convicine and isouramil. Patients with G6PD deficiency metabolize the above oxidants into free radicals that trigger the destruction of red blood cells.

Healthcare professionals need to be aware of this enzyme deficiency in their patients because certain drugs, infections, and of course, fava beans can trigger the hemolytic anemia in these patients. For example, trimethoprim (a component of the antibiotic Septra/Bactrim) should be avoided as should probenecid, nitrofurantoin and probenecid. For a complete listing of drugs to avoid go to the website: www.g6pd.org

Anthony Hopkins, in the Silence of the Lambs *(1991), won an Oscar for playing a cannibal. At the end of the movie he tells Clarice (Jody Foster) that he will be having his psychiatrist for lunch "with fava beans and a nice chianti."*

Fennel. Fennel is a vegetable related to parsley, dill and cumin. Every part of fennel is edible. Fennel is an excellent source of vitamin C, the body's primary water-soluble antioxidant that neutralizes free radicals. The vitamin C (10.4 mg per cup) found in fennel also contributes to its antimicrobial and immune boosting properties. One cup of fennel has 11 percent of the daily value for dietary fiber (2.7 grams), 10% daily value for potassium (360 mg), and 6% daily value for folate (23.5 μg). Fennel's fiber helps reduce cholesterol and reduce the risk of colon cancer. The potassium in fennel helps promote normal blood pressure levels, and the folate maintains the health of the nervous system and red blood cells, and may help to reduce the risk for cardiovascular disease. Fennel has only 27 calories per cup, so it's certainly a low calorie option.

Fennel is a major nutrient found in the Mediterranean diet of the present and the past. In Greek mythology, a fennel stalk carried the gods' gift of knowledge to man. The ancient Greek word for fennel is "marathon."

HISTORICAL HIGHLIGHT

Historically the fennel plant has been used to build courage before battle, to ward off evil spirits in medieval times, to stave off hunger during long Puritan church meetings (LOL), to serve as a digestive tonic and to cure bad breath.

Five-second rule. What is the five-second rule? "If a tasty treat spends less than five seconds on the floor it doesn't collect germs." True or not? We have all used the five-second rule at some point to justify eating a chocolate chip cookie that's touched a surface other than a clean plate. If you really think about it, the length of time a food item can remain on a surface, such as a floor, and still be deemed consumable is positively related to its desirability and negatively related to the perceived level of contamination of the surface on which is was dropped. For example, a piece of boiled cabbage dropped on a freshly cleaned kitchen floor is usually deemed inedible the moment it hits the floor, while a piece of chocolate may be deemed safe to eat even after several minutes on grass at a picnic. Actually the rule should be a "zero-second" rule…bacteria such as *Salmonella* can transfer onto food instantly on contact. As mentioned in Chapter A, the five-second rule when an apple drops in cow manure doesn't apply either. (Jillian Clarke, grad student, University of Illinois, Champaign-Urbana Campus. Dr. Paul L. Dawson, Clemson University)

> *Let's face it, the five-second rule is utterly redundant if you drop your sandwich on a pile of dog poop or your chocolate on a recently sterilized kitchen surface.* —Anonymous

FLATULENCE

Flatulence. "If we passed all of the gas we made, everybody would be farting a million times a day," says the guru of gas, Dr. Michael Levitt, M.D. and GAS-troenterologist extraordinaire, Director of Research at the Minneapolis Veterans Affairs Medical Center. (By the way, the field of GAS-troenterology is *not* named after the odiferous emission known as flatus. It is from the Greek word, *gaster,* which means "belly.")

The average American intestine processes 10 liters of gas every day. Ninety-nine percent of this gas is composed of nitrogen, oxygen, carbon monoxide, hydrogen, and methane. The nitrogen and oxygen come from swallowing air with meals and saliva. The typical swallow of saliva is accompanied by 15 ml of air. For people with a nervous habit of swallowing, that can add up to a significant bellyful of gas.

The zillions of bacteria found in your large intestine produce the other three gases—carbon monoxide, hydrogen, and methane. These bacteria are constantly champing at the bit for any morsel of food that sneaks past the small intestine. The food is fermented into gas, and a heck of a lot of it—10 liters, to be exact. However, we don't pass most of it (thank goodness), because a neighboring bacterium has the ability to consume it for personal use. If any gas is left over, it is expelled during a fit of laughter while reading this book, a coughing spell, a contest among close friends, while sitting on the throne, or just to impress the inebriated crowd that you're hanging out with. Of course, if you are an 8-year-old boy, this pastime provides endless hours of raucous entertainment.

For the record, the mean flatal frequency rate (the number of times one passes gas) is 13.6 episodes per day with no statistical differences attributable to age, gender, or any other discernible variables. The upper limit for the number of episodes, even for the most gaseous among us, is less than 25 per day. The average person releases between 500 and 2,000 ml of gas per day via the rectum, with an average volume of 90 ml per expulsion for women and an average of 125 ml for men. Note the gender difference with this statistic—once again; it appears as if this bodily function is one that the male of the species is particularly proud of.

The contents of the gaseous expulsion are generally rather benign. Hydrogen, nitrogen, oxygen, and methane have little or no odor. However, the unpleasant fumes are derived from trace amounts of sulfur in the intestine—residue from meats and cruciferous vegetables such as broccoli, cauliflower, cabbage, and Brussels sprouts.

HISTORICAL HIGHLIGHT

In the early 1980s, colonoscopy procedures led to a few mini-explosions when stray electrical sparks reacted with intestinal hydrogen. These slight mishaps prompted gastroendoscopists to require that patients fast prior to undergoing the procedure. Of course, some enterprising physiology students learned of this side effect of hydrogen meeting an electrical spark. That in turn "sparked" the late-night-fraternity-party-lighting-fart-frenzy.

What can be done about excess gas? Approximately 80% of patients complaining of excessive flatus can benefit from dietary changes. Recognize the "gas triggers" such as the cruciferous family of veggies, as well as onions, and hard-to-digest sugars such as lactose or fructose. These sugars are present in dietetic candies and sugar-free chewing gums. Also remember that chewing food thoroughly is better than gobbling, and that increasing water intake and exercise can improve digestion and reduce gas formation.

People with lactose intolerance also produce excessive amounts of gas. They have difficulty digesting milk or sugar due to the deficiency of an enzyme known as lactase. A breath test in the physician's office can pinpoint this problem. In such cases, dietary alterations and taking lactase (an over-the-counter product known as Lactaid) may reduce gas, though it won't solve the problem completely. (Kluger J. What a gas. *Discover Magazine.* 1995 (April):40–43; Satish SC. Belching, bloating, and flatulence. *Postgraduate Medicine* 1997;101(4): 26–278)

Flatulence treatment with over-the-counter and alternative carminatives. Over-the-counter products include simethicone, the active ingredient in Gas-X and Mylanta Gas. Simethicone breaks up gas bubbles and makes them easier to pass.

A carminative is an herb or preparation that prevents the formation of gas or facilitates the expulsion of gas from the GI tract.

Carminative herbs and spices known to prevent the formation of gas include chamomile, mint, ginger, and fennel. Coriander and oregano are also used to aid the digestion of foods that create gas. Plant-based enzymes including bromelain (from pineapple) and papain (from papaya) are available from health food stores for this purpose.

ASPARAGUS TIP

The more carbohydrates you consume, the more gas you will produce. The switch from carnivore to vegan is particularly hazardous to your relationships—especially when the traditional diet is switched to one containing increased legumes and carbohydrates of various sizes and shapes. However, have patience. After two to four weeks of complete social isolation, the excessive passage of flatus will diminish, and you can venture out in public once again.

Certain cultures have traditional food additives that help keep flatulence in check. For example:

Indian preparations: A spice called hing is routinely used in bean dishes to reduce excessive passage of flatus.

Mexican preparations: Black beans are always cooked with epazote, another carminative herb.

Chinese preparations: Fennel has traditionally been used in Chinese dishes for cases of "excess wind."

Capsules of activated charcoal will absorb gas (and unfortunately anything else coming down the pike, so to speak, including vitamins, minerals, and medicines). Speaking of activated charcoal, you can purchase your own charcoal filter cushion known as the flatulence filter, formerly the Toot Trapper. This cushion lasts for 18 months, and absorbs up to 90% of the odor generated by a plate of pinto beans.

The makers of Beano have received a bit of support from the scientific community, as well as whole-hearted support from the teeming masses. The sample size of the initial Beano study was small; however, the results packed a powerful punch. Nineteen volunteers agreed to two lunches of cornbread, and meatless chili made with beans, broccoli, cabbage, cauliflower and onions. At the first lunch, one half of the volunteers consumed the chili, while the others were given a placebo made of water and Worcestershire sauce. A week later, the volunteers' lunches were reversed. A few drops of Beano accompanied all of the lunches. This was a double-blind study, so neither the volunteers nor the researchers knew when each diner would receive the real thing. Beano's function is to inhibit alpha galactosidase, the enzyme that breaks down sugars.

HISTORICAL HIGHLIGHT

Consider the career of the French entertainer Joseph Pujol. Born in Marseilles in 1857, his stage name was "Le Petomane" (French for "to break wind"). Pujuol mastered the anal sphincter abilities of voluntary inspiration, retention, and voluntary exhalation, so to speak. To inhale, anal sphincter relaxation was combined with reduction of intra-abdominal pressure. He discovered that the tighter the sphincter during exhalation, the higher the pitch and the lower timbre.

He became known as the man with the musical anus, and his performances at the Moulin Rouge thrilled audiences for 22 years. Bird trills, twitters, and warbles would precede an early version of the game that we now know as "Name that Tune." Requests were honored for various songs and jingles of the day, including "Claire de Lune." The range of a Pujol symphony could extend from a brassy blare to a "violinistic tremolo." His solo falsetto was such a hit that nurses had to revive the female portion of the audience. The ladies laughed so hysterically that they developed "corset-induced" hysterical syncope and passed out. The grand finale was to blow out a candle from a one-foot distance.

HISTORICAL HIGHLIGHT

In 1781, Ben Franklin proposed that a scientific prize be awarded for the discovery of, "Some drug wholesome and not disagreeable, to be mixed with our common food, or sauces, that shall render the Natural Discharges of Wind from our bodies, not only inoffensive, but agreeable as perfumes."

Fast forward to 2012…sorry Ben, we're still working on it.

For six hours after each lunch the volunteers recorded the amount of abdominal pain, bloating and flatulence. Both groups reported the same amount of pain and bloating in the first four hours. The fifth hour was the clincher. The placebo group experienced almost four times the "flatulence events" of the Beano group—on average 1.9 events vs. 0.5 events per hour. One note: No one noticed a reduction in the smell factor. (Ganiats TB, et al. Does Beano prevent gas? A double-blinded crossover study of oral alpha-galactosidase to treat dietary oligosaccharide intolerance. *J Fam Pract* 1994 November;39(5):441–445)

Terry Graedon, a medical anthropologist, and her husband, Joe, co-authors of *People's Pharmacy*, suggest keeping a "fart chart." In other words, keep a food diary and a chart showing when you pass gas. Remember that it's important to consider not only what you just ate for breakfast, but also what you had 8–12 hours earlier.

FECES

Feces. The GI tract is home to more than 500 strains of bacteria—20 strains make up about 75% of gut bacteria. Any given normal stool specimen may contain as many as 1,000,000,000,000 bacteria per gram. Most of the nutrients from food have been absorbed on their journey through the GI tract. So a stool sample is 99% undigested fiber, the carcasses of billions of bacteria, and one kernel of corn.

We'll get to that kernel of corn in the next chapter—the GI transit time.

Stool also contains a bit of potassium, though not enough to cause a potassium imbalance with the normal number of stools per day. However, if a patient has copious amounts of diarrhea for a lengthy period of time they may experience a potassium deficiency. This is actually important in the world of fluid and electrolyte balance. Low potassium (also known as hypokalemia), can trigger cardiac arrhythmias (abnormal heart rhythms) that can result in death.

An interesting corollary to this: when a patient has too much potassium (also known as hyperkalemia), an attempt to lower the potassium by giving enemas containing Kayexalate and sorbitol is performed. Both of these drugs assist in the removal of excess potassium by triggering a drug-induced diarrhea.

Feces color and food. Can foods change the color of your feces? General Mills introduced a cereal in 1971 called Franken Berry. A dye in the cereal didn't break down when digested, resulting in magenta-colored stools. Pretty. The over-consumption of Oreo cookies can turn stools black. Green, leafy vegetables contain chlorophyll, which can change the stool to green. Foods with dark purple coloring like Kool-Aid, popsicles, and gelatin (JELL-O) can also result in rainbow-colored stools. Iron supplements or even foods that are rich in iron can also give stool a green tinge. Foods such as watermelon, tomato, beets, as well as foods containing red food coloring, can cause stools to be red.

HISTORICAL HIGHLIGHT

The meaning of the word "stool" has absolutely nothing to do with the "end-product" of digestion. A stool sample refers to a fecal specimen that has been produced while sitting on a closestool which has an appropriate hole in the middle of the seat. The stool is actually the means by which the sample was obtained. However, the clinical meaning has drifted somewhat, and we now use the term stool for the actual sample that we send to the lab for testing.

If you need time to think, ask older patients to describe their bowel habits. —Clifton Meador, M.D.

Fertility and dietary adjustments. Approximately one-quarter of women with fertility problems may be helped by dietary adjustments. Phytoestrogens (found in soy products, apples, carrots, and onions) may increase the length of the follicular phase of the menstrual cycle, resulting in fewer menstrual cycles over a lifetime. This translates into fewer eggs prepared for ovulation and fertilization. Women who have multiple risk factors for infertility may be more sensitive to subtle dietary influences. These women may want to avoid excessive intake of phytoestrogen-rich foods if they want to conceive. (*American Family Physician,* Quantum Sufficit, June 1996.)

FIBER

Fiber. When you hear, "Eat soluble fiber! Eat insoluble fiber!" just what exactly does that mean? Is there a difference in soluble vs. insoluble? If so, what is it and if so, which foods contain one or the other or both?

Insoluble fiber is the type of fiber that does not dissolve in water and basically zips right through the gastrointestinal tract to the toilet. This is the type of fiber that adds bulk to stool, causing it to push against the intestinal walls and move things right along during the process of elimination. A good source of insoluble fiber is wheat bran. Whole grains, flaxseed, and the skins of many fruits and vegetables are also sources of insoluble fiber. When insoluble fiber is absent from the diet, there's less stool, so the process of elimination slows to a crawl. When bulking up with this type of fiber, don't forget to add extra water as well. Water helps swell fiber, increasing its bulk.

The soluble fiber is referred to as water-soluble fiber and is the "sticky" fiber. It dissolves in water to a gel that binds cholesterol. This prevents cholesterol from being reabsorbed back into the bloodstream, thus reducing serum cholesterol levels. Soluble fiber comes from citrus fruits, dried kidney beans, psyllium, oats and oat bran, apples, and barley.

So, soluble fiber for the heart? Insoluble fiber for the bowels? Some foods have both soluble and insoluble fiber—you get a double bang for your buck. No one source of fiber is better than another source. Eat a variety of fruits, veggies, and grains totaling about 30 to 50 grams of fiber a day. The average American diet is 12–15 grams of fiber a day. Pump it up…but don't do it all at once. If you go from 15 grams to 50 grams you'll be sitting on the toilet all day. Gradually increase your fiber intake to get into the daily range of 30–50 grams per day.

Flaxseed. Flaxseed has three major therapeutic functions. It has anti-inflammatory properties, cholesterol-lowering effects and it's a natural laxative. One tablespoon of ground flaxseed is all you need to have your daily constitutional. Flaxseed also inhibits platelet function, so be cautious about its use if you are on other anti-platelet drugs or antiplatelet supplements including gingko, ginseng, glucosamine, garlic, omega-3 fatty acids, and vitamin E. Excessive bruising and mucous membrane bleeding may occur. (*Arthritis Today* 16 (5): 59, 2002)

Flaxseed, also known as linseed, has been used as food and medicine since ancient times. Hippocrates used it to relieve intestinal discomfort and it continues to be used for constipation today.

This nutty seed is recognized as the best plant source of alpha linolenic acid, the plant form of omega-3 fatty acids. It is also a great source of fiber and lignins, both of which are phytochemicals that help to prevent endocrine-related cancers including breast, endometrial, and possibly prostate cancer.

ASPARAGUS TIP

Quantifying the amount of fiber needed for heart disease risk reduction. For every 10-gram increment of fiber consumed per day, there is a 14 percent decrease in the risk of events such as a heart attack—and a 17 percent decreased risk of dying from coronary heart disease. (Mark Pereira, PhD, University of Minnesota, *Tufts University Health and Nutrition Letter,* June 2004).

Flaxseed ***oil*** is not a good source of fiber; ground flaxseed is. It's about one-third soluble fiber, which accounts for its cholesterol-lowering properties. The other two-thirds is insoluble fiber, which accounts for its laxative benefits.

Grind whole flaxseeds with a coffee grinder and sprinkle into cereal, yogurt, soups, and bread and pancake batters. If you mix whole flaxseed into cereal, make sure you chew it well or the full benefit will not be received. Ground flaxseed can be refrigerated for 30 days without turning rancid.

Flavonoids for anti-inflammatory effects. Foods that are high in the antioxidants known as flavonoids reduce C-reactive protein levels, a marker of inflammation. This, in turn, reduces the risk for disorders associated with chronic inflammation such as heart disease, Alzheimer's disease, and cancer. Data from 8,335 adults found lower CRP levels in people with the highest intake of flavonoids. Certain flavonoids were especially beneficial, such as quercetin (found in apples and onions), kaempferol (in broccoli and tea), and genistein (in soy). (*Journal of Nutrition,* April 2008)

Floaters vs. sinkers. One way to determine whether or not you have enough insoluble fiber in your diet is to observe the nature of the stool once it has made its final exit from your GI tract. Take a look at the stool (and don't tell me you don't look—everybody looks). If the stool is floating on top of the water (a "floater") in the toilet bowl, you can breathe a sigh of relief. You are consuming plenty of fiber in your diet. Stools float because of trapped gas from colonic fermentation of non-digestible fiber. What if your stool is torpedoing to the bottom of the toilet bowl? This is known as a "sinker" and you will need to bump up your fiber intake. You should eat at least 30–50 grams of fiber per day.

FOODBORNE DISEASE

Foodborne diseases—the numbers. Every day, about 200,000 Americans develop a foodborne illness. Of those, 900 are hospitalized and 14 die. According to the Centers for Disease Control and Prevention (CDC), one in every six Americans acquires food poisoning every year. The CDC also estimates that for every reported case of foodborne illness, 38 additional cases go unrecognized or unreported.

In testimony before the Senate, it was suggested to us that foodborne illnesses may now be the largest reason for emergency room visitations by Americans. It is a virtual plague. —U.S. Senator Robert Torricelli (D-NJ)

Foodborne illness. The top 5 foods regulated by the FDA for foodborne illness are as follows:

1) Leafy greens are responsible for 363 outbreaks involving over 13,000 reported cases of illness. Pathogens responsible for the outbreaks include *E.Coli, Norovirus,* and *Salmonella.* Most leafy greens are initially contaminated on the farm through contact with wild animals, manure, polluted water, or poor handling practices during harvest and processing.
2) Shell eggs are second on the list with 95% of illness being caused by *Salmonella.* Most types of *Salmonella* live in the intestinal tracts of animals and are transmitted to humans when feces contaminate a food item. Nearly 50% of all outbreaks linked to eggs come from inadequate cooking processes and improper holding temperatures.
3) Tuna and oysters combined account for about 400 known outbreaks of foodborne illness. Toxins from spoiled fish can lead to Scombroid poisoning. *Vibrio* cholera poisoning is the most common illness related to oyster consumption.
4) See above (3).
5) Potatoes. Seriously? Yes, seriously. Potatoes have been linked to 108 foodborne outbreaks since 1990. Potatoes are often cooked before consuming, so illnesses are likely related to cross-contamination from other food items. *Shigella* and *Listeria monocytogenes* are the primary bacteria responsible for illness. (Centers for the Science in the Public Interest and University of Minnesota School of Public Health, 2009)

Ok, so you may be asking, what about hamburgers, chicken, peanuts, and meat?

The USDA, not the FDA, regulates the production of animal meat products outside of fish, so they were not included in this study. Those will be covered in each chapter.

Foodborne illness—the bugs. Thirty-one pathogens are known to cause foodborne illness. The top five pathogens in the U.S. today are: *Norovirus* (58%), *Salmonella* (nontyphoidal)(11%), *Clostridium perfringens* (10%), *Campylobacter* spp. (9%), *Staphylococcus aureus* (3%). These five account for 91% of all foodborne illness.

The top five pathogens resulting in hospitalization are: *Salmonella* (35%), *Norovirus* (26%), *Campylobacter* spp. (15%), *Toxoplasma gondii* (8%), *E. coli* (STEC):O157 (4%).

The top five pathogens resulting in death include: *Salmonella* (28%), *Toxoplasma gondii* (24%), *Listeria monocytogenes* (19%), *Norovirus* (11%), *Campylobacter* spp. (6%).

Foodborne illness—the reasons. Is this increase in foodborne illnesses a new phenomenon? Yes, it appears to be. The CDC believes that the incidence of food poisoning has greatly increased during the past few decades for three major reasons.

1) We eat more uncooked fruits and vegetables, which is great. However, if improperly grown or handled, these foods can easily transmit unhealthy pathogens.
2) We also eat more imported food, often from countries with lower safety standards than ours. One fourth of our produce is imported from countries such as Mexico, Guatemala, and the Philippines, where crops are routinely irrigated with fecal contaminated water and workers have no place to wash their hands. In 2003 the FDA found that 4.4% of fresh produce imported to the U.S. contained harmful bacteria—about four times the rate of domestic produce.
3) Our highly centralized and industrialized food-processing system has become an ideal means for quickly spreading newly emerged and dangerous pathogens such as *E.coli O157:H7* and *Listeria monocytogenes* nationwide and around the world in less than eight days. When workers try to keep up with high-speed production lines, they commonly make mistakes. For example cow manure can contaminate beef, and once ground into patties it can be widely distributed throughout the meat. That cow manure may be contaminated with *E.coli O157:H7* and *Salmonella.*

Microbial count per gram of raw meat and the quality of the meat:

10x10 = 100 .... excellent condition
10x10x10x10 = 10,000 .... good, commercial quality
10x10x10x10x10x10 = 1,000,000........................rejected commercially
10x10x10x10x10x10x10x10 = 100,000,000 .... meat smells
10x10x10x10x10x10x10x10x10 = 1,000,000,000.............meat is slimy

(Schott, B. Schott's Food and Drink Miscellany. 2004.

As mentioned earlier, one of the great ironies of our food safety program in the U.S. is that our food-processing companies are centralized but the government agencies for food inspection are decentralized. More than 12 federal agencies are responsible for inspecting our food. Here are some government facts that would be hilarious if they weren't so absurd: the Food and Drug Administration (FDA) regulates pizza, but if that pizza has hamburger, sausage, or pepperoni as toppings, it falls under the jurisdiction of the USDA. The FDA regulates eggs, but chickens are regulated by the USDA. And, of course, we all know that any two government agencies have never seen eye to eye on anything, therefore efforts to reduce *Salmonella* in chickens and chicken eggs are often impeded.

The very young and the very old and the very immunocompromised are prime candidates for foodborne illnesses. Foods that are easily handled in our 30s, 40s, and 50s can be deadly in our 70s, 80s, and 90s. Older adults should consider a little more carefully whether the food they're eating could put them at risk for an infection from foodborne bacteria. In addition, immunocompromised groups such as transplant patients, cancer patients, diabetics, and patients with HIV or AIDS should also be cautious about where their foods come from, how they are handled, and how the foods are prepared.

Alfalfa sprouts, bean sprouts, radish sprouts, and mung sprouts are all high on the list for developing foodborne illnesses from *Salmonella* and *E.ColiO157:H7*. The high level of moisture needed for sprout growth provides the perfect environment for the pesky pathogens to persist and propagate. Since the sprouts are typically eaten raw, pathogens that can cause diarrhea or even kidney failure don't get killed. Washing, even thoroughly, doesn't rid them of all the pathogenic bacteria either. Fatal outbreaks of foodborne illness attributed to alfalfa sprouts have occurred not only in the U.S. but also in Japan, Finland, Norway, Australia, and Canada.

Deli meats and other ready-to-eat meats (hot dogs) and poultry products, smoked fish such as lox (smoked salmon), and refrigerated pâtés and meat spreads are perfect mediums for the culprit *Listeria monocytogenes*. Soft cheeses such as feta, brie, camembert, and blue-veined and Mexican-style varieties are also vulnerable to *Listeria*. Cooking can kill bacteria, but these foods are not generally heated at home after possible contamination at the processing plant. Symptoms of *Listeria* can range from gastrointestinal symptoms with cramping, nausea, vomiting, and diarrhea to life-threatening meningitis.

Caesar salad dressing, hollandaise sauce, eggnog, key lime pie (made with raw eggs), and any other dish made with unpasteurized raw eggs or under cooked chicken can contain *Salmonella*. Raw unpasteurized eggs (as opposed to eggs in bottled Caesar salad dressing, for example) may contain *Salmonella* bacteria, which can bring on garden-variety GI upset such as nausea and diarrhea, but can also lead to serious complications such as severe dehydration. Runny and sunny-side up eggs can also contain *Salmonella*. Eggs that are runny aren't exposed to enough heat to kill the bacteria that may be present, and the tops of sunny-side up eggs never make it close enough to the heat source to kill any bacteria that may be lurking.

Raw mollusks, including oysters, clams, and mussels, may be infected with *Vibrio vulnificus* or *Vibrio parahaemolyticus*. Either of these bacteria can cause symptoms ranging from stomach cramps to fever to severe dehydration to bacteremia (infection in the blood.) People who may have low stomach acid (the case with three out of 10 elderly people) are particularly vulnerable and should never eat raw mollusks.

ASPARAGUS TIP

Pound for pound, chicken is 200 times more likely to cause illness than seafood (except shellfish) and 100 times more likely to result in death from that illness. When shellfish are factored in, the numbers change. Raw and undercooked shellfish are 100 times more likely to cause illness than chicken and 250 times more likely to result in death.

The high salt content of ham provides an ideal environment for *Staphylococcus aureus.* It multiples readily in ham left at room temperature. Cooking does not destroy the toxins produced by *Staphylococcus aureus* that make you ill.

Foodborne organisms cause more than a third of the acute cases of gastrointestinal illness in the U.S.

Food safety. What do all of those "dates" mean on food packaging? "Sell By" date tells the store how long they can display the product. Meat and milk have a three- to seven-day grace period after the expiration date, assuming you are a normal person and store the above perishables in the fridge. The "sell by" date serves as a guideline for stores on when they should pull products from their shelves—not when you should indulge in that last drop of milk. Rather than being an indicator of the product's safety span, the date implies when a food's quality—its taste, aroma, and appearance—would be at peak conditions.

"Best if Used By" or "Use By" date tells you by when you should eat (or freeze) the product for best quality. It still might be fine to eat after the dates have expired, as long as it hasn't yet been opened or mishandled (not refrigerated properly). Typically you should eat a refrigerated food within three to seven days of opening it, though foods like hard cheeses and condiments last a lot longer. Just remember—when in doubt, throw it out or call the 800 number on the label to check just how long it's safe. (Environmental Nutrition, April 2009)

According to a survey in Parade Magazine, 33% of Americans admit to ignoring the expiration dates on foods and eating foods past the "use by" dates.

ASPARAGUS TIP

Use a solution of 1 tablespoon chlorine bleach per one gallon of water (or ¾ teaspoon of bleach per quart of water for a smaller size bleach solution) to wash kitchen countertops and kill harmful bacteria. (*CDC*, 2011) between the tines, which actually shield the food from the action of scrubbing. Take some extra time to wash the fork, especially those covered with fatty, sticky, gooey foods. (*Nutrition Action Newsletter,* November 2011)

FRENCH FRIES

French fries. French fries were invented in 17th-century Belgium as a substitute for, rather than accompaniment to, fish. When the rivers froze and fish couldn't be caught, potatoes were cut into fishy shapes and fried instead. The Dutch call chips *Vlaamsefrieten* (Flemish fries). The first recorded chip shop, Max et Fritz, was established in Antwerp in 1862. The Belgians often claim the term "French fry" came from British and U.S. troops exposed to their national delicacy during the First World War, but the expression "French fried potatoes" had been in use in America long before World War I.

French fries and fast food restaurants. Gotta have 'em? Then choose wisely. Here's a list to take with you to the next fast food restaurant.

- McDonald's French fries, small—2.4 ounces with 10 grams of fat, 210 calories, and 135 mg of sodium.
- McDonald's French fries, super-size thighs, oops, I mean fries—7.1 ounces with 29 grams of fat, 4.5 of which are saturated, 610 calories, and 390 mg of sodium. Ouch.
- Burger King French fries, small—2.6 ounces with 11 grams of fat, 230 calories, and 520 mg of sodium.
- Burger King King-Size French fries—590 calories and 30 grams of fat, 12 of them saturated, and an eye-opening, jaw-dropping 1,100 mg of sodium.
- Hardee's French fries (regular) and Jack in the Box French fries (regular) are neck-and-neck in the categories of ounces (4), calories (340–350), and fat grams (16). However, Jack-in-the-Box wins the sodium war hands down with 710 mg of sodium vs. only 390 mg for Hardee's. The clear winner (actually loser) for the sodium wars is Arby's Curly Fries, measuring in at 910 milligrams of sodium for a 3.8-ounce (small) order.

Did you know that the 1955 French fries served with a hamburger meal from McDonald's weighed in at only 2.4 ounces and 210 calories? Fifty years and 50 zillion pounds later, the French fries served with a Quarter Pounder with cheese weighs in at 7 ounces and 610 calories. Groan.

Frog legs. A British slur on the French, referring to their penchant for the gastronomic delicacy of frogs' legs.

Frozen vs. fresh. Did you know that frozen fruits and vegetables are sometimes more nutritious than fresh fruits and vegetables? Frozen green beans contain twice as much vitamin C as fresh ones that have been sitting for nearly a week on store shelves. Frozen and canned blueberries are just as nutritious as fresh blueberries. Blueberry growers freeze and can berries as soon as they are picked, allowing the berries to retain their potent antioxidant properties.

Fructose. Fructose is a simple sugar found naturally in honey, fruits, and some vegetables. A typical fruit contains 8 grams of fructose compared to a sugary soda containing 20 grams. The two main sources of fructose in the average American diet are table sugar (which is squeezed from beet and cane plants) and HFCS (high- fructose corn syrup) which is processed using enzymes that turn corn starch into glucose and fructose. Both table sugar and high-fructose corn syrup are almost identical in their chemical composition, and both, when consumed in excess have been shown to contribute to chronic health problems. We're all aware of the obvious foods that sugars have been added to—soft drinks and other sweetened beverages, cookies, and cakes. But added sugars are also found in not-so-obvious foods, such as salad dressings, ketchup, cereals, crackers, and bread. Take a look at the label because sugars may come with many aliases…including:

Beet sugar, brown sugar, cane sugar, corn sweetener, corn syrup, demerara sugar, fruit juice concentrate, granulated sugar, high-fructose corn syrup, honey, invert sugar, maple syrup, molasses, muscovado sugar, raw sugar, sucrose, syrup, table sugar, tagatose, and turbinado sugar. Deceptive to say the least.

The beverage industry is by far the largest user of high-fructose corn syrup. Canned, bottled, and the frozen foods industry is the second-largest user. (http://www.sweetsurprise.com/?q=learning-centr/hfcs-facts-and-stats/sweetener-consumption)

So what's the connection with high blood pressure, and is this an established fact? Traditionally too much salt and not enough potassium in the diet have been the culprits causing "essential hypertension." (Essential hypertension basically means that we essentially don't know what causes it…in other words, we are clueless ☺). But new, and I might add, preliminary, studies are pointing the finger at excess sugar in the diet as another possible cause. A study published in *Circulation* 2010 found that overweight adults with either stage 1 or borderline hypertension could lower their blood pressure if they drank one less drink sweetened with any type of sugar per day. A study in the *Journal of the American Society of Nephrology* (September 2010), found that adults whose diets included 74 grams or more of fructose daily had up to 77% higher risk for blood pressure problems compared to adults who consumed less than that amount.

So, if sugary drinks are reduced in the diet, will blood pressure decrease? It looks like the answer is a resounding yes. In another study, published in *Circulation* (June 2010), Louisiana State University researchers found that people who drank just one fewer sugary beverage a day significantly lowered their BP over 18 months. The study looked at 810 adults, ages 25 to 79, with borderline high blood pressure or stage 1 hypertension. The adults who reduced their intake by just one a day had a systolic drop of 1.8 mm Hg and a diastolic drop of 1.1 mm Hg. This association persisted even after controlling for weight loss, suggesting that obesity wasn't the only factor in lowering blood pressure.

Fatty liver disease is also a condition we're hearing more and more about today. In the "old days" if you had a fatty liver you were an alcoholic until proven otherwise. And generally, there was no "otherwise." It's a different world today. *Non*-alcoholic fatty liver disease has emerged with a vengeance and has the clever acronym of NAFLD. Researchers at Duke University have shown that individuals who ingest the greatest amounts of fructose have the highest risk of progression of NAFLD to serious complications including enlargement of the liver due to fat, as well as the formation of fibrous tissue—the precursor to cirrhosis of the liver. NAFLD is most common among patients with type 2 diabetes or patients who are overweight. A 2009 study in the Journal of Hepatology found that people with NAFLD consumed five times as many carbohydrates from soft drinks as those without the disease.

Consuming high amounts of HFCS may also predispose an individual to increased levels of uric acid and the development of gout. Ouch.

So how can the health risks from sugars and high-fructose corn syrup be minimized?

1) Beware of hidden sugars—read the label! Look for all of the possible substitutes for sugars.
2) Avoid prepared, prepackaged, or processed products that do not include an ingredient list.
3) Don't eat more than four fruits daily. (Yeah, I know that fruits are good for you, but the sugars in fruits count, too). And don't forget that fruit juice in a bottle, box, or can is high in added sugars.
4) Limit fructose intake to 25–35 grams per day. How do you know what the fructose content of food is? Hop online and go to the USDA Food Database at www.NAL.USDA.gov/fnic/foodcomp/search

5) Take a multivitamin with a little extra vitamin C per day (250 mg)
6) Keep an eye on restaurant foods—limit your intake of restaurant meals and takeout foods.
7) Uh-oh. You may actually have a sugar withdrawal with symptoms including headache, fatigue and an intense craving for sweets. Don't give in! Step away from the table…drink a large glass of water every time the craving hits.
(Johnson RJ, The Sugar Fix: The High-Fructose Fallout That Is Making You Sick, 2010, Rodale)

Fruitcake. Just what are those green "things" in fruitcake? Of course they're edible…but what are they? It's just candied fruit (usually either a cherry, pineapple, or citron) dyed with a non-toxic green dye. If the fruitcake is made with alcohol and properly stored, it can remain "edible" for years… and some say, even decades. Two thousand years from now a fruitcake will be found in a landfill—in perfect condition.

In 2003, comedian Jay Leno tasted a fruitcake reputed to have been baked in Ohio in 1878. His line? "It needs more time." In the mid-17th century, England's Long Parliament outlawed fruitcake and other desserts for being too "sinfully rich." Fruitcakes can't be flown into Canada because of their "dark matter-level density" and resistance to x-rays. Oh my. If you have a burning desire to learn all about fruitcakes—how to make, how to bake, how to eat, and just group support for being a fruitcake lover—go to FruitcakeSociety.org.

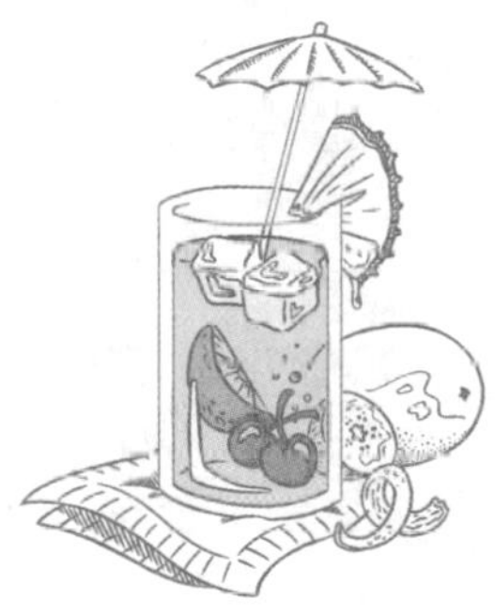

Fruity cocktails? The good news…adding booze to purees of blended fruit increases the level of healthy antioxidants…why didn't I think of that? So, all of you out there who love the froofru drinks with the strawberries and pineapple chunks, rejoice! You have just raised your antioxidant levels to a new high (no pun intended), along with your glass and along with your mood! Clink! (U.S. Department of Agriculture, 2007)

Fruits. The top 10 fruits that pack the most powerful punch. Tropical fruits are the clear winners in this contest. Paul LaChance, Ph.D., professor of Nutrition and Food Science at Rutgers University in New Brunswick, New Jersey, analyzed 31 popular fruits for eight vitamins and minerals—vitamin A, thiamine (B1), riboflavin (B2), niacin, folate, vitamin C, calcium, and iron. *And the top winners are:* guava, kiwifruit, papaya, cantaloupe, strawberries, mango, lemon, orange, passion fruit, and red currant.

Coming in a close second: raspberries and pears are full of fiber; apricots and bananas have loads of potassium; and apples are rich in flavonoids (plant chemicals that help protect the normal growth and differentiation of cells).

Fudge. According to the Oxford English Dictionary, the first definition of the word "fudge" was "nonsense or foolishness." A candy maker in Philadelphia was supervising his employees as they made caramels. Someone on the caramel line was having a bad day and instead of producing a chewy candy, the batch of caramels turned into a finely crystallized, nonchewy substance. The candy maker screamed, "FUDGE!" and now you know the rest of the story.

CHAPTER G

I stay away from natural foods. At my age I need all the preservatives I can get.
—George Burns

GARLIC

Garlic (Allium sativum). Garlic has been used for medicinal purposes since the earliest recorded history of food and medicine. In 1500 B.C. the Egyptians wrote that garlic had 22 medicinal uses, including for the prevention of heart disease, the prevention of fatigue, and the treatment of headaches,. The Greeks used garlic to protect the workers who built their pyramids. The literature doesn't discuss what garlic protected the workers from, only that they were protected when they consumed a daily clove of the garlic. Roman soldiers consumed garlic on long marches to boost their energy and endurance levels. Louis Pasteur identified the antiseptic properties of garlic in 1858. During World War II, garlic was used as a wound salve for its purported bactericidal effects.

Garlic is a member of the onion family. It contains more than 100 different sulfur compounds. The compound associated with its healing powers, as well as its odoriferous powers, is allicin. This compound is produced when garlic is crushed, cut, chopped, crunched or munched. Garlic powder also retains the medicinal allicin, as does cooked garlic. It appears as if allicin blocks certain enzymes associated with bacterial, fungal, and viral infections. Garlic's major vitamin contribution to the world of nutrition is vitamin C; its major mineral contribution is potassium.

The majority of studies on garlic's health benefits have been performed with garlic powder supplements. Supplements are not only more convenient for the average American, they are "generally" safer as well. Processing the garlic into the powder form removes any microbial contamination that may have been picked up in the soil (e.g., *Clostridium botulinum*). If a garlic tablet is chosen as a supplement, make sure it is enteric-coated. Enteric-coated tablets will bypass the stomach for metabolism reducing the risk of the proverbial "garlic breath."

Central California produces more garlic than any other state or country—an average of 250 million pounds per year. The garlic capital of the world is Gilroy, California, a 90-minute drive south of San Francisco.

Garlic's nickname is "The Stinking Rose." The name is derived from a British Social Club where patrons munched on garlic as they sipped on their favorite adult beverage.

Garlic and bleeding time. Even though garlic inhibits platelet aggregation (clumping), an overdose of garlic will not result in a hemorrhage. If platelets fail to aggregate, a blood test called the bleeding time will be prolonged. The normal bleeding time is 3–6 minutes. This would only be medically relevant if the individual is also on other platelet-inhibiting products such as gingko, glucosamine, grape seed extract, ginseng, and/or drugs such as aspirin, ibuprofen, or warfarin (Coumadin). Is there such a thing as a garlic overdose? Perhaps to friends in your up-close and personal environment, but basically the answer is no.

Garlic breath. When cutting into the garlic clove an enzyme is released that converts sulfur compounds in the garlic into ammonia, pyruvic acid, and the smelly compound known as diallyl disulfide. Diallyl disulfide is excreted in perspiration and in the air you exhale, which is why eating garlic makes you smell kind of "garlicky."

Researchers from Ohio State University have found that drinking a glass of milk after eating garlic can reduce the offending breath smell by 50%. Full-fat milk works better than skim milk, suggesting that it's the milk's fat that neutralizes the volatile compound. Parsley has traditionally been used for garlic breath. See chapter P. (Sheryl Barringer, Areerat Hunsanugrum, OSU, 2010).

In Wakefield, RI, citizens are banned from entering a movie theater within four hours after eating garlic.

Garlic and cancer risk. Research has demonstrated a protective role from the allium vegetables (garlic and onions) and the development of various cancers—including colon, prostate, esophageal laryngeal, oral, ovary, and renal. A high frequency of use of onions and garlic appears to be especially beneficial for oral and esophageal cancers. (Galeone C et al. Onion and garlic use and human cancer. *Am J Clin Nutri* 2006;84 (5):1027–1032; Kim JY, Kwon O. Garlic intake and cancer risk: An analysis using the Food and Drug Administration's evidence-based review system for the scientific evaluation of health claims. *Am J Clin Nutri* 2009;89(1):257–264)

Garlic guidelines. The World Health Organization (WHO) guidelines for general health promotion for adults is a daily dose of 2 to 5 grams of fresh garlic (approximately 1 clove), 0.4 to 1.2 g of dried garlic powder, 2 to 5 mg of garlic oil, 300 to 1,000 mg of garlic extract, or other formulations that are equal to 2 to 5 mg of allicin.

Supplements should contain the recommended standardized dose containing 1.3% of the active ingredient allicin, which provides the equivalent of approximately one fresh clove daily.

The caveat here is that many "fly-by-night" dietary supplement companies conveniently fail to add the active ingredient or they add such a small dose of the active ingredient that it does not provide one iota of health benefits. In fact, in one study of garlic supplements, 93% of the so-called standardized products were lacking sufficient amounts of allicin.

Garlic, raw or cooked? A plethora of controversy surrounds this $64,000 question. Most experts agree to disagree as to whether cooked or raw provides the most benefits. Literature from The Garlic Information Center states that cooked garlic still retains many of its active compounds and therefore, cooked garlic is still beneficial for health. One benefit of cooked garlic that no one denies—cooking can *reduce* the fairly annoying side effects and the pungent odor of raw garlic.

Cancer-fighting compounds that decompose on heating are called the allyl sulfides. That's why most experts advise that garlic be eaten in its raw form or in pill form to get the cancer protection benefits of garlic. Scientists at Penn State University have found a way to preserve the allyl sulfides during cooking. After chopping the garlic, let the garlic sit for at least 10 minutes prior to cooking. Having it sit for this period of time sets off a chemical chain reaction that dramatically boosts levels of the cancer-fighting allyl sulfides, allowing it to maintain its effectiveness when baked, sautéed, or microwaved.

Raw vs. cooked garlic as antibacterial supplements. It's a well-known fact that raw garlic has bactericidal properties; however, cooked garlic has not been "put to the test."

Thus, microbiologists from New Mexico State University in Las Cruces used several common types of food-borne bacteria, including strains of *Salmonella, Listeria,* and *Shigella.* She added raw garlic and cooked garlic to lab dishes where the bacteria was replicating with wild abandon. Within a day, bacteria-free zones surrounded the spots where either the raw-or-cooked garlic extracts had been placed. The dead zone for the raw extract was about twice as large as the dead zone surrounding the cooked garlic. The second test was similar but she grew the bacteria in a nutrient broth and then added raw vs. cooked garlic. The cooked garlic killed hundreds of millions of bacteria, but raw garlic killed about 10 times as many. The finding suggests that some of garlic's antibacterial components are heat stable; however, raw garlic is your best bet if you're in the "natural" mode to prevent food-borne illnesses.

Garlic (supplements), heart health, and cholesterol. In an October 2000 press release, the Agency for Healthcare Research and Quality (AHRQ) of the U.S. Department of Health and Human Services found that garlic supplements did not lower cholesterol for long enough periods to improve health, yet manufacturers of popular garlic supplements such as Kwai, One A Day, Nature Made and Centrum Herbals, claim that they do.

AHRQ evaluated 37 randomized trials that tested the effects of garlic supplements on cholesterol levels. Small reductions occurred when patients took garlic for one to three months, but not when they took it for six months or longer. Prolonged elevations of cholesterol promote vascular disease; therefore garlic supplements are useless in preventing the disease over time. Note: This report only studied garlic supplements, not fresh garlic. (www.ahrq.gov/news/press/pr2000/garlicpr.html)

A 2007 study compared the effects of raw garlic vs. commercial garlic supplements and basically found the same conclusions as the AHRQ study. None of the forms of garlic studied had statistically or clinically significant effects on LDL-cholesterol or other plasma lipid concentrations in adults with moderate elevations of cholesterol. Don't waste your money or your breath on garlic for cholesterol. (Gardner CD, et al. Effect of raw garlic vs. commercial garlic supplements on plasma lipid concentration in adults with moderate hypercholesterolemia: a randomized clinical trial. *Arch Int Med* 2007; 167(4):346–353)

Garlic (supplements) and immune function. Enteric-coated garlic supplements have been shown to boost immunocompetence, at least in mice. The phagocytic function of macrophages was enhanced, natural killer cells "killer" activity was boosted, and levels of cytokines increased—generally an overall boost in immune activity was significant. (Gu B, et al. Enteric-coated garlic supplement markedly enhanced normal mice immunocompetence. *European Food Research and Technology* 2010;230:1438)

Garlic supplements and HIV protease inhibitors. Garlic supplements can interact with the protease inhibitors used in many treatment regimens for patients with HIV (Human Immunodeficiency Virus). Many HIV+ patients are using garlic because of its purported benefits as an antiviral and immune-boosting supplement. As mentioned earlier, garlic has been shown to *temporarily* lower total cholesterol levels and to reduce triglycerides—both of which can be elevated with protease inhibitor therapy. Since the garlic the effect is only temporary, it's not very effective for lifelong therapy for HIV infection.

A new study shows that garlic supplements can lower the serum levels of the protease inhibitor saquinavir (Fortovase, Invirase) by approximately 50%. Whoa, just what you *don't* want to do. Researchers suspect that a substance in garlic speeds up cytochrome P450 (CYP3A4) enzymes that metabolize saquinavir and other protease inhibitors such as amprenavir (Agenerase), indinavir (Crixivan), ritonavir (Norvir), and nelfinavir (Viracept).

Garlic might also affect other antiretrovirals that are metabolized by this enzyme system found in the small intestine. These include delavirdine (Rescriptor), efavirenz (Sustiva), and nevirapine (Viramune).

This can be a very costly mistake! Ask HIV patients if they are taking garlic supplements, and if they are, explain that the supplements can be decreasing the effectiveness of their drugs.. Garlic found in food is not likely to cause the same problems. To be on the safe side, advise HIV patients to avoid consuming more than one clove of garlic per day on a regular basis and to completely avoid garlic supplements. (Piscitelli SC, Burstein AH, Welden N, et al. Garlic supplements decrease saquinavir plasma concentrations. 8th Conference on Retroviruses and Opportunistic Infections, Chicago Illinois, February 2001.)

Garlic supplements and other drugs. Also watch for transplant patients who might be taking garlic supplements along with cyclosporine (Neoral, Sandimmune). Reduced cyclosporine levels in these patients may cause transplant rejection. Women taking oral contraceptives while taking garlic supplements should use another form of birth control to avoid unwanted pregnancy. (Jellin JM, Gregory PJ, Butz R, et al. Natural Medicines Comprehensive Database. Stockton California: Therapeutic Research Faculty, 2010.)

Garlic, vampires and werewolves. Being a vampire or a werewolf may have a physiologic basis. A Canadian chemist has correlated the appearance and actions of vampires and werewolves with an extreme form of the disease known as porphyria, an inherited red blood cell metabolic disorder. Individuals with porphyria appear to have paws instead of hands and their lips and gums are so taut that their teeth become very prominent and fang-like. In the most severe cases, their teeth and bones will fluoresce in reaction to light. Their skin is hypersensitive to sunlight (hence, they abhor sunlight as vampires of lore traditionally did).

All porphyrias lack a specific enzyme required in the making of heme, the iron-compound responsible for making blood cells red and for the oxygen-carrying capacity of hemoglobin. The cells in most porphyria patients can produce heme, but are only able to make a certain amount. Since taking heme in any form (sucking blood for instance) turns off the heme pathway, this may treat one of the symptoms that patients complain about—severe abdominal pain. Since intravenous infusions of blood were not available in the Middle Ages, the next best thing was to drink a pint or so of blood.

Victims suffering from porphyria also react adversely to the chemical allyl disulfide in garlic—reputed in folklore to ward off werewolves and vampires. For sensitive porphyria patients, garlic may precipitate an attack. It is this link between garlic and porphyria that is considered to be the strongest proof that Count Dracula suffered from porphyria. Legend has it that Dracula and other vampires shied away from garlic. (Patient Dracula: did a medical condition cause Vlad the Impaler to suck blood and avoid garlic and sunlight? Porphyria symptoms could explain Dracula's behavior. *Medical Post.* July 15, 1997)

Gas stoves and asthma. Women who cook on gas stoves are two and a half times more likely to have asthma than women who cook on electric stoves. In addition, these women have twice the normal risk of wheezing, breathlessness, and waking up at night with shortness of breath. Nitrogen dioxide is the most likely culprit. It is a bronchospastic (triggering spasms of the bronchial tubes of the lungs) agent and is also found in the smoke of wood-burning stoves and secondhand smoke.

GERD

Gastroesophageal reflux disease (GERD). The lower esophageal sphincter (LES) is a physiological smooth muscle sphincter that separates the esophagus from the stomach. The sphincter opens and closes to let food into the stomach and to decrease the ability of acid from the stomach backing up (known as acid reflux) into the lower one-third of the esophagus. When acid reflux occurs, the individual will complain of a burning sensation under the sternum. The old name for this burning sensation was heartburn; the new name is gastroesophageal reflux disease, or GERD. Risk factors include the consumption of certain foods and beverages (fatty or highly acidic foods, caffeine, chocolate, alcohol, spicy foods, and tomato products), especially within 3 hours of reclining for the evening, body position (reclining, bending over), stress, smoking, obesity, and certain medications (nitroglycerin, beta-agonists for asthma, calcium channel blockers.) So, how about a big, spicy Mexican dinner accompanied by a couple of shots of Tequila, followed by a chocolate éclair, cup of coffee and a cigarette? Everyone with GERD has different triggers; however, the above mentioned triggers are the most common.

GERD capital of the world. According to American Demographics, Birmingham, Alabama wins this prize, with 72% of the adult population of this city claiming to have heartburn. The number two spot is held by Tucson, Arizona, with 62% of adults complaining of problems with acid reflux. Rounding out the top five are Minneapolis (60.5%), Miami (60%) and San Diego (60%).

Gastroesophageal reflux disease (GERD) and "alarm" symptoms. Three symptoms that indicate possible serious disease in patients with chronic GERD are

- difficult or painful swallowing
- hoarseness
- wheezing.

Patients with any of these alarm symptoms need further evaluation for GI problems such as hiatal hernia, erosive esophagitis, diffuse esophageal spasm, and peptic ulcer disease.

Gastroesophageal reflux disease and sleeping on the left side. In addition to chewing gum (see the end of this chapter), tell your patients to sleep on their left side when napping. It appears as if GERD is more pronounced in individuals who sleep on their right side, so logically, one should roll over and try the left side. Gastric acid takes longer to clear from the esophagus of right-sided sleepers compared with those who sleep on their left side, back or stomach. The lower esophagus bends to the left, and when sleeping on the left side gravity straightens out the curve, making it easier for acid to flow out of the esophagus. Advise your patients to sleep on their left side and to use a pillow behind the back to maintain this position.

Gatorade. In 1965, Dr. Robert Cade was studying the effects of heat exhaustion on the football team at the University of Florida. He analyzed the body fluids lost during sweating and came up with the formula for the drink within 3 minutes. The formula tasted just like urine—he added lemon to mask that urine flavor. Since the University of Florida's mascot is the alligator or shortened to the Florida Gators, he combined his name (ade) with that of Gator and voilá! The name Gatorade had its origins. By 1983 it had become the National Football League's official sports drink and by 1985 the first head coach received the official "Gatorade shower." In other words, after winning a football game the New York Giants poured a huge container of Gatorade over their head coach, Bill Parcells. Fast forward to 2009. Gatorade rebranded its name to just G.

Gender-related cravings. There are a few interesting studies on gender-related food issues, and the findings aren't really surprising. Using PET scans, researchers have shown that men are able to voluntarily suppress their hunger more effectively than women. Annoying. Gender differences were also found regarding comfort food choices. When it comes to foods that bring psychological comfort, men chose a big hearty meal, while women tend to devour snacks that require little or no preparation--including chocolate, ice cream, and candy. (Wang G, et al. PNAS. 2009;106:1249–1254; Wansink B. *Physiol Behav.* 2003;79:739–747)

Whoever could make two ears of corn or two blades of grass grow upon a spot of ground where only one grew before would deserve better of Mankind, and do more essential service for his country than the whole race of politicians put together.
—The King of Brobdingnag Gulliver's Travels by Jonathan Swift, 1727

Genetically modified or genetically engineered foods. This is one of the most controversial topics in the world of food science today. Should we or should we not genetically engineer or genetically modify foods?

The proponents of genetically modified foods would certainly agree with The King of Brobdingnag on this one. The benefits of genetically engineered plants include: insect resistance, herbicide resistance, virus resistance, delayed fruit ripening, altered oil contents, and pollen control. In other words, scientists can develop foods that resist disease, that can travel around the world without spoiling, and can provide more bang for the buck, so to speak.

How do scientists develop all of the characteristics of genetically engineered foods? They take genetic material from various organisms and modify it in a way that does not occur in the natural world. When genetically modifying a product, a small piece of genetic material or DNA, from one plant or animal is inserted into the genetic material of another plant or animal, transferring the desired trait. The plants and animals involved may not even be genetically or species-related. For example, a gene found in cold-water fish confers tolerance for cold. This makes sense. How else would a halibut live off the coast of Alaska without turning into a fish-sicle? In order to survive it developed a gene that provides a type of "antifreeze" substance in the blood to prevent the fish from freezing. The use of this specific antifreeze gene is not being used on any current crops at this time.

The GMO (genetically modified organisms) were introduced into crops commercially in 1994 with the first genetically modified tomato. The modification involved removing an enzyme that caused the tomato to ripen too fast. The removal of the enzyme was supposed to allow more time for the tomato to ripen on the vine and still have a long shelf life in the grocery store. The tomato was not successful and as of today there are no genetically modified tomatoes in the U.S. and European nations. The most common genetically modified foods today are soy and corn crops. The most recent USDA data as of July 2010 indicates that 86% of all corn in the U.S. is genetically engineered. Many processed foods containing soybeans or corn have also been grown from genetically modified seeds. In fact, more than half of the U.S. soybean crops grow from genetically modified seeds and approximately 60% to 70% of packaged grocery products contain some genetically modified components. Potatoes, rice, papaya and squash have been genetically engineered to repel insects and resist disease.

The opponents of genetically modified food products refer to them as "Frankenfoods." They are concerned that the technology is not precise enough to avoid causing unwanted traits to be passed to a new plant form such as antibiotic resistance, or that it might cause health problems, including allergies. They cite the October 2000 recall as a perfect example of what can happen with genetically modified foods. Taco shells containing the StarLink brand of corn were pulled from grocery shelves because the corn was specifically developed to kill crop-destroying caterpillars. The corn was not approved for human consumption. Somehow it made it's way into taco shells. This protein had the potential to cause allergic reactions in humans and hence the recall.

How do you know if the food you are consuming is genetically modified? You don't. The government does not require any special labeling for genetically modified foods unless the food differs in safety, composition or nutritional quality compared to its natural counterparts. At this time, no food currently falls into this category. At least that's what the U.S. Government says.

This is currently undergoing a "re-evaluation" by the U.S.D.A. as consumer groups are pressuring the government to label all GMO-containing foods. Labeling is required in over 40 countries throughout the world. Until that time, how do you know if you are eating a genetically-engineered food?

You don't. But there are some clues: Nix processed foods. The soybean oil and high-fructose corn syrups all come from genetically modified crops. Purchase organic products and a GM food will not pass your lips. A new label is also being used on non-GMO modified foods. It says non-GMO Project—Verified and it indicates that the food has been tested and meets the standards of a GMO-free product. (Environmental Working Group, www.justlabelit.org, www.nongmoproject.org, *Environmental Nutrition* July 2010, June 2012)

Genetically modified foods as vaccines. In 1991 the World Health Organization challenged scientists to create a simpler, safer, cheaper way to vaccinate children. Scientists accepted the challenge. Syringes and needles are so expensive to developing countries, why not make an edible vaccine? Since plants produce a myriad of proteins, the scientists decided to attempt to engineer plants to produce specific proteins from a pathogen to stimulate the body's immune response.

The first plant considered for an edible vaccine was the potato plant. Potatoes grow in many areas around the world, they are cheap to grow, and they are easy to store and ship. So the scientists inserted the gene from a specific protein in the cholera bacteria into the genes of the potato plant. The result was a genetically modified potato that stimulated the immune system. Stay tuned. Bananas are also on the list for use as an edible vaccine.

Genetically modified potatoes may also hit your local fast food restaurant in the near future. When a potato is fried, the oil that it is fried in replaces the water in the potato. Hence, many fast food restaurant French fries are harbingers of saturated and trans fats. But, the starchier the potato, the less oil it soaks up and obviously the less fat consumed by the consumer. McDonald's pays a premium price for the 3.2 billion pounds of starchy potatoes it uses every year. Potatoes that are full of starch make crisper, less greasy fries. Scientists are attempting to develop potatoes with even more starch so they will soak up even less oil.

Ghrelin, the hunger hormone. Our bodies rely on a host of involuntary cues to regulate food consumption.In 1999, researchers discovered a hormone that contributes to strong feelings of hunger. The hormone was dubbed "ghrelin" after the Hindu word for "growth." Research has demonstrated a variety of diet and lifestyle factors that modify the body's production of ghrelin and other eating-related signals.The name's initial letters also reference ghrelin's role as a growth hormone releasing factor—"ghre." It is produced by the primarily by the stomach and secondarily by the intestine to stimulate growth hormone release from the pituitary. This in turn stimulates hunger. It is the only appetite stimulant made outside the brain. It spikes approximately thirty minutes prior to a meal and returns to normal after eating. Clinically, when volunteers are given shots of ghrelin they become ravenous and eat 30 percent more than they normally would. Ghrelin levels rise in dieters who lose weight and try to maintain the weight loss. It's as if their bodies are trying to regain the fat they have lost. Interestingly ghrelin levels drop sharply in patients who have had gastric bypass surgery, possibly explaining why their appetites sharply decline after the surgery.

GI TRANSIT TIME

GI (gastrointestinal) transit time in humans. Let's get back to that kernel of corn in your feces. And don't tell me you don't look—everyone looks!

(See Chapter F (feces) if you're confused about where I mentioned the kernel of corn.) Food digestion and elimination should actually be completed within a certain time frame for gastrointestinal health. This is where the GI transit time comes in. What is the GI transit time? It's a fancy way of explaining how long it takes food to travel from the mouth to the toilet. In humans, the residues of a high fiber, low fat meal typically make the big splash around 18 hours after the initial bite. The normal range is 18–72 hours. The residues from a high fat, low fiber meal may not see the white walls of the porcelain bowl for 3–10 days.

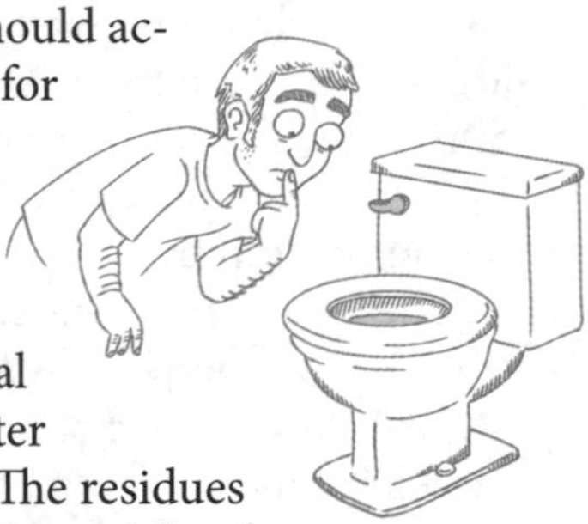

Let's compare humans to hummingbirds and snakes. It takes only one hour for the nectar consumed by a hummingbird to make its way into the great hummingbird toilet in the sky. For the big snakes, (anacondas, boa constrictors and pythons), transit times may be measured in days or weeks. It takes about 12–14 days to process a rat through the GI system of your basic rat-consuming python. Read on for the fascinating travels through a big snake gastrointestinal system.

GI transit time in snakes. Humans consume small meals at regular intervals several times a day. In other words, our 16–22 feet of intestinal tubing is working most of the time and doesn't have to adapt to a very wide range of food intakes. This makes our intestines' responses modest in scope and difficult to study and analyze. Enter the anaconda, boa constrictor and the four python species of the Old World and Australia. These giant snakes are notorious for consuming humongous meals at long and unpredictable intervals. Since their meals are so massive, their intestinal responses must be equally huge, making these responses quite amenable to study as models of our own digestion.

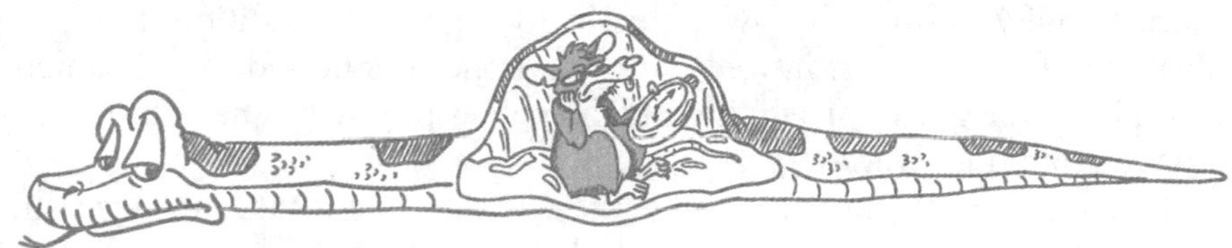

The largest snake on record is a 37-foot anaconda. The longest snakes can be as thick as a man's waist and weigh several hundred pounds, most of it muscle. The muscles allow the snakes to squeeze their prey to death. The victims, interestingly enough, don't suffer broken bones and tend to retain their original shape while sliding through the snake's GI tract. Case in point: a 14-year-old Indonesian boy was swallowed by a reticulated python and his body was still intact and recognizable in the snake's stomach when the snake was killed and cut open two days later.

Swallowing a human being is not an everyday occurrence in the life of the reticulated python, and there are only a few authenticated cases. You can breathe a sigh of relief if you are an adult male—all cases have been small children or small women. These unfortunate individuals had to have been unconscious for some reason, as they would never have cooperated while the snake devoured them for over an hour.

Do you remember how your mother used to admonish you for not chewing your food thoroughly? Well, snakes don't chew their food—they just swallow it whole. The biggest prey on record is a 130-pound antelope swallowed by an African rock python. Another record-breaking case involved an Asian reticulated python gulping down a 28-pound goat and a 39-pound goat at one sitting. Two days later the same snake consumed a 71-pound ibex.

Are you impressed yet? How about a few comparisons in terms of relative body weights? Sheer gluttony in a human being may result in consuming a few pounds of food at one sitting, and 10 pounds would be practically unheard of. Eating 10 pounds would be under 10% of our body weight. By comparison, a giant snake regularly consumes 20% of their unfed body weight and, if particularly ravenous on any given day, it can easily eat 6 – 96% of their body weight. Let's open the Guinness Book of World Snake Records—a viper swallowed a lizard 1.6 times its body weight. What would that equate to in the Guinness Book of World Human Records you might ask? It would equate to a 140-pound male downing a 35-pound T-bone and occasionally swallowing a 224-pound side of beef.

So, if snakes only swallow foods whole, why bother having fangs? Snakes bite their prey but they don't chew it. The bite merely anchors the prey so that the prey cannot wiggle back out of the snake's mouth. Ugh. The fangs actually curve back toward the snake's stomach, so once the fangs engage it is virtually impossible to disengage.

The snake's jaws can open to an angle of 130 degrees, as compared to the human ability to open the jaw a measly 30 degrees. In addition, the lower jawbone of the snake is hinged with two bones connected by a ligament. This allows for greater flexibility, which enables the snake's head to literally stretch around its prey.

One major problem with a huge meal is the time it takes to digest the food. The digestive process of the snake has to compete with the microbes of the GI tract of the swallowed victim. Dead animals begin to putrefy as their own bacteria begin to break down their bodies and release toxic chemicals. So, the bigger the victim is the greater the risk of a prey rotting in the snake's stomach.

This brings us to a simple explanation of why snakes enjoy basking on a rock out in the sun, and why they coil up to conserve heat. Heat speeds up the digestive process and reduces the probability of putrification of the devoured prey. An Indian python, fed a rabbit, completed digestion in 4–5 days when kept at a temperature of 82° F; however, when the temperature was reduced to 71° it took 7 days, and when the temperature was reduced to 64° it took 14 days. In fact, if the temperature gets too cool, the snake will refuse to eat anything at all.

The interval between swallowing and defecating may be quite lengthy (approximately 12–14 days to digest a rat), but the time between feedings may be even longer. Pregnant female rattlesnakes may go one and a half years without a meal. Zoo snakes have been known to refuse food for over two years. Snakes in the wild have feeding intervals of weeks to months. So the three square meals per day in the human population certainly doesn't apply to the snake population, nor does the got-to-have-it daily bowel movement that obsesses a significant percentage of the human population.

When a python swallows a mouse, its intestine doubles or triples in weight overnight. Each cell of the intestinal lining enlarges and produces longer finger-like villi to increase the surface area for digestion. By analogy, a 150-pound man would have to add six pounds to the weight of his intestine overnight. The snake has a 60-fold increase in the amount of enzymes produced for digestive purposes. In addition, it has a 3,600% increase in oxygen consumption as compared to the human's 20% increase in oxygen consumption after a meal. The cost of making extra intestine and digestive enzymes is so high that the snake uses approximately one-third of the energy it gets from the mouse's body just to consume the mouse. Wow.

Gin and tonic dermatitis. It's not the gin and it's not the tonic that causes that itchy rash. However, it's that oh-so-tasty lime squeeze that can trigger the sunburn-like dermatitis. This may be especially hazardous for your backyard bartender, since sunlight tends to trigger this photosensitivity reaction. Limes, celery, or parsnips are all culprits. Any taker's for a gin and tonic with a twist of parsnip? (*Internal Medicine News.* October 1, 2006)

Ginger (Zingiber officinale). Ginger has been used for medicinal purposes in China for more than 2,500 years to treat indigestion, nausea, and motion sickness. The Chinese were obviously privy to the fact that ginger's major function targeted gastrointestinal motility. Today it is recommended for the treatment of dyspepsia, colic, flatulence, nausea/vomiting, fluid retention, motion sickness, and morning sickness. The anti-vomiting properties of ginger are thought to be mediated through local action on the stomach mucosa, not through central brainstem mechanisms. Is ginger safe for pregnant women? Yes. (*Am Fam Physician* 2007; 75:1689; Jellin JM, Gregory PJ, Butz R, et al. *Natural Medicines Comprehensive Database.* Stockton California: Therapeutic Research Faculty, 2010.))

In studies of morning sickness and vomiting, women who took between 1,000 mg and 1,500 mg of ground ginger (about ½ to 1 teaspoon worth), divided into several doses over the course of the day were unlikely to experience morning sickness. Stomach pain may occur in some patients with this dose. More than 6,000 mg per day can cause ulceration of the gastrointestinal tract. (Nutrition Action Healthletter, October 2007)

Ginger also stimulates the secretion of stomach acid, aiding in digestion and reducing gas, bloating and nausea. Ginger can be taken by drinking ginger tea, taking a 300 mg capsule or 20 drops of the liquid form two or three times daily, ideally prior to meals. (Wu, KL. Et al. *European Journal of Gastroenterology and Hepatology,* May 2008)

Gingivitis (inflamed gums). It takes 16-24 hours for the bacteria in the mouth to produce the plaque that contributes to gingivitis and periodontal disease. Therefore, brushing after every meal to prevent plaque is an unnecessary expenditure of time and energy. If you brush properly in the a.m. and p.m. and throw in one flossing episode with either, plaque problems will be history.

Ginkgo (Gingko Biloba). Gingko, also known as the Maidenhair Tree, is the oldest living tree species. Gingko trees have existed for over 200 million years. This herb is especially popular in Europe, where it is one of the most prescribed and lucrative of all herbal products.

Gingko improves blood flow in the peripheral circulation and has been shown to improve the symptoms of peripheral vascular disease. (American Heart Association, 2010)

Even though gingko also improves blood flow to the brain, studies have not been encouraging as far as improvement in memory, for mild cognitive impairment, or for the prevention of any form of dementia, including Alzheimer's dementia.

Gingko's side effects can be clinically significant in some patients. Gingko has potent platelet-inhibiting effects and may cause bleeding in patients who are also on other drugs that inhibit clotting. There have been several reports of spontaneous subdural hematomas (bleeding in the subdural space) with chronic use of gingko combined with aspirin. (Jellin JM, Gregory PJ, Butz R, et al. *Natural Medicines Comprehensive Database.* Stockton California: Therapeutic Research Faculty, 2010; Borins M. What to tell your patients about herbs, *Hospital Medicine,* August 1999).

Ginseng. American ginseng was used traditionally by Native Americans as a stimulant and as a treatment for headaches, fever, indigestion, and infertility. Laboratory studies in animals have found that American ginseng is effective in boosting the immune system, and as an antioxidant. Other studies show that American ginseng might have therapeutic potential for inflammatory diseases.

Preliminary studies have shown that taking American ginseng may lower the steep rise in blood sugar after a meal in patients with type 2 diabetes. The dose was three grams prior to eating; however, one gram will probably do the trick. Is this enough to run out and start gobbling American ginseng? No. First of all, the ginseng used for the study is not available as an over-the-counter herbal product. Second, the studies are preliminary and the sample size was a whopping 19 patients. So, hold off on the ginseng until more research has been completed. It's promising, but too early to recommend for clinical practice. (Vuksan V et al. American ginseng reduces postprandial glycemia in nondiabetic subjects and subjects with type 2 diabetes mellitus. *Archives of Internal Medicine* 2000;160: 1009; Jellin JM, Gregory PJ, Butz R, et al. *Natural Medicines Comprehensive Database.* Stockton California: Therapeutic Research Faculty, 2010).

GLUCOSAMINE

Glucosamine for osteoarthritis. Glucosamine is one of the most widely used complementary therapies for osteoarthritis. Unfortunately, studies show mixed results with the form most often used—glucosamine sulfate. This form of glucosamine scored a three out of five on the effectiveness scale for osteoarthritis. Some research has shown that glucosamine may be effective for reducing the pain and progression of knee arthritis; however, if no benefit is observed after a three-month trial, there will likely be no benefit with continuing the supplement.

Glucosamine and shellfish allergies. Glucosamine is a compound that occurs naturally in the human body. However, the glucosamine in dietary supplements is extracted from shellfish. So, ask your patients if they have a shellfish allergy prior to recommending it for osteoarthritis.

Gluten. What is gluten? After starch has been extracted from wheat flour, gluten is the residue that is left. This is made up of multiple proteins that are distinguished by their solubility and extraction properties. For example, the alcohol-soluble fraction of wheat gluten is wheat gliadin. It is the protein component that is primarily responsible for the mucosal injury that occurs in the small bowel of patients with celiac disease.

Gluttony, a famous case of. The average dinner eaten by King Louis XIV of France: four plates of soup, a whole pheasant, a whole partridge, two slices of ham, a salad, mutton with garlic, pastry, fruit, and hardboiled eggs. On autopsy it was discovered that the King's stomach was twice the size of a normal stomach.

Glycemic Index. The glycemic index (GI) is a measure of the rapidity of carbohydrate absorption after a meal or serving. The glycemic index ranks are based on the average blood sugar responses to 50 grams (g) of carbohydrates from an individual food, including cereals, pastries, vegetables and fruits, and comparing that increase in blood sugar to the increase seen after eating 50 g of white bread or 50 g of pure glucose. Eating high glycemic index foods triggers a rapid and sustained increase in blood glucose and insulin demand. Of all foods consumed, rice contributes to the highest glycemic load. Potatoes and bananas are also high on the GI list. Chocolate actually has a lower glycemic index than a banana or a potato. There is a God. Foods with high fiber content are low on the list. The glycemic index is easy to figure out when eating a single food cooked in a specific way.

Combining foods and cooking methods can alter the GI quite a bit. Mix milk and butter into mashed potatoes, and the glycemic index actually drops because the fat of the butter slows the absorption of the starchy potato. Bake the potato instead of boiling it, and the GI changes again. Some of the principles behind the GI approach— like choosing high-fiber foods, which have a lower GI—are sound, but the index itself is confusing and unreliable.

Studies have shown that eating a diet with a low glycemic index can reduce the risk of a woman developing diabetes and cardiovascular disease. Other studies have shown that kids can lose weight when using foods with low glycemic indexes. (Krishnan S et al. Glycemic index, glycemic load and cereal fiber intake and risk of type 2 diabetes in U.S. black women. *Arch Intern Med* 2007 Nov 26; 167:2304; Villega R et al. Prospective study of dietary carbohydrates, glycemic index, and incidence of type 2 diabetes mellitus in middle-aged Chinese women. *Arch Intern Med* 2007 Nov 26; 167: 2310)

Glycemic index of foods. Each food is assigned a glycemic index number from 0 to 100, with a high GI number over 70 signifying a rapid rise in blood sugar accompanied by an equally rapid surge in the release of insulin. Pure sugar serves as a reference point and has a glycemic index of 100. The glycemic index hypothesizes that the faster the release of insulin from the pancreas, the more pounds you pack around your middle. In theory, the more weight you pack around your middle, the higher your risk for type 2 diabetes as well as other chronic conditions including hypertension, certain types of cancer including endometrial cancer and postmenopausal breast cancer, and Alzheimer's dementia.

Foods with a low glycemic index, less than 55, stimulate a much slower release of insulin. Examples of foods with glycemic indexes less than 55 include lentils (28), soybeans (18), apples (38), peaches (42), skim milk (32), heavy, mixed grain bread (30–45), All-Bran cereal (42), low-fat yogurt (33), and a chocolate bar (49). Foods with a glycemic index greater than 70 tend to be low-fiber, highly refined carbohydrates such as white bread (70), Corn Flakes (84), jelly beans (80), Gatorade (78), and watermelon (72). Some foods considered in the "gray zone," between good and bad are bananas (55), ice cream with full fat (61), and a Mars Bar (65). The diet book, Sugarbusters! By H. Leighton Steward et al., is based on eliminating foods with a high glycemic index. Jenny Craig is also based on the glycemic index of foods with a dose of portion control thrown in.

Before rushing off to the bookstore to buy various diet books on low glycemic index diets, remember that high glycemic foods are not the only culprit in an ever-increasing waistline, or in the development of type 2 diabetes. In theory the GI is a good idea, in practice it leaves much to be desired.

Gourmand syndrome. Swiss researchers have reported on a brain disorder in a small percentage of patients who have suffered strokes, brain tumors, and head trauma. In each case, the damage has produced a persistent behavioral effect—a craving for fine foods. As of today, none of the patients has requested a cure for this condition.

The first patient described with this syndrome was a 48-year-old man who had been hospitalized with a stroke. CT scans pinpointed the area to a small region around the middle cerebral artery in the right frontal lobe. He also suffered a temporary weakness on the left side of the body. His main concern, however, was not the temporary inability to ambulate, but with the lousy hospital food. Since this complaint is universal in all hospital patients, his fixation on the hospital food was basically ignored. However, when the neuropsychologist asked him to keep a diary of his thoughts, the man exhibited an inordinate preoccupation with food. Before the stroke, he had an overwhelming interest in politics as a political journalist, and very little interest in fine dining. After the stroke, he dumped the political scene and became a columnist for fine dining.

The second patient with gourmand syndrome, a businessman hospitalized for a right-sided, middle cerebral artery stroke, exhibited a new found "lusting" after food. After studying 723 more patients having a similar area involved, the researchers identified 34 more instances of gourmand syndrome. Most of the patients exhibited additional symptoms attributed to right-sided frontal lobe damage, including weakness on the left side; however, the weakness disappeared for the most part, but the passion for food remained. Most of these patients became preoccupied with shopping, dining rituals, and food preparation. None of the patients became overweight as a result of their fine dining cravings. (*Science News* 1997; 151)

Gout. Gout is on the rise in the U.S. and many researchers are blaming it on the obesity and hypertension epidemic. Historically gout was known as the "disease of kings," since only the wealthy and privileged who had the means to overindulge in food and drink, were affected. However, in the U.S. over the past half century the prevalence of gout has more than doubled with over eight million American adults with this condition. Men bear the brunt of this illness, with gout being 9 times more common in men than women. In the U.S. it occurs in approximately 840 per 100,000 people. Gout often affects men in their 40s and 50s and is more common in postmenopausal women.

Gout results from the deposit of urate (uric acid) crystals in a joint or the shedding of crystals from deposits in the synovial tissue of the joints, causing an acute inflammatory response. Gout may be due to the overproduction of urate, its undersecretion by the kidneys, or both. Although the terms uric acid and urate are used interchangeably there is a difference depending on the pH (acidity or alkalinity) of the body fluid (serum (alkaline) vs. urinary tract (acidic). But for the purposes of this book, either term can be used. Serum uric acid levels greater than 7 mg/dl are associated with an increased risk of gout. If the serum uric acid levels are greater than 9 mg/dl, symptomatic gout develops within 5 years in about 20% of men.

There are many causes for the accumulation of uric acid—age, obesity, diet, booze, and medications (diuretics). Obesity is associated with an increased urate production and decreased urate excretion, whereas alcohol primarily reduces urate excretion. Gout occurring in men *under* the age of 30 or in *pre*menopausal females should prompt a thorough metabolic and renal investigation.

The initial manifestation is usually a painful attack of arthritis in one joint (monoarticular arthritis)—and for unknown reasons it's usually the big toe joint. The joint is swollen, red, and intensely painful. Gout can also present in the ankle, knee or other joints.

Can gout be prevented? Most likely the answer is yes. Genes may play a role in predisposing to gout, and at this point genes cannot be modified, but

HISTORICAL HIGHLIGHT

The treatment of gout in Tudor times was as follows: Boil a red-haired dog in oil, stir in a few worms as well as the marrow from pig bones and apply the mixture to the affected part. There was no citation in the literature as to whether this concoction was effective.

limiting weight gain, reducing alcohol intake, decreasing high fructose corn syrup and red meat can all help to reduce the risk of developing gout.

Can dietary changes reduce gout flare-ups? Eating foods rich in a compound called purine can produce increased levels of uric acid, thus increasing the risk for gout. The purine content of food reflects its nucleoprotein content and how fast the food grows. Foods containing many nuclei (e.g., liver) have many purines, as do rapidly growing foods such as asparagus.

Foods high in purines include anchovies, beer, fortified wines, brewer's yeast supplements, clams, goose, gravy, herring, lobster, mackerel, meat extract, mussels, red meat, organ meats (liver), oysters, sardines, scallops and shrimp. Asparagus, beans, cauliflower, lentils, mushrooms, peas, oatmeal and spinach are also high in purines. Vegetable-based purines do not significantly affect serum uric acid levels, whereas meat and shellfish increase the risk of gout and gout flare-ups. Don't forget foods containing high-fructose corn syrup can do the same. Good grief. Dairy products have been shown to decrease the incidence of gout.

The purine content of the diet usually does not contribute more than 1 mg/dl to the serum uric acid concentration. Restricting purines in the diet has the greatest benefit for patients who have a low uric acid clearance from the kidneys.

What foods are low in purine? Low-purine foods include butter, polyunsaturated margarine, other fats, cream soups made with low-purine vegetables but without meat or meat stocks, fruit, nuts, peanut butter, milk, milk products, eggs, refined cereals and cereal products, white bread, pasta, flour, tapioca, cakes, sugar, sweets, and gelatin, water, pure fruit juice, cordials and carbonated drinks.

(Zhu Y, Pandya BJ, Choi HK. Prevalence of gout and hyperuricemia in the US general population. *Arthritis & Rheumatism,* July 28, 2011 (online).DOI:10.1002/art.30520; Harmon J, Gout on the rise as Americans gain weight. *Scientific American* 2011 July 28, 2011 (online); Dadig B, Wallace AE. Gout: A Clinical Review. *Clinician Reviews* 2011 (July):29–35; Choi HK, Atkinson K, Karlson EW, et al. Purine-rich foods, dairy and protein intake and the risk of gout in men. *N Engl J Med.* 2004; 350:10931103)

Graham crackers. The Reverend Sylvester Graham, a 19th century self-proclaimed nutritionist and naturalist, led a crusade against refined white flour. Graham advocated the use of only whole coarse grain flour for baking. His name became attached to "graham bread" and "graham crackers," also referred to at the time as "digestive biscuits." Seems like Graham was on to something back in the 19th century.

Grapes. Grapes are perfect for winemaking. They have enough sugar to produce a product that has 10% alcohol and they have enough acid to inhibit the growth of pathogens during the fermentation process. One ton of grapes will make 170 gallons of wine.

Will one glass of nonalcoholic grape juice substitute for one glass of wine's health benefits? Both grapes and red wine contain flavonoids that protect the heart. The July 2000 issue of the *American Journal of Clinical Nutrition* provides an answer to the question. The researchers suggest that a daily glass of grape juice is just as effective for heart protection as a daily glass of wine.

A study by Lekakis et al. also found significant arterial vasodilation when test subjects with coronary artery disease were given a red grape polyphenol extract vs. placebo. The effect lasted for 60 minutes. They concluded that the polyphenolic compounds from the red grapes acutely improved endothelial function (vasodilatory properties) in patients with coronary artery disease. (Lekakis J, et al. Polyphenolic compounds from red grapes acutely improve endothelial function in patients with coronary heart disease. *Euro J of Cardio Prev & Rehab,* 2005; 12:596–600)

A study by Chaves, et al. found that the consumption of grape products equivalent to 1.25 cups of fresh red grapes caused significant improvement in arterial blood flow within three hours of consumption. When patients consumed this dose of red grapes two times a day for three weeks, significant vasodilation continued as did total antioxidant activity. In addition, consuming grapes with a high fat meal completely prevented high-fat-induced vascular dysfunction. High fat meals cause a 50% reduction in blood flow—grapes can negate that effect. Hmmm. Should we suggest a "chaser" of 1.25 cups of red grapes after consuming a Big Mac with fries? (Chaves AA, et al. Vasoprotective endothelial effects of a standardized grape product in humans. *Vasc Pharm* 2009 (Jan/Feb); 50:20–26)

GRAPE SEED EXTRACT

Grape seed extract. Historically grape seeds have been dismissed as useless. However, increasing data indicates that these seeds may contain a tremendous number of antioxidants. According to the National Center for Complementary and Alternative Medicine, grape seed extract is used for cardiovascular disease, diabetes, neurologic conditions, vision problems, and wound healing.

ASPARAGUS TIP

If you get a "mustache" from drinking grape or cherry juice, you can quickly wipe it off with a bit of toothpaste dabbed on a washcloth.

The mechanism of action results from the high concentration of phenolic compounds, or proanthocyanics, which are known to provide high levels of antioxidants. Grape seed also contains a significant number of essential fatty acids. Linoleic and oleic polyunsaturated fatty acids together compose nearly 90% of the oil in grape seed.

In addition, grape seed extract has vasodilatory and antiplatelet properties. It appears to increase the release of nitric oxide from both endothelial cells and platelets. Releasing nitric oxide lowers systemic blood pressure and maintains normal elasticity and tone of blood vessels.

Grape seed extract may also have a role in fighting breast and prostate cancers. When grape seed extract was added to prostate cancer cells, 16% more cells died compared with only 2.4% in the untreated cells. In a breast cancer study grape seed extract blocked aromatase, the enzyme that converts androgen to estrogen. This is the same effect that "aromatase inhibitors" have when used to treat breast cancer. Grape seed extract might be useful in the prevention and treatment of estrogen-receptor positive breast cancer. (Kijima I, et al. Grape seed extract is an aromatase inhibitor and a suppressor of aromatase expression. *Cancer Res.* 2006; 66:5960–5967; Sego S. Grape Seed. *Clinical Advisor.* 2010; February: 120–122)

Grape seed extract and drugs. Grape seed extract can interfere with prescribed drugs. Grape seed extract is a potent inducer of one of the enzymes in the liver that metabolizes drugs. As a result it can cause a decrease in drug levels of such common medications as warfarin, acetaminophen, calcium channel blockers, and tricyclic antidepressants. (Memorial Sloan-Kettering Cancer Center. Grape Seed. www.mskcc.org/mskcc/html/69243.cfm)

GRAPEFRUIT

Grapefruit. One-half of a pink grapefruit has 1 gram of dietary fiber, 320–780 IU of vitamin A (up to 15.6% of the RDA for a man, and up to 19.5% of the RDA for a woman), and 47 mg of vitamin C (78% of the RDA). White grapefruit isn't quite as nutritious. One-half of a white grapefruit has 1 gram of dietary fiber but only 10 IU of vitamin A, and 39 mg of vitamin C. Pink and red grapefruits are also rich in the carotenoid, lycopene. Lycopene appears to reduce the risk for heart disease. Another substance in grapefruit, D-limonene, is a member of a family of plant chemicals that also appears to protect against the development of cancer. Remember foods that are high in vitamin C also help to absorb iron from iron supplements or foods that are rich in iron. The other benefit of grapefruit and other foods that are high in vitamin C, is the promotion of wound healing. Vitamin C is necessary for the conversion of proline to hydroxyproline, an essential component of collagen. Collagen is the "glue" that holds skin, bones, and tendons together.

Grapefruit, grapefruit juice and drugs. Concomitant administration of either grapefruit or grapefruit juice can increase the plasma concentration of numerous drugs, resulting in adverse clinical effects.

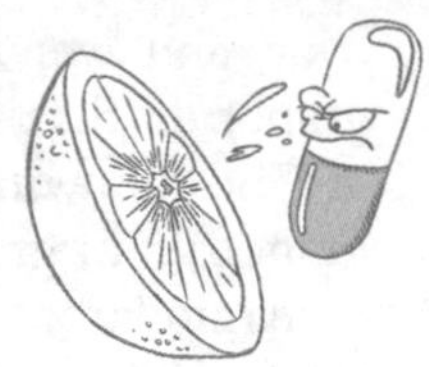

PHARMACOLOGY 101. In order to understand this interaction, a brief review of Pharmacology 101 is necessary. Drugs are metabolized via an enzyme system primarily located in the liver and the small intestines. The enzymes responsible for drug metabolism are referred to as the cytochrome P450 (CYP) "family" of drug-metabolizing enzymes. This "family" of enzymes is designated as CYP 1A2, CYP 2C9, CYP 2C19, CYP 2D6, CYP 3A4, and P-glycoprotein—a drug transporter. If you had to pick the ONE family member that does the lion's share of the work, CYP3A4 would be the chosen one. Approximately 50–60% of all drugs are handled by this enzyme. Grapefruit juice inhibits the CYP 3A4 of the intestinal enzyme system, which of course makes perfectly good sense, as grapefruit must traverse the intestines as it makes its way through the body. One important caveat to consider: there is a large ***individual*** variation in the effect of grapefruit juice on intestinal enzyme metabolism. In other words, individuals may have different responses to grapefruit juice based on their CYP 3A4 concentration. Unfortunately those individuals will remain anonymous until the establishment sees the necessity of testing everyone for pretreatment levels of intestinal CYP 3A4. And that's not going happen any time soon, so to be on the safe side and to avoid toxicity, it's easier to say ***NO*** to grapefruit juice when taking any and all drugs and that means ***NO*** to grapefruit as well.

What is it about grapefruit and/or grapefruit juice? Grapefruit juice contains several hundred compounds including the flavonoids, furocoumarins, and furanocoumarins. The furanocoumarins appear to be the component involved in grapefruit-drug interactions. Furanocoumarins inhibit intestinal CYP 3A4; however, the inhibition does not affect the 3A4 enzyme in the liver; therefore grapefruit juice does not inhibit the same drugs given intravenously.

Who's at risk for this potentially serious and in some instances fatal interaction? The elderly, of course. Why? Because they take the most drugs!

So, how long does this drug/grapefruit interaction last? *"Can I have grapefruit in the morning and take my drugs at lunchtime? NO.* The maximum effect on drug metabolism appears to be within 24 hours of grapefruit consumption, but reduced drug metabolism can occur to a lesser degree for 3 to 7 days. Therefore, separating the interacting drug from the intake of grapefruit juice by a couple of hours will NOT avoid or diminish the interaction. How much grapefruit or grapefruit juice does it take to cause the interaction? Just one 8 ounce glass or one grapefruit can affect drug levels; however, as a friendly reminder, this interaction depends on the patient, the drug, and even the variety of grapefruit. Once again, it's easier to say NO to grapefruit than it is to predict who, what, when, where, and how much.

The following is a list of potential and known drug interactions with grapefruit or grapefruit juice:

Amiodarone (Cordarone, Pacerone) is a cardiac drug prescribed for patients with atrial fibrillation. Amiodarone has a narrow therapeutic to toxic ratio. In other words, for this drug to have the desired effect, the drug level is one step away from being toxic to the patient. Yikes. Using amiodarone with grapefruit juice can raise blood concentrations to toxic levels even when using therapeutic, nontoxic doses of the drug. The half-life of amiodarone may double in elderly patients when grapefruit juice is ingested, providing a greater potential for the adverse effects of pulmonary (lung) toxicity, hypotension (dangerously low blood pressure), and cardiac arrhythmias. The obvious recommendation here is to avoid using Amiodarone in patients who are clueless to this potential fatal interaction or who may not comprehend the toxic potential of this interaction.

Concomitant use of grapefruit juice with the erectile dysfunction drug, sildenafil (Viagra—aka the "Pfizer riser") may demonstrate two adverse effects. First of all, grapefruit juice may delay the maximum concentration of sildenafil by 15 minutes. The implications of this delay are quite obvious—she's ready, willing and able, and you're *not.* Avoiding this combination may be in the best interest of your sex life, gentlemen. The second effect could increase the serum concentration of the drug resulting in the adverse effects of hypotension (dangerously low blood pressure) and reflex tachycardia (a response of the heart to the low blood pressure with a rapid heart beat). This interaction could presumably occur with the other erectile dysfunction drugs known as vardenafil (Levitra) and tadalafil (Cialis—the "weekend warrior") as well.

A 50% increase in the serum concentration of cilostazol (Pletal), occurs when taken with grapefruit juice. Pletal is a drug used in patients with peripheral arterial disease or diminished blood flow to the feet. This may result in adverse side effects secondary to extremely dilated blood vessels, including severe headaches and heart palpitations. It is recommended that the combination of grapefruit juice and cilostazol be avoided.

The famous cholesterol lowering drugs, the "statins," are one of the top prescribed classes of drugs in the world. Simvastatin (Zocor), lovastatin (Mevacor), and atorvastatin (Lipitor) are all metabolized by the intestinal enzyme CYP 3A4. Taking grapefruit juice with any of these three statins may increase the risk of statin-induced myopathies (muscle aches and pains) and rhabdomyolysis (muscle breakdown). Of the three, lovastatin and simvastatin have the strongest risk for interacting with grapefruit juice. Grapefruit juice can actually increase the bioavailability of simvastatin (Zocor) by 300%. Atorvastatin (Lipitor) has a moderate risk of toxicity with grapefruit juice. If the patient insists on guzzling grapefruit juice, substitute either pravastatin (Pravachol), fluvastatin (Lescol), or rosuvastatin (Crestor). These three statins are not affected by grapefruit juice and will not cause potential toxicity.

U.S. and Canadian prescribing information advises avoiding grapefruit in patients on certain blood pressure drugs known as calcium channel blockers. Specifically, nisoldipine (Sular), nifedipine capsules (Adalat, but not Procardia XL), felodipine (Plendil), verapamil (Calan, Verelan) interactions may result in toxicity with grapefruit juice. Substituting amlodipine (Norvasc) for any of the above would negate the concern about calcium channel blocker side effects including painfully swollen feet, tachycardia (a dangerously rapid heart beat), hypotension (low blood pressure), and debilitating headaches.

Certain benzodiazepines interact with grapefruit juice. The benzodiazepines that interact with grapefruit juice include diazepam (Valium), midazolam (Versed), quazepam (Doral), and triazolam (Halcion). Watch for increased sedation with these four drugs if grapefruit juice is consumed at the same time. Chooses alprazolam (Xanax) if a benzodiazepine is necessary and grapefruit juice continues to be ingested.

Prescribing information for the immunosuppressants cyclosporine (Neoral, Sandimmune) and tacrolimus (Prograf) advises avoiding grapefruit juice because of significantly increased bioavailability and serum concentrations. Signs of toxicity with cyclosporine include nephrotoxicity (kidney dysfunction), hepatotoxicity (liver dysfunction), and increased immunosuppression. Signs of toxicity for tacrolimus include hypertension (increased blood pressure), tremor, headache, and insomnia. This interaction is theoretically possible with sirolimus (Rapamune) as well. (Bressler R. Grapefruit juice and prescription drug interactions. Geriatrics 2006;61(Nov):12–8; Lilja JJ, Kivisto KT, Neuvonen PJ. Duration of effect of grapefruit juice on the pharmacokinetics of the CYP3A4 substrate simvastatin. *Clin Pharmacol Ther* 2000;68 :384 90; Takanga H, Ohnishi A, Murakami H, et al. Relationship between time after intake of grapefruit juice and the effect on pharmacokinetics and pharmacodynamics of nisoldipine in healthy subjects. *Clin Pharmacol Ther* 2000;67:201–14; Libersa CC, Brique SA, Motte KB, et al. Dramatic inhibition of amiodarone metabolism induced by grapefruit juice. *Br J Clin Pharmacol* 2000;49(4):373–88; Jetter A, Kinzig-Schippers M, Walchner-Bonjean M, et al. Effects of grapefruit juice on the pharmacokinetics of sildenafil. *Clin Pharmacol Ther* 2002;71(1):21–9; Potential drug interactions with grapefruit. Pharmacist's Letter/Prescriber's Letter 2007;23(2)230204. Pletal (cilostazol) package insert. Otsuka America Pharmaceutical, Inc. Rockville, MD. Available at: http://www.fda.gov/cder/news/cilostazol/cilo_label.htm. Accessed July 20, 2006; Lilja JJ, Neuvonen M, Neuvonen PJ. Effects of regular consumption of grapefruit juice on the pharmacokinetics of simvastatin. *Br J Clin Pharmacol* 2004;58(1):56–60 ; Kantola T, Kivisto KT, Neuvonen PJ. Grapefruit juice greatly increases serum concentrations of lovastatin and lovastatin acid. *Clin Pharmacol Ther* 1998;63(4):397–402; Yasui N, Kondo T, Furukori H, et al. Effects of repeated ingestion of grapefruit juice on the single and multiple oral-dose pharmacokinetics and pharmacodynamics of alprazolam. *Psychopharmacology* (Berl) 2000; 150:185–90)

Grapefruit juice and kidney stones. Women can significantly reduce their risk for kidney stones by drinking wine and tea. Yes! Using data from the Nurses' Health Study, researchers from Brigham and Women's Hospital and Harvard School of Public Health and Medical School showed consumption of tea, coffee (with and without caffeine), and wine can reduce the risk of kidney stones.

After controlling for a zillion variables, the researchers found one cup of coffee or tea daily and/or one glass of wine decreased the risk of kidney stones by 8% (tea and coffee) and by 59% (wine). Clearly the drink of the hour here is wine, wine, fruit of the vine.

On the other hand, consuming grapefruit juice had just the opposite effect. One eight ounce glass of grapefruit juice daily increased the risk of kidney stones by 44%. Clearly the drink not to choose is grapefruit juice. (Curhan GC, et al. Ann of Intern Med April 1, 1998;128(7):537–540)

Green-Bean Casserole—America's favorite casserole. America's favorite casserole dates back to 1955, when a chef named Dorcas Reilly created it for a Campbell's soup cookbook to promote Campbell's products. By 2003, more than 20 million families reportedly served the dish at Thanksgiving.

Greenhouse gases from food—the environmental impact of foods. First, let me say, it's not the food per se, that contributes to the greenhouse effect—it's the way we raise our animals for consumption in the U.S. that contributes to degrading our environment and consuming our natural resources. What do I mean by the way we raise our animals? We have industrialized agriculture by consolidating and concentrating all of the animals into specific areas.

The U.S. now produces 9 *billion* animals for food each year. Specifically 100 million hogs, 35 million head of cattle, and a tad more than 8 billion broiler chickens per year. That's one million chickens per hour, 24 hours a day, 365 days per year.

So, what's the cost to the environment by raising animals "in bulk," so to speak? It takes approximately seven pounds of grain to produce one pound of beef, and 6.5 pounds of grain to produce one pound of pork. Chicken, the most efficient environmentally friendly animal, takes 2.6 pounds of grain to produce one pound of meat.

OK, so we use lots of grain to feed the nine billion animals. Here's the catch—it requires water to produce the grain that feeds the animals that feed the humans. Our water resources are not infinite. To grow the seven pounds of grain to produce one pound of meat requires 840 gallon of water. Yes, I said 840 gallons of water. This is clearly not sustainable, as our water tables for irrigation are declining throughout the country.

Here's an interesting breakdown of the percentage of greenhouse gases from food in the U.S. from the various food products:

Beef and pork	29%
Dairy products	17%
Cereals/carbs	10%
Fruit/veggies	10%
Chicken/fish/eggs	10%
Beverages	9%
Oils/sweets/condiments	6%
Other	10%

And, I'm not finished yet with the environmental impact of meat production. What goes in one end has to come out of the other end, and we're talking "animal waste solids" or "pig poop" and "cow-a-dunga," so to speak. Our industrial agricultural system produces about one ton of animal waste solids (that's the poop after the water has been extracted) for *every* person in the U.S. per year. That's 40 times more than the amount of human waste produced per year. The result? Whereas we used to use animal waste solids as fertilizer, the majority of it is now polluting our surface water, soil, and air. (Just drive through a major hog-producing state for a whiff if you don't believe me.) (Robert Lawrence. Director, Center for a Livable Future, Johns Hopkins Bloomberg School of Public Health, Baltimore MD, October, 2011)

GREEN TEA

Green Tea. (See Chapter T for an extensive discussion of teas.)

Green tea (brand name, Veregan) for genital warts? Really? Convince me…The FDA has approved the marketing of sinecatechins for the treatment of external and perianal warts. Sinecatechins are derived from the water extract of green tea leaves. It is a mixture of catechins and other green tea components as well as caffeine, theobromine, and theophylline. Each gram of Veregan contains 150 mg of sinecatechins.

Just exactly how does it work against genital warts? Actually nobody knows. The results of some studies suggest that the major sinecatechin, epigallocatechin (ECGC) induces apoptosis (preprogrammed cell suicide) and inhibits telomerase activity. Telomerase is an enzyme that helps to repair DNA. No enzyme? No repair mechanism and therefore no continued growth of the warts.

Compared to placebo, Veregan demonstrated complete clearance of warts. The median time to clearance was 10 weeks in one study and 16 weeks in another. Recurrence rates 12 weeks after complete clearing were 6.8% with Veregan. (*The Medical Letter* 2008 Feb 25; 50 (1280):15 – 16)

St. Lawrence, the patron saint of those who grill. The annual feast day of St. Lawrence is August 10. St. Lawrence was roasted alive on a spit, but faced death heroically, telling his torturers, "Turn me over— I'm cooked on that side."

Grilling temperatures to kill the bugs. According to the FDA, the minimum safe temperature for various types of foods, however they are cooked, is as follows (in degrees Fahrenheit):

Ground beef, ground veal, ground lamb, and ground pork...... 160°
Beef, veal, lamb (steaks, chops, and roasts)............................... 145°
Pork (roast and chops).. 145°
Ham, uncooked.. 160°
Ham, precooked.. 140°
Ground chicken and turkey.. 165°
Whole chicken and turkey.. 165°–180°
Chicken breasts... 165°
Chicken thighs and wings... 180°
Poultry stuffing (cooked alone or in the bird)........................... 165°
Egg dishes and casseroles.. 160°
Leftovers.. 165°

Reheated soups and gravies should be brought to a rolling boil; all other leftovers should be hot and steaming.

The only way you can safely know if the meat is cooked to the desired temperature is to use a thermometer. Just eyeballing the meat doesn't do the trick. Pressing your finger into the meat doesn't do the trick. A digital thermometer is best for measuring the temperature after the meat comes out of the oven or off the grill. The digital thermometer only needs to be inserted a half an inch and it records the temperature in just 10 seconds. For measuring the foods while they are still in the oven, use either a liquid-filled or bimetal oven-safe thermometer.

ASPARAGUS TIP

If you are nervous about under-cooking fish, here's a helpful hint from the May 2000 *Nutrition Action Newsletter.* Measure the thickness of any fish fillet at its thickest point. Cook it 10 minutes per inch. It doesn't matter if you are baking, broiling, grilling, steaming or poaching the fish—the 10 minute per inch rule reigns.

Grocery bags. The flat-bottomed paper bag was invented by Margaret Knight (1838–1914), one of the first American women to be awarded a patent. She was working in a paper bag factory after the Civil War when she saw the need for a different kind of bag. The factory only made flat bags shaped like envelopes that were unsuitable for bulky items. She actually invented the machine that made the flat-bottomed paper bag. She was brilliant. And she didn't stop with that one patent. She continued inventing and received 27 total patents. The barbeque spit is another patent held by Margaret Knight.

Guaiac test for occult blood in the stool (Fecal Occult Blood Test, FOBT). Certain foods can interact with the guaiac test for hidden (occult) blood in feces. The active ingredient in the guaiac slide test is alpha-guaiaconic acid, a chemical that turns blue in the presence of blood. Foods containing peroxidase, a natural chemical that also turns alpha-guaiaconic acid blue, may produce a false positive test. In other words, the individual will have a positive test without hidden blood in the stool. Foods causing false positive tests include: Artichokes, broccoli, carrots, cauliflower, cucumbers, lamb, mushrooms, oranges or other citrus fruits, radishes, turnips and vitamin supplements that contain more than 250 mg of vitamin C. These foods should be eliminated from the diet for three days prior to testing for blood in the stool using this method.

GUM

Gum. Chewing gum is as old as the ancient Greeks and Mayan Indians. Both cultures reported that they chewed on various substances, such as paraffin, for breath freshening purposes, tooth cleansing purposes, and just for the heck of it. Modern commercial chewing gum got its start in the 1860s with the discovery of *chicle,* a rubbery substance derived from the sapodilla tree, which grows in tropical climates. Chicle was popular because it was smooth, springy and held its flavor well. Most gums are now made from synthetics, rather than the real chicle…but you can certainly guess where the name Chiclets comes from. (*US Berkeley Wellness Letter,* June 2004)

Gum chewing and peristalsis after surgery. How about using good old-fashioned chewing gum to kick-start the bowel after gastrointestinal surgery? A prospective, randomized study of 34 patients who underwent elective colectomy (removal of either all or part of the colon or large intestine) found that the group who chewed gum after the surgery had the best post-operative outcomes.

The gum-chompin' post-op group chewed gum three times a day for 1 hour until discharged. One of the first signs of a bowel starting to function is the production and passage of flatus (gas). The first passage of flatus occurred at 65.4 hours post-op in the gum-chewing group. The non-gum-chewing group didn't "break wind" until 80.2 hours after the surgical procedure. Listen up, insurance companies—if you want to save a few thousand bucks on hospital costs you might want to spring for a pack of Orbit. Jean cartoon with girl holding a package of gum and a star on teeth) (Noblett HD. Bowel management after surgery. *ADVANCE for Nurse Practitioners.* February 2010;45–51)

Gum chewing and the afternoon cravings for sweets. Chewing sugarless gum throughout the afternoon can curb consumption and craving of sweets and make people feel more energetic and alert throughout the evening. Participants in the study were asked to periodically chew sugarfree gum during a three-hour stretch after lunch one day. Researchers found that, on average, chewers ate some 60 fewer calories of sweets in the mid-afternoon, when compared with a gum-free day. Chewers also reported feeling steadier energy levels during the afternoon, vs. flagging levels on the day without gum. (Experimental Biology Meeting in New Orleans April 19, 2009)

Gum chewing and GERD (Gastroesophageal reflux disease). Chew gum to stimulate saliva—it helps to neutralize the gastric acid that is refluxing from the stomach into the lower esophagus. Drink fluids between meals, not with meals. Combining fluids with foods increases the likelihood of reflux.

Gum chewing and weight loss. People who continuously chew sugarless gum burn 11 calories more per hour than people who sit still and do nothing. This translates into a weight loss of about 10 pounds over a year, if calorie intake stays the same. (Levine J, Baukol P, Pavlidis I. The energy expended in chewing gum [letter]. *The New England Journal of Medicine.* Dec 30, 1999;341(27): 2100)

Gustatory rhinitis—the "Salsa Sniffles." Gustatory rhinitis, also known as the "Salsa Sniffles," occurs when one snarfs down meals containing chili peppers, horseradish sauce, onions and other spicy hot foods. These sniffles and drips are due to over-stimulated parasympathetic (cholinergic) nerves that supply the glands in the nasal passages. Fluid production is turned on and the drip begins.

Anybody who believes the way to a man's heart is through his stomach flunked geography.

—Robert Byrne

Haggis. Haggis is a traditional Scottish dish is made from the stomach, heart, liver and tongue of a sheep, chopped with onions, seasoning, suet, and oatmeal, and then boiled in a bag made of the sheep's stomach. Haggis anyone?

Halimeter. This device measures the level of bacteria in the mouth. Used exclusively in "fresh breath" clinics, the halimeter is the first step in determining the cause and severity of halitosis. Once the level of bacteria has been measured, tongue scrapers, tooth irrigators, and other bacteria-removing devices are employed to rid the oral cavity of bugs that contribute to bad breath, also known as halitosis. Read on for a primer on halitosis.

Halitosis—facts, fiction, and fixes. First, the facts. Your mouth contains 1,600 billion bacteria(over 600 species of bacteria)—all of which have adapted to living in this moist, tropical environment. Bad breath usually develops during sleep when the salivary glands slow production to just under 10 milliliters an hour. During waking hours the salivary glands produce approximately 1,000 milliliters of saliva or 60–70 ml per hour.

The bacteria thrive on remnants of meals, dead squamous cells from the inside of the cheeks, and mucus from post nasal drip. They survive by snipping off pieces of sugar from glycoproteins. Once the sugar is consumed, the protein is exposed in its entirety as a polypeptide fragment. Other types of bacteria break down the polypeptides into individual amino acids and eventually foul-smelling sulphur compounds with names like hydrogen sulfide and methyl mercaptan are formed. Foul-smelling nitrogen-containing compounds are also formed with nasty names like skatole and indole—both of which smell like the distal portion of the gastrointestinal tract. Two other nitrogenous gases have names that provide clues to their foul-smelling properties in the breath—putrescine (decay, putrid) and cadaverine (corpses).

Most bacteria prefer the back of the tongue as their dining area. As mucus from the nose drips onto the back of the tongue, bacteria thrive on this sticky substance for hours to days. Bacteria also thrive in the crevices between the teeth and the gums, where food particles become lodged during a meal. One way to get rid of bacteria in the mouth is to provide a sticky, oily substance that they can adhere to. Once the bugs stick, the product can be expelled—as in a mouthwash. One mouthwash does this beautifully—Dentyl pH, marketed by Blistex in the United States.

Let's dispel a few myths:

1) Bad breath comes from the stomach. No, bad breath comes from the mouth most of the time.
2) Mouth sprays reduce bacteria for hours. Wrong. Mouth sprays only mask halitosis for a few minutes.
3) If a mouthwash stings or foams it's a good one. Not necessarily.

Tips for a fragrant breath.

1) Gargle mouthwash with your tongue sticking out, allowing the mouthwash to reach the back of the tongue.
2) Don't use mouthwash right after brushing. Toothpaste contains a foaming soap, which takes some of mouthwash's effective ingredients out of commission by binding to them.
3) The best time to use mouthwash is before bedtime, so that it is active all night.
4) Clean your tongue. Scrape your tongue before bedtime.
5) Visit your friendly dentist twice a year.
6) Avoid coffee and alcohol.
7) Eat a good breakfast with rough foods.
8) Floss every day. The time of day is irrelevant. Just do it.
9) To increase salivary flow and decrease halitosis, eat an orange or grapefruit between meals. It gives your mouth's natural cleansing system a boost. (Fisher R. A breath of fresh air. *New Scientist.* September 22, 2007;50–52)

Halitosis treatments in various cultures.

Do all cultures throughout the world have halitosis? Yes, it's a universal phenomenon. And, all cultures have their own ways of combating the problem. Brazilians chew cinnamon bark, Iraqi's chew cloves, and giant guavas are used in Singapore to combat bad breath.

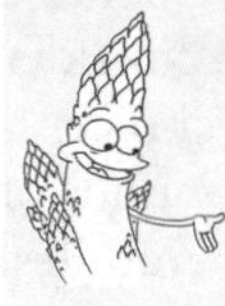

ASPARAGUS TIP

If halitosis persists after scraping the back of the tongue with a teaspoon, try a nonprescription tablet of bismuth subgallate from the American Foundation for Preventive Medicine, P.O. Box 1144, Indianapolis, IN 46202.

Halitosis and gender. Hormonal fluctuations also play a role in the development of halitosis. Women have more of a problem during ovulation. The increase in estrogen causes the blood vessels in the gum surrounding each tooth to contract, forming a crevice that allows fluid to pool, attracting bacteria. You would think this phenomenon would be counterproductive to the spirit of procreation.

Ham. The term "ham" is used loosely; however, it technically refers to the hind leg of a pig, from the shank to the hip. You can define hams further by the type of pig, to the curing method, to the smoking time, and to the region in which the ham is made. For example, *country ham* is the result of a long curing process in which the ham is smoked over fragrant hardwoods and aged for up to one year. No water is added during the process, resulting in a highly flavored, very salty ham. You can dine on a delicious slice of this ham at any roadside diner in the southern part of the U.S. If you drive through Smithfield County, Virginia, you may recognize the home of the premier cured and processed *Smithfield* country ham. *Prosciutto* is an Italian ham that is salted and air-dried but not smoked. It is usually served in paper-thin slices and wrapped around a delicious piece of cantaloupe. *Canned ham* is made from either a whole piece of meat, or it is "formed" from smaller pieces of meat. It is brine-cured, pressed, and molded, often with the addition of gelatin to help retain the natural juices. *Cottage ham* or *smoked Boston shoulder* comes from the neck and shoulder of the pig, not the leg. It has also been called the *daisy ham. Fresh ham* is another term that refers to a cut from the shoulder of the pig. It is uncooked and has a delicate pork flavor that lacks the smokiness or saltiness of cured hams. *SPAM* is the number one canned luncheon meat sold around the world—the word SPAM is the combination of two words—Spiced Ham, or SPAM. More cans of SPAM have been sold that there are people on this earth. See Chapter S for more on this popular luncheon meat.

HAMBURGER

Hamburger heaven. Hamburgers and cheeseburgers account for 76% of all the beef sold in restaurants. Steak accounts for just 5%. The average American eats 67 pounds of beef per year. Of the 67 pounds of beef, approximately 28 pounds are ground beef, or hamburger. That is the equivalent to a Quarter Pounder from McDonald's every three days. Although we consider hamburgers our meat of choice here in the U.S., it's not the best choice. It contributes more than 60% of the saturated fat we get from our 67 pounds of beef. It also most contributes to the many extra pounds around our middles, as well as to quite a few clogged arteries supplying hearts, brains, kidneys, and feet. (USDA, 2009. http://www.newdream.org/food/beef_health1.php)

If you had to pick a single food that inflicts the most damage on the American diet, ground beef would be a prime contender. Whether it's tacos, meatloaf, lasagna, or the ubiquitous hamburger, Americans stuff themselves with ground beef without a second thought about its consequences."

—Nutrition Action Newsletter, September 1999.

Hamburgers on the grill. Flip those burgers every 60 seconds for safety's sake. While all cooking methods reduce the levels of *E. Coli O157:H7* in raw ground beef, turning the patties every minute does it faster. As a bonus, your burgers will cook faster. The frequent-flipping method cooked the burgers in 8 eight minutes compared to a 16-minute cooking time when the burgers were turned over just once after five minutes of cooking.

HISTORICAL HIGHLIGHT

The hamburger. Although the esteemed *Oxford English Dictionary* traces the first reference to the hamburger to 1889, the residents of Seymour, Wisconsin beg to differ. As the story goes, 15-year-old Charlie Nagreen arrived at the Seymour-Outagamie County fair in 1885 in an ox-drawn wagon with plans to open a food stand that sold fried meatballs. Well, fried meatballs weren't "in" that year, and no one seemed to be interested. Actually the problem was in the presentation—it's hard to stroll around the fairgrounds eating meatballs. So Charlie decided to flatten the meatballs. He plopped the flattened meat in between two pieces of bread and voila! Hamburger. Charlie became a legend in his own right. He returned to the Seymour-Outagamie County Fair every year after that for 65 years, and made the rounds at all of the other county fairs in Wisconsin. Seymour's claim to fame is the 5,520-pound grilled hamburger patty made in 1989 to celebrate the centennial (based on the *Oxford English Dictionary's* definition, which is of course still in dispute). If you're driving through Seymour, Wisconsin, visit the four-story, hamburger-shaped shrine, the Hamburger Hall of Fame, Seymour, Wisconsin.

Hamburgers, holes and White Castles—the scoop on "Sliders." At last, the answer to why White Castle hamburgers have five holes per patty. The holes were introduced in 1946 (twenty-five years after the first White Castle restaurant was up and running in 1921 in Wichita, Kansas), for a very important reason. The holes allow the steam and grease from the grill to escape up to the upper bun, which cooks atop each patty. This release of steam and grease eliminates the need to flip over the meat in order to cook it evenly. How simple is that?

Hamburgers, test tube burgers. The first test-tube stem cell sliver of hamburger has been produced by a Dutch physiologist, Mark Post of Maastricht University. Granted it cost about $330,000 to produce an entire hamburger, but hey, what's $330,000 when you're talking about a major medical miracle of stem cell burgers? Dr. Post says that at some point in the future using stem cells from an adult cow will offer a better way than traditional farming to satisfy the world's taste for meat. Researchers estimate that within the next 50 years meat production will have to double worldwide to meet the demands of the growing population. (*The Week*, March 9, 2012)

Hand washing. "With the possible exception of immunization," says Ralph Cordell, an epidemiologist at the Centers for Disease Control and Prevention in Atlanta, "hand-washing is the most effective disease-preventing measure anyone can practice."

Studies have shown that a single hand can carry around 200 million organisms, including bacteria, viruses, and a few fungi thrown in for good measure. It takes a full five minutes of hand washing to cleanse 99% of the most dangerous bacteria from the fingernails, thumbs, palm creases, and backs of the hands. Surgeons have the time to do this; the rest of us do not. So, if you want to wash off 95% of the bugs lurking in the nooks and crannies of your hands, wash to the tune of "Happy Birthday " sung twice—or about 20 seconds. (CDC, http://www.cdc.gov/cleanhands/)

E.coli and other intestinal bugs are the first to go with soap and water—they're zapped after about five seconds of handwashing. Plain soap and water also "uncoat" the flu virus in about 9.5 seconds, rendering it incapable of infecting cells of the respiratory tract.

The real cleansing is done by the friction and force of rubbing your hands together along with the soap. The temperature of the water doesn't really matter: It takes 160 degrees to kill bacteria, which would be fine if you want third-degree burns on your hands. Another 10 seconds of vigorous rubbing with a towel also helps as the friction rips the microbes off your skin. (Doug Power, Professor of Food Safety, Kansas State University, Manhattan, KS. 2012)

Another interesting tidbit—the hand you use the most, the dominant hand, is often under-washed. If you're right-handed, your left hand is usually cleaner. So make sure you shake the *left* hand of any man exiting the washroom, if you are so inclined to be shaking hands with a man who has just exited the washroom. Studies have also shown that men only wash their hands 74% of the time after using the washroom. You might want to think twice about using that particular moment as a meet and greet.

Don't use the antibacterial soaps that are advertised on TV. Many of the big household product companies tout the benefits of triclosan, an antibacterial chemical that kills bacteria on contact. The studies demonstrating the effectiveness of antibacterial soaps typically tested them by having people scrub for 60 to 90 seconds or longer, or four times longer than the usual scrub-a-dub-dub. Only one study has actually compared washing with soap and water to washing with triclosan. Volunteers washed for 30 seconds at a time, six times a day for five days in both groups. Bacterial counts on the hands of both groups were the same.

The FDA is considering a ban on triclosan. Studies in rats have shown hormonal disruption, including thyroid suppression and estrogen increases. Triclosan may also increase the resistance to bacteria. (Williams, G. The Biology of Hand-Washing, *Discover Magazine.* December 1999; 36-38; *Nutrition Action Newsletter,* November 2011; (*Toxicology Science,* 2010;117:45)

HEMOCHROMATOSIS

Hemochromatosis. Hemochromatosis is the most common inherited disorder in the United States, with one out of every 200 to 300 people affected, men more severely than women. Hemochromatosis results from the genetic predisposition to absorb too much iron from food. The average American without the hemochromatosis gene absorbs approximately 10% of the iron they ingest, whereas individuals with hereditary hemochromatosis may absorb as much as much as 30% of the iron ingested. The body can't use or eliminate this additional iron so it's stored in the liver, heart, and pancreas. Over time patients with hemochromatosis may accumulate five to 20 times as much iron as normal. Stored iron acts as an "oxidant" and damages these organs leading to life-threatening conditions such as cancer, diabetes, heart failure, and cirrhosis of the liver. Signs and symptoms usually manifest between the ages of 30 and 50 in men and after 50 in women. Prior to menopause women lose iron every month with menstruation. Women usually don't develop symptoms until after menopause, when they no longer lose iron with menstruation or use increased amounts of iron during pregnancy.

The medical treatment for hemochromatosis is phlebotomy—the removal of blood on a regular basis. The frequency depends on the age of the patient, overall health, and severity of the disease. The goal is to reduce iron levels to normal.

Hemochromatosis and dietary concerns. What are the dietary changes that can be helpful?

What to avoid:

- Avoid iron supplements and multivitamins containing iron.
- Avoid vitamin C supplements, especially with food. Vitamin C increases the absorption of iron.
- Avoid cooking with iron skillets.
- Avoid prune juice. A cup of prune juice has 3 mg of iron (37 percent of the recommended daily allowance for men and 17 percent for premenopausal women)...do I really need to tell anyone to avoid prune juice? At least anyone under the age of 70?
- Avoid ironing. (hahaha...just seeing if you're paying attention)
- Avoid eating raw shellfish. Hereditary hemochromatosis increases the risk of infections, especially those caused by certain bacteria in raw shellfish.
- What to do: There are three dietary changes that can be made.
- One dietary practice that has been shown to help is drinking tannin-rich black tea which hinders the absorption of iron. In a European study, when people with hereditary hemochromatosis drank tea with meals for one year, body iron stores were reduced by about one-third compared to the control group that drank plain ol' water.
- Green tea extract is a potent iron-chelating agent as well. It helps to remove excess iron from the liver.
- Take 300 mg of elemental calcium with a meal that contains iron. This has been shown to reduce the amount of iron absorbed by 40 percent.
- None of these dietary remedies completely takes care of the problem and phlebotomy is still necessary. (Kaltwasser JP, et al. *Gut,* 1998; www.cdc.gov; accessed 2011; digestive-system.emedtv.com)

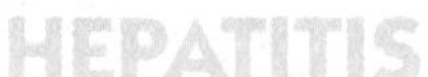

Hepatitis A virus. Hepatitis caused by the hepatitis A virus (HAV) is contracted through contaminated food or water. Young adults and children in institutional settings and travelers in countries with minimal sanitation are at greatest risk for infection; small epidemics have been seen among persons eating at restaurants where the food handlers haven't paid close attention to hand hygiene after using the restroom.

The course of the illness is usually mild, with the acute stage resolving in about two weeks and complete recovery within eight weeks. When traveling to countries with poor sanitation, consider the hepatitis A vaccine to develop immunity or the immunoglobulin to HAV for acute protection. Also, use good clinical judgment about the foods you choose and the water you drink, depending on the country.

In November 2003, a month after filing for Chapter 11 bankruptcy, Chi-Chi's was hit with the largest hepatitis A outbreak in U.S. history, with at least 4 deaths and 660 other victims of illness in the Pittsburgh area, including high school students who caught the disease from the original victims. The hepatitis was traced back to raw green onions from Mexico that were served at the Chi-Chi's at Beaver Valley Mall in Monaca, Pennsylvania, about 30 miles northwest of Pittsburgh. While the sickness was not linked to the cleanliness or staff of the restaurants themselves, Chi-Chi's took a hit from the outbreak: by mid-2004, Chi-Chi's only had 65 restaurants, less than half of the number from only four years before. Although Chi-Chi's settled the hepatitis A lawsuits by July 2004, the outbreak sealed the fate of the already-bankrupt company.

Hepatitis C. Hepatitis C is not considered a foodborne illness; however, people with this form of chronic hepatitis should take a few dietary precautions. If a person has developed cirrhosis of the liver as a chronic complication of hepatitis C, it is recommended that they avoid raw seafood, iron, and limit or avoid vitamin A supplements. In addition, certain herbal products have been found to be toxic to the liver and should be avoided at all costs in patients with chronic liver disease. These herbal supplements include chaparral, comfrey, germander, jinbuhuan, mistletoe, nutmeg, ragwort, sassafras, senna, kava, and tansy.

If a multivitamin is part of the daily routine, make sure it's iron-free. The best bet for patients with Hepatitis C is to consume a diet high in fresh vegetables and fruits, making sure that appropriate safety precautions are taken while washing the vegetables and fruits. It is controversial as to whether or not animal protein should be eliminated from the diet. Most patients can eliminate animal proteins from their diet; however, patients with HCV who are co-infected with HIV cannot. Animal proteins are necessary to keep the immune system healthy in order to fight the HIV infection. (*National AIDS Treatment Advocacy Project Handbook 2010,* NATAP, 580 Broadway, Suite 1010, New York, NY, 10012, www.natap.org)

Hiccups. Excessively large meals or drinking carbonated beverages cause the stomach to distend, pushing against the diaphragm and irritating the phrenic nerves. The irritation of the diaphragm causes a spasm and hiccups result. Acid reflux into the esophagus can also be a cause of the hiccups.

How about treating hiccups? There's lots of folklore out there about how to treat hiccups—some work, some don't, but everyone attempts one or two of these remedies at some time during an episode of hiccups. Drinking water through a straw while holding your ears closed with your fingers is one of them. This appears to interrupt the "arc" of nervous signals that travel from the diaphragm to the brain. Gargling, which activates the throat muscles,

ASPARAGUS TIP

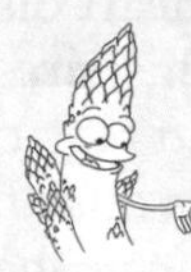

Anyone who has severe or frequent hiccups lasting longer than 48 hours should visit their friendly health care professional for a more extensive workup as to the cause.

may have a similar effect. Scaring the "bejesus" out of someone may also kick the diaphragm back on the right track. Sometimes these methods work, sometimes they don't.

Fun fact about hiccups

Hiccups are very common in the fetus and are easily recognized on ultrasounds during pregnancy. Hiccups appear before breathing movements as the fetus develops and are also common in newborns but gradually disappear over the next few months.

High-Density Lipoprotein (HDL). If you remember from the cholesterol segment in Chapter C, HDL, the "good" cholesterol, has three properties that help protect the cardiovascular system. It removes excess LDL-cholesterol from the blood, is it an anti-oxidant and it has anti-inflammatory properties. Studies focusing specifically on HDL have found that low HDL levels are an independent risk factor for coronary artery disease, especially in high fat consuming cultures such as ours in the U.S. Now, as more and more compelling data are reported, it is necessary to focus on ways to increase HDL levels. Here are some pearls you should know about HDL:

.....The risk of coronary artery disease in women is more closely related to the low HDL than to elevated LDL levels.

.....The risk of coronary artery disease increases by 2–3% for every 1 mg/dl decrease in HDL.

.....For every 21-mg/dl increase in HDL, people are 50% less likely to develop albuminuria (protein in the urine). (Diabetes Care January 2006)

.....The many causes of low HDL include genetic disorders, obesity, cigarettes, drugs, and dietary influences. The major dietary influence that decreases HDL is trans fats. Trans-fatty acids are commonly used in baked goods like cakes, pies, cookies and French fries.

.....Moderate exercise (walking a minimum of seven miles per week) does not raise HDL levels significantly. However, intense exercise (running a minimum of seven miles per week) does increase HDL.

.....The positive effects of moderate alcohol intake on heart disease are numerous. Moderate alcohol intake boosts HDL. One study found that men who abstained from alcohol had an average HDL of 38 mg/dl while those who drank more than 14 drinks per week (two per day) had an average HDL of 46.2 mg/dl. Kick it back, Jack.

.....Replacing saturated fat calories with carbohydrates has a negative effect on HDL levels. However, replacing saturated fats with monounsaturated fats

(olive oil) maintains HDL levels and also lowers the incidence of heart disease. Patients with isolated low HDL levels should be cautioned against drastically cutting total dietary fat and should instead be encouraged to replace saturated fat with monounsaturated fats such as olive oil and canola oil.
.....Life-style changes (more exercise, smoking cessation, moderate alcohol consumption) increase HDL by about 10–15%.

Holiday heart. Heart attacks (aka, myocardial infarctions or acute coronary syndromes) occur in a seasonal pattern. A research team from UCLA examined the month-by-month death rate from myocardial infarctions over a 12-year period. They found that the death rate stayed relatively stable through November and then increased dramatically after Thanksgiving, peaking around New Year's Day. The incidence of heart attacks increased by 33% in December and January.

The assumption could be made that the winter trigger for heart attacks would be cold weather and subsequent coronary vasoconstriction resulting in an increased work load on the heart. However, upon closer scrutiny of the data, the authors of the study realized that even in warm areas such as southern California, where the temperatures rarely dip below 50° F (10° C) even on the coldest day of the year, there was still an increase in the number of heart attacks.

The second theory blames the good ol' American way of overindulging during the holiday season—lots of booze, fatty foods, and salt to make the season bright. A heavy meal quadruples the risk for a heart attack. It temporarily raises blood pressure, which can rupture cholesterol-laden plaque already present. A heavy meal also increases insulin, which can make coronary arteries less relaxed. The increased stress of the holiday season increases cortisol levels, which in turn increase blood glucose and increase the stickiness of platelets, making platelets more likely to trigger clot formation. (*Circulation* 2000; 1(02) Supplement: 612.)

Note: Just in case you were wondering, the lowest-risk month for heart attacks is June, with September second and July and August coming in third and fourth.

HOMOCYSTEINE

Homocysteine: Yet another important risk factor for heart disease. Homocysteine is a naturally occurring amino acid found in serum. It cannot be obtained from the diet. Instead it is biosynthesized from methionine via a multistep process. This normal metabolic process depends on adequate amounts of 22 vitamins belonging to the B family; however, the most important members of the family in terms of homocysteine levels are B6, B12, and folic acid. Deficiencies of any of the three nutrients may lead to excess homocysteine, as defined by a level of greater than 12mmol/L, which in turn may promote the development of atherosclerosis. It is estimated that 5–10% of the American population has elevated homocysteine levels.

How does excess homocysteine promote heart disease? Excess homocysteine inhibits an important enzyme in the smooth muscle cells of the walls of the arteries. The enzyme, glutathione peroxide, is necessary to prevent vascular smooth muscle proliferation, which has been shown to contribute to the development of fatty plaques in the arteries. In addition, elevated levels of homocysteine may also impair the release of the potent vasodilator nitric oxide. Reduced nitric oxide contributes to the process of fatty plaque formation by elevating intra-arterial pressure. The third consequence of elevated homocysteine levels is the activation of protein C, which subsequently triggers the clotting cascade. (Lonn E, et. Al. Homocysteine lowering with folic acid and B vitamins in vascular disease. *N Engl J Med* 2006; 354 (15):1567–77)

Should all patients be tested for homocysteine levels? No, this is not currently recommended; however, it may be appropriate to obtain the homocysteine level in patients with premature heart disease who do not have traditional risk factors such as smoking, hypertension, elevated LDL-cholesterol, low HDL-cholesterol, obesity, and a sedentary life-style.

The American Heart Association has not yet designated elevated homocysteine as a major risk factor for cardiovascular disease. Therefore, they don't recommend that everyone take folic acid and vitamin B6 and B12 supplements to reduce the risk of heart disease and stroke. However, the American Heart Association does recommend eating a balanced diet rich in foods containing folic acid. Citrus fruits, tomatoes, vegetables and grain products are excellent sources of folic acid. Since January 1998, wheat flour has been fortified with folic acid to add an estimated 100 mcg per day to the average diet. The recommended daily value is 400 µg per day for folic acid. For more information log on to the website for the American Heart Association—www.amhrt.org.

Homocysteine and Alzheimer's disease. Recent studies have implicated high levels of homocysteine in association with Alzheimer's disease. Researchers in England followed 164 patients diagnosed with Alzheimer's disease. Compared with age- and sex-matched controls, those with Alzheimer's had significantly lower levels of nutrients that reduce homocysteine—folic acid (folate) and B12. This study doesn't actually prove that elevated homocysteine contributes to an increased Alzheimer's risk, or that B12 can help prevent the disease. However, it does contribute to a growing body of evidence that Alzheimer's disease is a type of vascular disease and shares risk factors with other vascular conditions. (Folate and homocysteine in the cerebrospinal fluid of patients with Alzheimer's disease or dementia: a case controlled study. *European Neurology.* 2011)

The pessimist is someone who can look at the land of milk and honey and see only calories and cholesterol. —Quote magazine

---

Honey. Have you ever thought about how a honeybee makes honey? Or did you just think that a jar of honey magically landed on the shelf at the grocery store. It takes a colony of around 80,000 bees living together in one large beehive. The bees collect nectar from plants in their mouths, which mix with enzymes in the bee saliva to turn it into honey. They fly back to the beehive where they deposit the honey into the walls for storage. The fluttering of their wings reduces the moisture content of the honey. The 80,000 bees have to collectively visit approximately 2 million flowers in order to make just one measly pound of pure honey. Pretty amazing, eh?

Honey and wound care. The use of honey dates back 3,500 years ago in an Egyptian medical text. It was described in the Koran as "a drink of many colors wherein there is healing for all people." Honey was first used for wound healing centuries ago by the Greeks and Egyptians. It continued to be a popular remedy until it fell out of favor when antibiotics became widely used in the 1960s. The pendulum is swinging back to the use of honey for topical wound care as more and more pathogens are becoming resistant to current antibiotics.

Honey has been shown to be effective on a variety of wound types, including venous stasis ulcers, pressure ulcers, burns, surgical wounds, necrotizing fasciitis (the "flesh-eating disease), diabetic foot ulcers, split-skin grafts, and extravasation wounds from various chemotherapeutic agents. Arterial leg ulcers have not been shown to improve with honey. (Acton C. Medihoney: a complete wound bed preparation product. *Br J Nurs* 2008;17:244–48)

Honey from New Zealand, extracted from the pollen of the manuka shrub *(Leptospermum),* has been shown to have potent antibacterial properties in addition to the usual hydrogen peroxide activity of all honeys. The phytochemicals responsible for this nonperoxide activity have not been definitively identified but have been termed Unique Manuka Factor (UMF). In particular, Manuka honey has antibacterial effects against some pretty nasty bacteria, including Methicillin-resistant *Staphylococcus* aureus (MRSA), *E.coli,* and *Helicobacter pylori.*

All forms of honey, including *Medihoney* and honey purchased at the supermarket, have antibacterial properties. A University of Wisconsin Professor Jennifer Eddy, MD, is testing the standard supermarket honey for the treatment of diabetic foot ulcers. The use of supermarket honey offers promising results as a low-cost remedy for not only preventing foot ulcers, but also speeding healing and reducing the need for repeated courses of antibiotics.

Researchers in the Netherlands also investigated the antimicrobial properties of a "medical-grade" honey produced by bees in an enclosed greenhouse environment. In vitro studies of bactericidal (bacteria-killing) activity demonstrated a 40% solution of honey killed all bacteria present—including methicillin-resistant *Staphylococcus aureus* (MRSA), vancomycin-resistant

E. faecium (VRE), and multi-drug resistant gram-negative rods. They also swabbed the foreheads of 42 volunteers with honey and covered the areas with a patch for 48 hours. Compared with control patches without honey, the honey-covered patches were culture-negative for bacteria significantly more often.

The use of medical-grade honey *(Medihoney)* ensures that the honey is not contaminated with bacteria as grocery-store honey might be. *Medihoney* dressings for wound care have been approved in the U.S. and Canada since 2007. The promising news—honey might one day be used as a topical microbicide or even as a treatment for wounds that are infected with a variety multidrug-resistant organisms. (Kwakman PHS et al. Medical-grade honey kills antibiotic-resistant bacteria in vitro and eradicates skin colonization. *Clin Infec Dis* 2008 Jun 1; 46:1677; Honey for wound care. *Pharmacist's Letter/Prescriber's Letter* 2008;24(12):241212)

So how does honey work? It's thought to promote wound healing by promoting the granulation of tissues. It promotes epithelial cell growth by providing a moisture barrier to help keep the wound hydrated. Enzymes and hydrogen peroxide in honey can help in debriding the wound as well. Honey also has anti-inflammatory effects, reduces the swelling or edema surrounding the wound, and reduces the amount of wound secretions. Honey also has a low pH or acid pH which helps to correct the higher alkaline pH of wounds and promotes healing. The lower the pH the more the antibacterial and antifungal activity. The pH of honey is 4.4. As a few points of reference, the pH of the acid in the stomach is 2, the pH of urine is 6, and the pH of blood is 7.4.

Honey for hangover headaches. Here's a tip for preventing and/or managing a hangover headache: Eat some honey. Spread it on a cracker or over some toast, before or after the alcohol, and you may prevent the inevitable headache from being "over-served." Honey supplies fructose, which helps the body metabolize alcohol and reduce hangover symptoms. If you do wind up with a headache, even after this prudent advice, drink fluids containing minerals and salts to alleviate the dehydration from the alcohol. For example, a cup of bouillon replaces fluids and does not cause nausea. And the vasoconstrictor effects of a quick hit of coffee help to shorten the duration of the headache. (National Headache Foundation. Prevention and treatment for hangover headaches. Archive for June, 2009. Accessed June 24, 2010)

Honey is a no-no in infants.
See Botulism, honey, and infants in Chapter B.

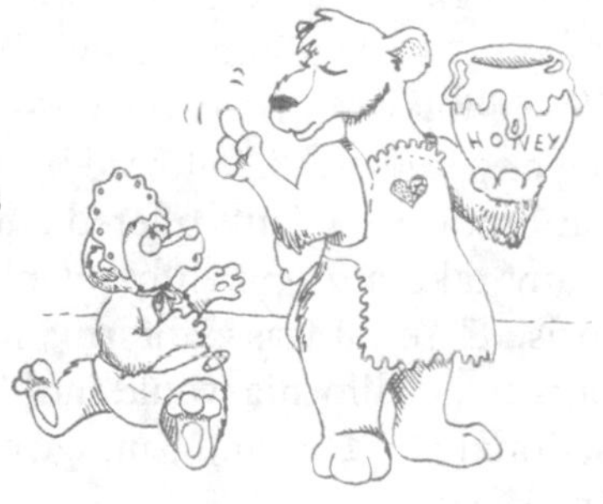

Honey is the only food that does not spoil. Honey found in the tombs of ancient Pharaohs has been tasted by archeologists and found to still be palatable.

Honeymoon. One of the customs of the day 4,000 years ago in far-away Babylon, was for the father of the bride to supply the new son-in-law with all the mead he could drink for the first month of marriage. Since mead is a honey beer and because the calendar was based on the cycle of the moon, this period was referred to as the "Honey Month," or what is commonly known today as the "Honeymoon."

Hospital food. Just the mere mention of hospital food sends chills up and down the spine…and now, a study has given us another reason for those chills, besides the obvious. A national survey of 57 university hospitals found that the menus at only 7% met all the federal dietary guidelines. Of menus for patients with no dietary restrictions, 40% served too much fat, and more than half poured on the salt. So much for practicing what we preach.

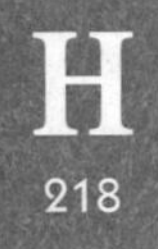

HOT DOGS

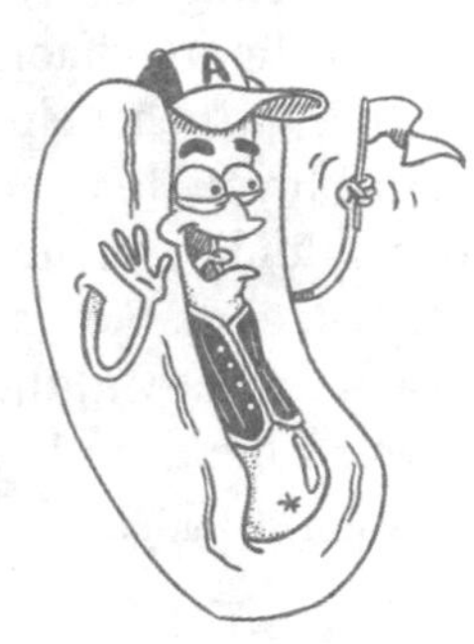

Hot dogs. What would a summer be without hot dogs? What would a baseball game be without hot dogs? The connection between baseball and hot dogs has a 100-year history. The origin of the connection is unknown, but it is a well-established fact that hot dog stands have ruled ball parks for more than a century. Baseball fans ate 21,233,839 hot dogs in major league parks during the summer of 2010, according to the National Hot Dog and Sausage Council. In fact, string all those "dawgs" together and you can link Yankee Stadium in New York with the Dodgers Stadium in Los Angeles. Speaking of those two cities—Los Angeles is the highest hot dog consuming city in the U.S. followed by New York City.

The San Francisco Giants offered a tofu hot dog for two years but didn't get too many takers. Apparently people who eat tofu are not big baseball fans. Surprised? Yes, it was California for gawd's sake. If any state would go for tofu burgers, California would rank right up there in the top three.

The National Hot Dog and Sausage council has its own name for the tofu frank—The Weakest Link.

HISTORICAL HIGHLIGHT

The National Hot Dog and Sausage Council states that European immigrants first brought hot dogs to the United States from Germany and Austria in the 1800s. The frankfurter was nicknamed dachshund dog because of its resemblance to the little extended-length canine. Legend has it that the term "hot dog" was coined at the Polo Grounds during a baseball game around 1906. Concessionaire Harry M. Stevens couldn't sell ice cream and soda on a cold day in April, so he had his vendors load up on sausages and holler, "Get your red hot dachshund dogs!" It just so happened that a cartoonist for the *New York Journal* was at the park looking for an idea and penned an illustration of a real dachshund in a bun with the caption, "Get your hot dogs!" As the story goes, the cartoonist, Tad Dorgan, couldn't spell dachshund, so he shortened the caption to just "hot dogs." Unfortunately, no one can find the cartoon by Tad Dorgan, so the story has been disputed. Now the ballpark and hot dog historians are back at the drawing board as to the origins of the hot dog.

During hot dog season, Memorial Day to Labor Day, Americans typically consume seven billion hot dogs or 818 hot dogs every second. (National Hot Dog and Sausage Council, 2011)

A hot dog at the ball park is better than a steak at the Ritz.
— Humphrey Bogart

HISTORICAL HIGHLIGHT

Humble pie. Where did the term, to eat humble pie, originate? This saying dates back to the eighteenth century. The men of the house were given the best meat of any meal (filet, T-bone, sirloin) and of course, the women and children ate the umbles or leftovers: the tongue and the entrails (intestines). The leftovers were baked in an umble pie, hence the name.

Hypertension—tips for lowering systolic blood pressure.

- For every 20 pound weight loss—5 to 20 point reduction
- Follow the DASH diet (see Chapter D)—8 to 14 point reduction
- Exercise daily (30 minutes brisk walking)—4 to 9 point reduction
- Limit sodium to no more than 2300 mg—2 to 8 point reduction
- Limit alcohol (less than 2 drinks/day for men, 1 drink per day for women)—2–4 point reduction

(Joint National Commission on Hypertension VII; 2008)

Hypoglycemia. Hypoglycemia (low blood sugar) is the most common endocrine emergency seen by primary care practitioners. It frequently occurs in patients receiving insulin treatment with tight control of their diabetes and in older patients receiving a sulfonylurea drug such as glyburide or glipizide. Another common group are people who have nonspecific symptoms including fatigue, concentration difficulties, anxiety, and dizziness. Most patients with hypoglycemia are self-diagnosed. A glucose tolerance test (GTT) is actually needed to diagnose this condition and the patient will need a workup by the primary care practitioner or endocrinologist to determine the cause of the hypoglycemia.

Clinical hypoglycemia is defined using the following criteria:

.....Central nervous system symptoms including confusion, aberrant behavior, seizures, and coma. Other symptoms may include headache, slurred speech, tremors, tachycardia (rapid heart rate), and the inability to concentrate.

.....Mental efficiency (mild confusion) declines as blood glucose falls below 65 mg/dL (3.9 mmol/L)

.....Hormonal defense mechanisms (epinephrine and glucagon) are activated when blood glucose drops below 55 mg/dL (3.0 mmol/L), producing the typical hypoglycemic symptoms of shakiness and dysphoria

.....Significant symptoms occur with a simultaneous blood glucose level equal to or less than 40 mg/dL (less than 2.2 mmol/L)

.....Relief of these symptoms by the administration of glucose.

The longer the patient has diabetes, the less obvious are the signs and symptoms of hypoglycemia. Patients who have had diabetes for more than 10 years may not manifest with the classic signs listed above. Instead, numbness and/or tingling (around the mouth especially), yawning and or a feeling of "heaviness" in the legs may become primary symptoms.

Ten to fifteen grams of a fast-acting carbohydrate will increase the blood sugar most rapidly. The recommended source for the fast-acting carbohydrate is 8 ounces (1 cup) of skim milk. If skim milk isn't handy, four ounces (½ cup) of fruit juice will do, as will 6 or 7 pieces of hard candy or 4 ounces (½ cup) of regular soda (not diet soda).

One common mistake is to add 5 packs of sugar to an 8-ounce glass of orange juice. This definitely is "overkill" as far as a sugar dose is concerned. Another common mistake is to use ice cream or a chocolate bar to treat the hypoglycemia. As tasty as both of those happen to be, the large fat content of these foods slows the absorption of the sugar so that the blood glucose level does not rise as rapidly, putting the patient in danger of prolonged hypoglycemia.

It's like slurping up two pounds of T-bone steak and a buttered baked potato through a straw.

—Jane Hurley of the Center for Science in the Public Interest discussing Cold Stone Creamery's "Oh Fudge!" milkshake.

ICE CREAM

Ice cream headache. An ice cream headache is triggered when a cold substance hits the hard palate. Ice cream drastically cools the mouth, triggering vasodilation to increase blood flow and warm up the area. As the blood moves in to warm up the mouth, the trigeminal nerve endings are irritated. The pain peaks in approximately 25–60 seconds, and the skin temperature in the forehead falls almost two degrees Fahrenheit. The treatment? Eat your ice cream slowly.

Ice cream fun facts:

.....The origin of ice cream sundaes. Ice cream sodas were quite popular in the late 1800s. Ice cream sodas were made with a mixture of sweet cream, syrup, and carbonated water. In October 1874 a man named Robert Green was selling soda fountain drinks when he ran out of sweet cream. A quick thinker, he decided to use ice cream instead, hoping that no one would notice the substitution. It seems as if everyone noticed. His profits jumped from $6.00 per day selling the traditional cream soda to $600.00 per day for the soda with ice cream added.

The ice cream drink became so popular that religious leaders declared it sinful. By the 1890s some cities and towns passed laws prohibiting the sale of sodas on Sunday. For this reason the ice cream sundae was invented. (It was spelled with an "ae" so as not to offend the leaders of the Church.)

The largest ice cream sundae on record weighed 24.5 tons. The sundae was made by Palm Dairies Ltd, under the supervision of Mike Rogiani in Edmonton, Alberta, Canada, on July 24, 1988. (Guinness World Records, 2001)

.....The origin of Häagen-Dazs ice cream. One fine morning in 1959, Rose and Reuben Mattus had an epiphany. America needs a luxury-brand ice cream—let's create one and let's come up with a name that tags it as a luxury dessert. Reuben had visions of Danish milkmaids dancing in his head and ladling out cream. He blurted out a nonsense name that sounded rather Danish. And that name just so happened to be Haagen-Dazs. Voilà! What was missing? An umlaut—turning the brand into Häagen-Dazs. Never mind that the Danish language doesn't use umlauts in their alphabet, but *hey,* we're talking about a new exciting product—so authenticity isn't really an issue. Reuben came up with the recipe and Rose was the marketing guru. Reuben's ice cream was 15% butterfat, used real egg yolks, and contained a myriad of natural ingredients, such as Belgian chocolate, vanilla beans from Madagascar, and coffee from Columbia. Mmmmm—good...and the rest is history. By 1983, Häagen-Dazs had sales of $115 million per year. Pillsbury scooped the company up for a cool $70 million, umlaut and all. The company is now owned by Nestlé. Rose continued to eat her very favorite flavor, vanilla, until she died at 90. So who says 15% butterfat reduces longevity?

The scoop: One pint of vanilla Häagen-Dazs ice cream = 2/3 stick of butter, or 1,080 calories and 72 grams of fat with 82 grams of sugar.

.....In Sutherland, Iowa, citizens may not carry ice cream cones in their pockets.

.....In Halstead, Kansas, residents must refrain from eating ice cream with a fork in public.

Inflammation. Various foods can either contribute to inflammation or decrease inflammation throughout the body. Is inflammation bad for you? Yes, and no. Don't you hate ambivalent answers like that? When you ask that question to a group of cardiologists, oncologists, and rheumatologists, the answer will be a resounding yes. Inflammation in the blood vessels contributes to cardiovascular disease and atherosclerosis. Inflammation in the joints contributes to various types of arthritis, including osteoarthritis and rheumatoid arthritis. Inflammation has been shown to be a precursor to various cancers. Barrett's esophagus is an inflammation of the lower third of the esophagus and a precursor to cancer (adenocarcinoma) of the lower third of the esophagus. Hepatitis C viral infection of the liver causes chronic hepatitis and an increased risk of cancer of the liver. Ulcerative colitis and Crohn's disease have been shown to increase the risk for cancer of the large and small intestine. And, those are just a few examples. Sooooo...

A 2006 review published in the *Journal of the American College of Cardiology* found that a dietary pattern high in refined starches, sugar, saturated fats and trans fats and low in fruits, vegetables, whole grains, and omega-3 fatty acids increased inflammation. Mediterranean diet patterns (see Chapter M), with high fruits and vegetables, fish, whole grains, and wine have been linked to lower levels of vascular inflammation.

So do you want to reduce "generalized inflammation" in your body? Head for the B aisle at the grocery store—beans, berries, and broccoli. Then swing by the fish tank and take some salmon home. Stop by the tomato and grape aisle, grab a sweet potato out of the bin, and head home for a heart-healthy, cancer-preventing, joint pain-free, anti-inflammatory diet.

INSECTS

Insects as food. The European Union has allocated 4.2 million Euros to research and promote the eating of insects as a cheap, low-fat protein source. A contest in the September 30, 2011 issue of *The Week* magazine asked its readers to name the first French or Italian restaurant to specialize in serving insect entrees on the menu. The winner:

.....Beetle Jus (Jerry Gilbert, Hillsborough, N.J.)

.....2nd place: Le Moulin Roach (Hans Naumann, Orlando, FL)

.....3rd place: Beetlemangia (Joe Prenoveau, Baltimore, MD)

Insect fragments in grains. First let me point out that it's practically impossible to keep insects out of grain silos, so zero tolerance is not possible. The government knows this but has set standards to regulate the tolerable level of insect fragments per 50 grams of grain.

The current process is to do a gross inspection by spreading out grain kernels and eyeballing them for whole insects or insect fragments—the wing, torso, leg, etc. To pick out the smaller segments, testers mix up an elaborate concoction, shake it up, filter off what floats to the top, dry the extract, and study it under a microscope. Just so you realize the complexity of the job, "It takes six months of training to become an insect-fragment counter," says Dr. Barrie Kitto, Chief Insect-Fragment Counter. I can only imagine the intensity and stress of the six-month course.

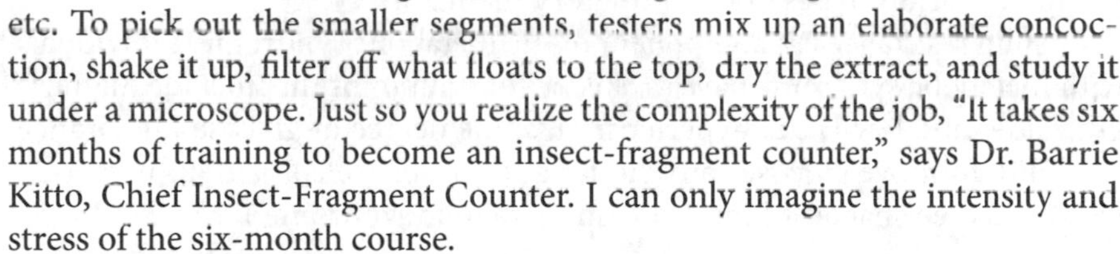

Current federal standards allow 75 insect fragments per 50 grams of grain, but here's the clincher: contrary to the usual thinking *size does not matter* when we're talking insect fragments. Three-fourths of a large maggot or just a measly wing tip of a fruit fly is immaterial in the world of federal standards. The number of fragments is the issue. Yikes.

The ol' eyeball technique is obviously a bit outdated. A new assay is currently being tested to determine the number of insect fragments in grain products. The new assay measures myosin, a muscle protein present in in-

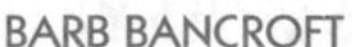

sects at all life stages regardless of size or shape. When an extraction fluid is added to grain or foods containing the myosin, the mix turns green. The deeper the hue, the greater the amount of myosin found in the grain. The greater the myosin, the more insect fragments present.

Insulin resistance 101. Insulin is produced by the beta cells of the pancreas. Muscle tissue, liver tissue and fat tissue all have insulin receptors. When insulin is secreted into the blood in response to a meal the insulin binds to the insulin receptors on muscle, liver and fat tissue and glucose is transported into the cells to use for energy. Pretty straightforward, eh?

With insulin resistance, the pancreas secretes plenty of insulin, but tissue receptors are resistant or unable to use the insulin to transport glucose into the tissues. Glucose levels in the blood rise, the pancreas attempts to compensate by releasing increased amounts of insulin, the tissues continue to resist the insulin and a vicious cycle ensues. In the early stages of insulin resistance, the excess insulin manages to keep the blood glucose in check; however, the glucose level is usually in the upper range of normal. As insulin resistance progresses and insulin levels continue to increase, blood sugars will rise to above normal levels. Other metabolic changes also occur. Triglycerides levels increase, HDL-cholesterol levels decrease, and levels of small, dense LDL-cholesterol increase. High insulin levels also trigger the release of angiotensin, a hormone that "tenses your angios" or vasoconstricts your arteries, thus raising blood pressure to hypertensive levels. All of these changes contribute to an increased risk of atherosclerosis and heart disease.

What causes insulin resistance? One of the major causes of insulin resistance is an overabundance of visceral fat around the waistline. Visceral fat in the belly is now considered by your friendly endocrinologist as a "new" organ. The visceral fat cells are not only resistant to insulin, but they also pump out various types of inflammatory mediators.

Insulin resistance is a component of the metabolic syndrome. Individuals with metabolic syndrome have a "cluster" of symptoms that include high triglycerides and low HDL, hypertension, some degree of glucose intolerance (inability to move glucose into the fat and muscle cells), and an increased waistline. (See chapter M for more on metabolic syndrome.)

Interstitial cystitis and foods to avoid. First of all, what is interstitial cystitis (IC)? IC is a painful condition of the bladder that involves both bladder overactivity and chronic neurogenic inflammation. In addition, central nervous system pathways supplying the bladder are sensitized and interact to perpetuate the chronic pain.

To treat IC, avoidance of bladder irritants is required. Common bladder irritants include caffeine, chocolate, alcohol, fruit including strawberries, or-

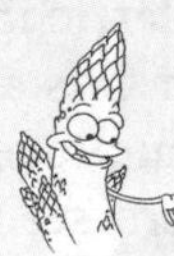

ASPARAGUS TIP

The small and large intestines process, at about one inch per minute, forty tons of food over the course of 70 years.

anges and tomatoes (yes, a tomato is a fruit), carbonation, vinegar, tea, vitamin B complex, chilies and spicy foods. Although cranberry juice has been commonly recommended in the past for patients susceptible to urinary tract infections, it is *contraindicated* in women with IC because its acidity irritates and aggravates bladder pain. If a patient inadvertently ingests a bladder irritant, she can take Prelief twice a day on that same day, or a daily teaspoon of baking soda in eight ounces of water. (Hornick L, Slocumb JC. Treating chronic pelvic pain. *ADVANCE for Nurse Practitioners* 2008 February: 44–54)

Intestines and absorption. The small intestine is a coiled tube extending from the stomach to the ileocecal valve, where it joins the large intestine. Its average length in the living adult is five meters, approximately 16½ feet. However, it elongates after death, because of the loss of smooth muscle tone. In an interesting postmortem study of 109 adult subjects, the intestine ranged from 3.35–7.16 meters (10.99–23.49 feet) in women and 4.8–7.85 meters (16.01–25.75 feet) in men, the average being 5.92 meters (19.42 feet) in females and 6.37 meters (20.9 feet) in males. Length was correlated with the height of the individual, but was independent of age. The large intestine is approximately two meters or 6.56 feet. The total surface area of the intestines is more than 100 feet, or five times the area of the body's skin.

Iodine. Iodine is a mineral necessary for the health of the thyroid gland. Iodine deficiency can lead to an enlarged thyroid (goiter), hypothyroidism, or both. Hypothyroidism due to iodine deficiency is rare in developed countries because of the amount of iodine we consume in iodized salt. The recommended daily intake of iodine is 150 μg for all adults. One-quarter of a teaspoon of iodized salt contains 95 μg of iodine, more than half of your daily needs. Other food sources of iodine are cod, tuna, salmon, shrimp, and haddock. What about sea salt? Sea salt comes in two forms—iodized and non-iodized. So if you are strictly a sea salt fan, make sure to look for the iodized form in your grocery store.

IRON

Iron absorption. In order to absorb iron from food, it is best to serve iron-containing foods (such as prunes) with meat or a food high in vitamin C. Meat increases the acidity of the gastric juice, and iron is absorbed better in a more acidic environment. Vitamin C changes iron from ferric iron to ferrous iron, a more easily absorbed form. Of course, vitamin C is also known as ascorbic acid, providing the acid to help in the absorption process.

Also, taking iron supplements with a food rich in vitamin C increases the absorption of iron from the supplement. Ferrous gluconate has been shown to be better absorbed as a supplement and a lot easier on the stomach. Use 100 mg of vitamin C or a glass of orange juice or any citrus juice to boost absorption. And, take it on an empty stomach. (Dr. Andrew Weil, Self-Healing. September 2007)

Iron deficiency and cooking with iron. Cooking foods in an iron pot or skillet can significantly increase iron absorption from the foods you eat. This is especially true for foods with high acidity such as tomatoes. For example, one serving of spaghetti sauce normally has less than one milligram of iron, but when cooked in an iron skillet that amount can increase six fold. (Hint: You have to have enough strength to lift the iron skillet if you're going to be cooking with cast iron.)

Is this a piece of good news or would it be considered hazardous to your health? It would certainly be of benefit for individuals needing extra iron, and that includes growing kids and pregnant moms. But for men as well as older women who are not at risk for iron deficiency, it is not beneficial. In addition, it would not be prudent to cook with an iron skillet if you have been diagnosed with the hereditary disease known as hemochromatosis (see Chapter H). Patients with hemochromatosis accumulate excess iron which can result in serious manifestations of iron overload in organs including the liver and the heart.

An Ethiopian study confirmed the benefits of cooking with iron pots. In a February 27, 1999 *Lancet* study, researchers compared 195 children who ate food cooked in aluminum pots with 207 children whose food was cooked in iron pots. After one year, blood tests demonstrated that the iron-deficiency anemia rate decreased from 57% to 12% in the group using the iron pots but only from 55% to 39% in the aluminum pot group. The children whose families used iron pots also grew slightly more, and none experienced iron overload. (Adish AA et al. Effect of consumption of food cooked in iron pots on iron status and growth of young children: A randomized trial. *The Lancet* 1999 (February 27);353:712–717)

Iron deficiency and restless legs syndrome (RLS). It has been estimated that one-fourth of the patients with restless legs syndrome (RLS) have an iron deficiency. Low dopamine in the striatum of the brain is the presumed mechanism for restless legs syndrome. Iron is a necessary co-factor in the brain for the synthesis and regulation of dopamine receptors, and thus for the amount of dopamine available in the synapse. Iron and ferritin have also been found to be abnormally low in the cerebrospinal fluid of RLS patients.

(Hening W et al. Impact, diagnosis and treatment of restless legs syndrome (RLS) in a primary care population: the REST (RLS epidemiology, symptoms, and treatment) primary care study. *Sleep Med* 2004;(5):237–2 46); Ekbom K, UlfbergJ. Restless legs syndrome. *J Intern Med* 2009;266 (5):419–431.)

Iron deficiency and tea drinking. Can tea drinking cause iron deficiency anemia? Yes. Tea reduces the absorption of iron in the GI tract. A study performed in Israel evaluated 122 infants aged 6–12 months. The percentage of tea-drinking infants with iron-deficiency anemia was 32.6% compared to 3.5% for the non-tea drinkers. The tea drinkers had significantly lower levels of hemoglobin as well. Iron-deficient adults should be aware of this fact as well. The iron-deficient adult should wait one to two hours after a meal before drinking tea or remove tea from the diet altogether. (Merhav H, et al. Tea drinking and microcytic anemia in infants. *American J Clinical Nutrition* 1985;41:1210–1213; Alleyne M, Horne MK, Miller JL. Individualized treatment for iron-deficiency anemia in adults. *The Am J of Med* 2008;121 (11):94 –948)

Iron and multivitamins. (See chapter M)

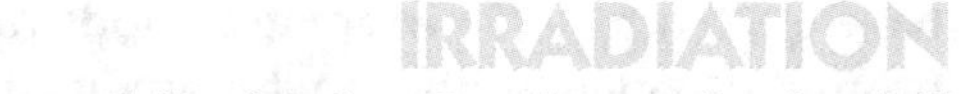

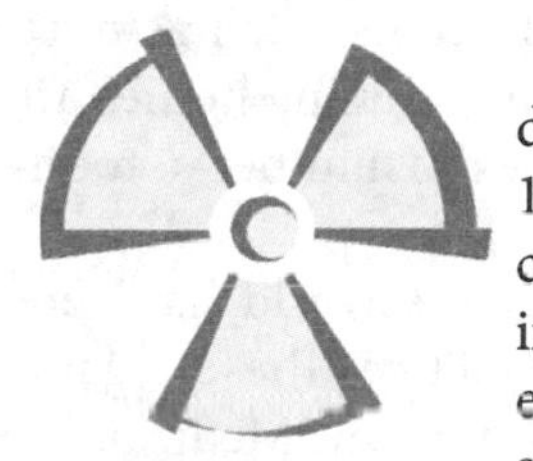

Irradiation and food safety. Irradiating food to kill disease-causing pathogens was first recommended in 1904 and first tested in the 1920s and 1930s. This process has been approved in the United States for killing or inactivating bacteria, fungi, parasites, and other creepy, crawly critters in flour, grains, fruits, eggs, sprouting seeds, vegetables, spices, poultry, beef, and pork. For example, irradiating chicken can destroy *Salmonella* and *Campylobacter jejuni,* as well as other chicken-borne pathogens. Irradiation can also kill *E. coli O157:H7.*

Before you go ballistic and deny the benefits of irradiating food, consider the following numbers: Every ***day,*** about 200,000 Americans develop a foodborne illness. Of those, 900 are hospitalized and 14 die (5,110 per year). According to the Centers for Disease Control (CDC), 48 million Americans acquire food poisoning every year. Irradiating food can prevent many of these illnesses.

Now, for some questions about food irradiation. Is this the same type of irradiation used in cancer patients to zap cancer cells? Yes. Is this type of irradiation safe and effective for foods to be consumed by humans of all ages? Yes. Do irradiated foods cost more money? Yes. Do foods that are irradiated lose their nutrients? No. Is this type of irradiation being used for all of the foods that it has been approved for? No. Allow me to explain each question.

Yes, this is the exact same type of irradiation used to destroy cancer cells. Irradiation is capable of destroying pathogens that lurk outside and inside fresh or frozen meat and chicken, strawberries, dried spices, and any other source of contaminated food. The irradiation works in one of three ways: it destroys the genetic code of the pathogen, it can disrupt the cell membranes of the pathogen, or it inactivates essential enzymes necessary for growth and reproduction of the pathogen.

Yes, this type of irradiation is quite safe. It kills the unwanted pathogens; however, it does not make food radioactive, just as external radiation does not make a patient radioactive. Food irradiation does not result in DNA mutations, nor create cancer-causing chemicals in food as some of the consumer naysayers proclaim. Irradiation alters the chemistry of the food just about as much as if it were heated or sun-dried.

Numerous studies have been performed on the safety of irradiated foods. The U.S. Army has performed studies on three generations of mice, rats, and beagles with nary a mishap. These research subjects developed no more cancer or inherited diseases than their control counterparts that were chowing down on canned foods or frozen, non-irradiated foods. Human research has demonstrated similar results. In addition, many tertiary care centers have elected to serve irradiated foods to their most severely immunocompromised patients—those who are at high risk of infections, such as burn patients and recipients of organ transplants. In addition, nursing homes are also choosing to use irradiated foods in order to reduce the number of food-borne infections in their elderly residents.

Numerous agencies and organizations throughout the world have endorsed irradiation as a completely safe and effective practice. These organizations include the World Health Organization, the American Medical Association, the American Public Health Association, and most amazing one of all, our very own Food and Drug Administration (FDA), a historically cautious agency that requires approximately 10 bazillion studies and 20 bazillion pages of documentation. The FDA has determined that the process is safe and effective in reducing or eliminating harmful bacteria on a variety of foods.

If you know that the food you buy is free of contamination from disease-causing microbes, if you prepare it on clean surfaces with clean utensils, and if you then cook it to just the right temperature, you probably have no need to buy irradiated food. However, for the individual writing this blurb on irradiated food, who isn't as squeaky clean as all that, or who needs to eat in a fast-food restaurant on more than one occasion, irradiation can offer real benefits.

Does irradiated food cost more money? Of course it does…what kind of a question is *that?* A few extra pennies per pound maybe a wise investment for anyone who has a compromised immune system, as well as for very young children and very old adults. For everyone else, including those who are currently reading this very informative section, it offers extra protection that will prevent days of gastrointestinal distress and protect your health for future decades.

No, irradiated foods do not lose any of their nutritional value. Not one iota.

No, irradiation is not being used for all of the foods that it has been approved for.

If you prefer to avoid irradiated foods, simply check the package label. All foods that have been irradiated must carry the international symbol for irradiation, the "radura," as well as the phrase, "treated by irradiation" (or "with irradiation"). You can also choose organic foods. Radiation is not acceptable under the rules of the USDA National Organic Program; thus, foods labeled "organic" cannot be irradiated.

A two-pound turkey and a fifty-pound cranberry. That's Thanksgiving dinner at Three-Mile Island. —Johnny Carson

---

ISOFLAVONES

Isoflavones. Most of the theorized health benefits from soy foods are attributed to isoflavones, a type of naturally occurring plant hormone, or phytochemical. (See Chapter P for more on phytochemicals) Isoflavones belong to a large group of antioxidants called polyphenols, and a subgroup named flavonoids. The chemical structure of isoflavones is similar to that of human estrogen, and isoflavones can both decrease excess estrogen in the body and increase estrogen activity—a paradoxical response to be sure. The two most common types of soy isoflavones are genistein and daidzein.

CHAPTER J

Jello—an edible substance best comprehended as having the taste of a politician's promises and the consistency of his spine; sweet, but nonexistent.

—Gordon Bowker

Jam. Jam is a preparation of fruit cooked in sugar syrup. The art of jam making began in the Middle East and was introduced into Europe by the Crusaders, who had discovered sugar cane and certain previously unknown fruits. A zillion fruits can be made into jam—bilberry jam, green tomato jam, pear jam, peach jam, apricot jam, strawberry jam, raspberry jam, toe jam (ha! Just checking to see if you're reading all of the jams), plum jam, red currant jam, rhubarb jam, watermelon jam, mango jam, haw jam, elderberry jam…ok, ok. You can add spices to enhance the flavor, or you can also add a little alcohol such as rum or kirsch.

Marmalade and jam are one and the same; however, it appears as if there are two origins for the word marmalade. The name may have come from the Portuguese *marmelo,* meaning jam. It may also be that Joao Marmaloado (1450–1510) made the first breakfast "jam" by boiling oranges with sugar.

Jambalaya. This specialty dish of N'awlin's (New Orleans) was inspired by Spanish paella. Jambalaya is made of highly spiced rice, chicken, and ham. Various ingredients can be added including sausage, peppers, tomatoes, okra, prawns, or oysters.

HISTORICAL HIGHLIGHT

To treat jaundice in Tudor times it was recommended that one should drink a pint of ale containing nine drowned head lice every morning for a week. Fall on your knees and shout hallelujah if you're happy that you are *not* living in Tudor times.

Jejunum. The jejunum is the middle portion of the small intestine, between the duodenum and the ileum. It is about eight feet in length and comprises about two-fifths of the small intestine. It is derived from the word jejune, which means deficient or lacking in nutritive value. The jejunum was originally thought to be empty, and certainly lacking in nutritive value after death, hence, the name. The jejunum specializes in the absorption of carbohydrates and proteins.

Jellies. Only fruits rich in pectin are suitable for making preserves, or jellies (apples, bilberry, red currants, mulberries, quinces, etc.). Vegetarians and vegans beware: Dessert jellies are made with gelatin or with calf's foot jelly.

Jello. Jello has been in the history books since the Middle Ages. You probably won't be so enamored with this jiggly slab of amorphous gelatin once you have heard how it's made. If you don't want to know, stop now. If you're interest has been piqued, here goes. Animal remains, primarily bones, cartilage and tendons are boiled for several hours. After boiling, the parts are strained and discarded. The liquid sets for 24 hours, after which the fat is skimmed from the top. What's left is gelatin—a colorless, odorless, and tasteless thickening agent added to packaged and preserved foods. It wasn't named jello until around 1897 when a carpenter named Pearle Wait invented a flavored gelatin dessert that his wife named jello. JELL-O is the official registered name and is now owned by Kraft Foods.

Jelly beans. Jelly beans are bean-shaped, brightly colored candy with a hard sugar coating and a firm gelatinous filling. Jelly beans have absolutely no nutritive value whatsoever, except that they are full of sugar calories. Ronald Reagan's love for jelly beans was a source of amusement for the average American during his tenure as President of the United States. He started eating them soon after he became the Governor of California in 1967, supposedly to help him break a pipe-smoking habit. His favorite jelly bean flavor was licorice. (Jacob M. and Jacob M. What the Great Ate. Three Rivers Press, 2010)

Jicama. Pronounced "hik-ah-mah," jicama is a root vegetable that is often eaten raw. It's crunchy with a slightly sweet taste, and yummy. Jicama is low in calories, has absolutely no fat, and is a great source of vitamin C and fiber. Shred it and add it to your salad or cook it along with a slew of other root vegetables for a delicious side dish or main dish for dinner.

Juicy Fruit gum. What are the four predominant flavors in Juicy Fruit gum? Lemon, orange, pineapple, and banana.

Jujube. The jujube is an oval olive-size fruit with a smooth, tough red skin; soft, sweet yellowish or green flesh; and a hard seed in the middle. The jujube tree and its fruit, which originated in China have been used medicinally for hundreds of years. Some Far East countries export jujubes, either fresh or dried, they are also known as "red dates."

Junk foods. Americans eat 50 percent more junk food than they did 20 years ago, including 45 bags of potato chips a year per person, 120 bags of French fries, and 190 candy bars. (*The Week,* May 24, 2002) The average American gets one-fourth of his/her calories from junk foods. One-third of all American adults get 50% of their calories from high-calorie, nutrient-poor foods like ice cream, cakes, cookies, candy, chips, and soft drinks. More weight is gained as more junk food is consumed. Although people who eat junk food take in more calories, it doesn't mean that they get the appropriate nutrients. Most junk-food junkies have lower blood levels of vitamins A, E, C, and B12, folate, and carotenoids. (Kant AK. Consumption of energy-dense, nutrient-poor food by adult Americans: Nutrition and health implications. The third National Health and Nutrition Examination Survey, 1988–1994. *American Journal of Clinical Nutrition 2000* (October);72:929, 2000.)

CHAPTER K

For what we are about to receive,
Oh Lord, 'tis thee we thank,"
Said the cannibal as he cut a slice
Of the missionary's shank
—E.Y. Harburg (1898–1981)

KALE

Kale. Kale has been cultivated for over 2,000 years in the Mediterranean region. It was a staple in Scotland where every kitchen had a "kail pot" for cooking. One of its major attributes is its ability to grow in the winter, so the Scottish had their kail pots up and running all year long. It's also known as borecole (no, that's not a misspelling of broccoli), and it's a member of the cruciferous family. It's a "non-heading" cabbage like collards and bok choy.

Its health benefits escalate when it's steamed. Chopping and chewing release the chemical compounds known as the sulforaphanes (same chemicals are in broccoli) which help clear carcinogens from the body. The lutein and zeaxanthin protect the eyes, the vitamin K helps protect the bones.

One cup of raw, chopped kale contains:
34 Calories, 10,302 IU of vitamin A (206% of the DV), 80 mg of vitamin C (134% of the DV), 547 mg of vitamin K (684% of the DV), lutein and zeaxanthin 26.5 mg, and manganese 0.5 mg (26% of the DV).

Kava (Piper methysticum). Kava is made from the root of a perennial shrub native to the South Sea Islands. When taken in liquid form it provides a sense of euphoria and well-being. The native islanders considered the shrub a sacred plant. It was used by the islanders in just about every ritual imaginable—from celebrating wedding ceremonies and the birth of an infant nine months later, to paying homage at the death of a family or tribal member.

ASPARAGUS TIP

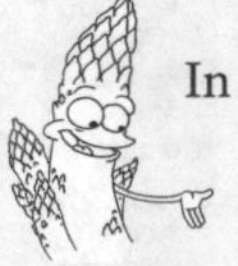

In 2002 the FDA issued a warning that taking kava supplements has been linked to a risk of severe liver injury—including hepatitis, cirrhosis, and liver failure. (FDA 2002; http://nccamnih.gov/health/kava/ataglance.htm; http://www.fda.gov/Food/ResourcesForYou/Consumers/ucm085482.htm)

In religious ceremonies, the tribal members chewed the kava root in order to prepare it for liquid consumption. Once chewed, it was spat into a bowl and mixed with coconut oil. You'll be happy to know that significant progress has been made in the preparation of kava in today's world. The root is now ground by mechanical means and the active ingredients, the kavalactones, are extracted. The kavalactones are then added to beverages, capsules, tablets, and topical solutions.

Kava appears to be a natural remedy for anxiety, fatigue, insomnia, asthma, urinary tract infections, and menopausal symptoms. So, if the anxiety, fatigue, urinary tract infection, and insomnia caused by menopausal symptoms triggers an asthma attack, kava is the herbal product for you. Topically, kava has been used as a numbing agent. Today, kava is used primarily for anxiety and insomnia.

It should not be used by patients with depression as it may trigger an increased risk for suicide. Obviously, it should be used with caution, and the patient population should be carefully screened before recommending kava for use. Kava is best reserved for patients with situational anxiety that prefer an herbal approach vs. a pharmaceutical approach. If used for anxiety, the individual should take the herb in the morning; if used for insomnia, the individual should take kava in the evening. Advise patients not to take kava in addition to prescribed anti-anxiety drugs, sedatives, or with alcohol. See above, FDA Warning.

Kentucky Fried Chicken. This finger-lickin' formula for the original fried chicken containing 11 herbs and spices was originally mixed on the floor of Colonel Harland Sanders back porch 66 years ago. Only the Colonel knows what else was on that floor of his back porch. Today, the complete formula is kept under lock and key in a bank vault in Louisville, Kentucky. Since this is the best kept secret in the U.S. today, two separate companies are used to blend the spices, so neither possesses the complete recipe.

KETCHUP

Ketchup. Two tablespoons of ketchup have 30 calories and 380 mg of sodium, as well as 6 mg of the antioxidant lycopene. Lycopene has been touted as a powerful antioxidant with cardioprotective benefits and possible cancer prevention benefits. However, in order to consume enough lycopene from ketchup for heart and cancer prevention benefits, you would trigger heart failure from the amount of sodium overload. Fast forward to Chapter L for the section on lycopene for better sources of this antioxidant.

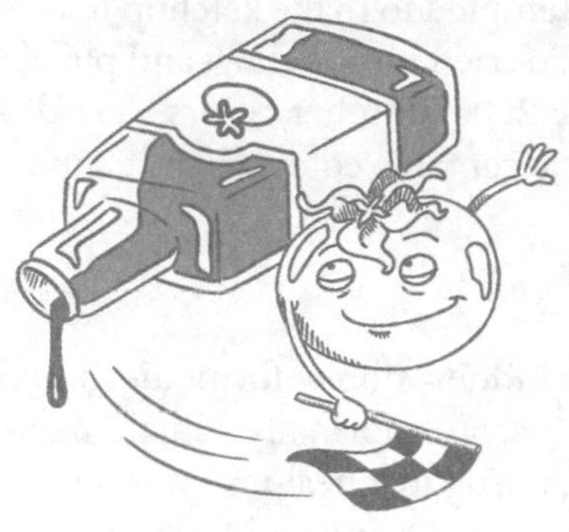

Our government has passed legislation that regulates the flow of ketchup. It has been mandated that ketchup must exit the glass bottle at .028 miles per hour. If the viscosity of the ketchup is too thin, and the speed is greater than .028 mph, the ketchup is rejected for sale.

Tomato tips:

.....Dr. Archibald Miles of Cincinnati, Ohio patented pills called "Dr. Miles' Compound Extract of Tomato" in 1837. This extract was touted to cure everything from athlete's foot to cholera, indigestion to diarrhea, and even baldness. He sold them to over 100,000 customers. It didn't cure a thing, of course, but it tasted delicious. In fact, it tasted so good that it continues to be popular today under its modern name: Ketchup.

.....The Heinz plant in Fremont, Ohio makes more ketchup than any other factory in the world. The company estimates it produces 4.1 million 14-ounce bottles every day.

.....Ohio is the fifth largest producer of fresh and processed tomatoes, after California, Florida, Georgia, and Virginia.

Shake and shake
The catsup bottle,
None will come,
And then a lot'll.
—Richard Armour (1977)

Why are kids so fond of ketchup? Children are the main consumers of ketchup. Why? The flavor of ketchup is designed to be attractive to small children because they detect sweetness more readily than other tastes. Commercially produced ketchup may contain up to 30% sugar, derived both from the natural sweetness of tomatoes and from added sugars. The second reason children (and adults) love ketchup is the color—the bright red color of tomato ketchup is intensely attractive. Red foods are perceived as being sweeter or richer.

Remember when the Heinz Company attempted to make ketchup in other colors? Green comes to mind, but they also tried pink, yellow and purple. None of these other colors caught on, so by 2006 all other colors were discontinued. Clearly the red color is the only acceptable color when it applies to ketchup.

Kidney stones—an overview. How are kidney stones formed? Kidney stone formation usually begins with a little dash of normally soluble materials, such as calcium, oxalate, phosphate and/or magnesium ammonium. These normally soluble materials supersaturate the urine and form crystals. Over time the crystals aggregate (clump) and these clumps grow into stones. Most kidney stones are composed of calcium and oxalate. Other stones form with calcium and phosphate. A third type of kidney stone is composed of magnesium ammonium and phosphate (known as struvite stones) and still another type of kidney stone is called a calcium carbonate apatite kidney stone. The last two types of kidney stones are usually associated with bacterial urinary tract infections that produce the enzyme urease.

Who gets kidney stones? Approximately 12% of the average American male population and 5% of the average American female population will develop at least one episode of symptomatic kidney stones by their 60s. The incidence of kidney stones increases with age and it's higher in Caucasians than African-Americans. There is a significant regional variation in kidney stone formation with the highest prevalence in the Southeastern part of the United States.

Does fluid intake make a difference? Yes…the time-honored recommendation for reducing the risk of kidney stones is to take two or more liters of fluids per day. Women who drink six or more 8-ounce servings of fluids per day have a 62% reduction in the risk of developing kidney stones. And not just any fluids. (see below) This approach increases urine flow rate and decreases the urine solute concentration—both mechanisms prevent kidney stones. In warmer climates, inadequate fluid intake causes dehydration, which increases the acidity of urine and stone formation. The southeastern U.S. is hot and has an increased rate of kidney stones.

Certain fluids have been associated with a high risk of kidney stones—these include soft drinks and tea. The southeastern U.S. drinks the most tea in the nation adding to the increased risk of kidney stones in this geographic area. Grapefruit juice has been shown to increase the risk of kidney stones by 44%. Why? It may increase the alkalinity of the urine or it may be an unexpected source of oxalate. Coffee, and alcohol, especially wine, have been

negatively associated with kidney stones. In other words, drink coffee and wine, hold the tea and grapefruit juice.

Vitamin C as a supplement (greater than 1000 mg/day) increases urinary oxalate levels and calcium oxalate stone formation. If you are predisposed to kidney stones you will want to throw out your vitamin C supplements. What were you taking them for anyway? You should be getting the majority of your vitamin C from food sources.

Large amounts of animal protein predispose patients to increased urinary levels of calcium and uric acid and subsequent kidney stones. High salt diets have opposing effects on calcium—reabsorption of sodium and water creates a favorable concentration gradient that allows for passive reabsorption of calcium in the renal tubules. On the other hand, a high-salt diet also creates a volume-expanded state, which in turn decreases sodium reabsorption in the proximal tubule. This leads to increased urinary calcium excretion. If there's more calcium in the urine, there's a greater chance for stone formation.

Until a few years ago, it was believed that too much calcium in the diet could aggravate or predispose individuals to kidney stones. This is ***not*** the case. Restriction of dietary calcium *promotes* calcium oxalate stone formation. The decreased availability of calcium in the intestine leads to increased absorption of and excretion of oxalate that would otherwise bind with the calcium. So, if you have kidney stones, can you drink milk? Yes.

Some vegetables, such as spinach and rhubarb, as well as peanuts, cashews, and almonds, all have high oxalate content and should be avoided in an individual with a history of kidney stones. (Massey LK, Kynast-Gales SA. Substituting milk for apple juice does not increase kidney stone risk in most normocalciuric adults who form calcium oxalate stones. *Journal of the American Dietetic Association* 1998; 164:98(3):303–309; von Unruh GE, Voss S, Sauerbruch T, Hesse A. Dependence of oxalate absorption on the daily calcium intake. *J Am Soc Nephrol.* 2004;15:1567–1573. Lerma EV. A comprehensive look at kidney stones. *The Clinical Advisor.* August 28, 2009. www.clinicaladvisor.com; Curhan GC, Willett WC, Knight EL, Stampfer MJ. Dietary factors and the risk of incident kidney stones in younger women. *Archives of Internal Medicine,* 2004;164:885–891; Curham GC, Rimm EB, Willet WC, Stampfer MJ. Regional variation in nephrolithiasis incidence and prevalence in among United States men. *J Urol.* 1994;151:838–841)

Kiwifruit. Kiwifruit is about the size of a large egg, with a greenish-brown, hairy skin. The plant actually originated in China (hence, it's real name, the Chinese gooseberry), but most of us associate the kiwifruit with New Zealand and Australia. It was introduced into New Zealand in the early 1900s and in the 1940s it was renamed after New Zealand's national symbol—the plump, flightless kiwi bird. It is also currently cultivated in California, western France, and Israel. Kiwifruit has the vitamin C of a Florida orange (65 mg), the potassium of one half a medium banana (242 mg), the fiber of a half-cup of corn flakes and the calorie content of a large egg (70). Don't forget, kiwifruit made the top ten list for the most powerful fruits. Would you like to download a few recipes with kiwifruit? Go to www.zesprikiwi.com/recipes.htm.

Knorr. Carl Heinrich Knorr was a German industrialist who, after marrying his second wife in 1838, set up a small industrial plant for roasting coffee and chicory. You might wonder why he waited until he married his second wife—she had the money. Anyway, his business was profitable but didn't really take off until his two sons took over after his death. They expanded the business and began to manufacture peas, lentils, small green French beans (haricot vert), and sago flours, which were marketed in packets. These were the precursors of the current packet soups that you can find on grocery store shelves, still bearing the family name, Knorr.

Kohlrabi. Ok, so I'm guilty of trying to fill up the K chapter. It's a stretch, but it's also a cruciferous vegetable for you to add to your repertoire. Kohlrabi means "cabbage-turnip," and it belongs to the cabbage family. It's packed with fiber, vitamin C, iron, and potassium. In fact, one-half cup of kohlrabi has 16% more potassium than one-half cup of orange juice. So a bowl of kohlrabi in the morning to accompany your piece of whole grain toast and cup of coffee is a perfect way to start your day. Sure it is.

Kohlrabi, like the other cruciferous vegetables including cauliflower, Brussels sprouts, broccoli, and cabbage, contains natural cancer-fighting chemicals. These chemicals, known as isothiocyanates, assist in the inactivation and elimination of carcinogens.

Don't forget that all cruciferous vegetables contain goitrogens, substances that cause the thyroid gland to enlarge or develop a goiter. These goitrogens inhibit the ability of the thyroid gland to produce thyroid hormones, which causes the thyroid to enlarge to compensate and produce more hormones. This does not pose a problem for healthy adults eating a large amount of cruciferous vegetables. However, individuals with an established thyroid problem or who are taking thyroid medications should be aware of this interaction.

Krill oil. Krill are miniscule shrimp-like crustaceans eaten by whales, seals, penguins, squid, and fish. Krill oil, like all fish oil, contains EPA and DHA, the marine-based omega-3 acids known for their numerous health benefits.

The big question? Is Krill oil better than regular fish oil for cardioprotection and all of the other health benefits? There's some evidence that maybe 20 or 30 percent more EPA and DHA is absorbed from krill oil than from regular fish oil. However, is that enough to warrant the 10 times greater cost of krill oil vs. regular fish oil? Regular fish oil comes from herring, sardines, and menhaden. Menhaden, what's thaaat? Menhaden fish are defined as "the most important fish you have never heard of." If you have a moment, Google menhaden and you'll be amazed.

Claims abound when it comes to krill oil. Claims include that krill oil can lower cholesterol, alleviate symptoms of PMS, and reduce symptoms of arthritis. This is all wonderful news except that all of the research was funded by the company that manufactures krill oil. (Neptune Krill Oil, Canada) Interestingly, krill oil does lower cholesterol, but only in combination with a statin drug such as atorvastatin (Lipitor). Krill oil, by itself, doesn't lower cholesterol any better than a placebo pill. (*Nutrition Action Newsletter,* June 2011)

Kuru (koo'roo). Kuru is a rapidly progressive neurological disease that is invariably fatal. The disease affected mostly adult women and children of both sexes belonging to the Fore (FOR-ae) tribe of New Guinea. Kuru is transmitted by the practice of ingesting tissue from an infected loved one who has died (ritual cannibalism) and rubbing infected tissues over the bodies of the women and children kin to the victim. The men of the Fore tribe rarely ate the dead and if they did partake, it would only be the red meat. The women and children, however, ate everything from the liver to the small intestines to the heart. In fact, even the feces was eaten, mixed with plants and cooked in banana leaves. If the dead loved one was a man, his penis, considered a rare delicacy, was delivered with great care to the wife for her personal consumption. A dying member of the Fore tribe bequeathed various body parts to his/her favorite kin in advance. "Their bellies are their cemeteries," remarked one of the observers of the Fore tribe. In fact, "I eat you" was a Fore greeting. That greeting may have been a bit unsettling to a visiting anthropologist in New Guinea in the 1940s and 1950s.

As this practice continued, more and more Fore women died of the fatal disease known as kuru. Kuru meant shivering—with cold or with fear—and by 1950 kuru was killing women in every Fore village. Once the shivering began, the women progressed through a series of neurological symptoms primarily consisting of gait problems and mental decline. They eventually lost their ability to walk and swallow, and died of complications due to pneumonia and dementia. The flesh of those who died of pneumonia was considered especially delicious, and was eaten by the children and

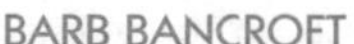

the female members of the family. Thus, the disease was passed from family member to family member.

The Fore tribe of New Guinea no longer practices cannibalism. Of course, there aren't many Fore members left—you can't propagate a species if there are no women. The incidence of kuru has fallen dramatically and is nonexistent at this time.

Kumquat. The kumquat is a citrus fruit originally from China and now cultivated in the Far East, Australia, and the United States. It resembles a small orange, the size of a quail's egg, and has a sweet rind and a sour flesh. It is packed with vitamin A, potassium and calcium.

The most remarkable thing about my mother is that for thirty years she served the family nothing but leftovers. The original meal has never been found.

—Calvin Trillin

Lactase. Lactase is an enzyme synthesized by bacteria in the large intestine that hydrolyzes lactose into two sugars, free glucose and galactose. Both sugars are absorbed rapidly and completely via the normal small intestine. The rate of lactase synthesis is high from birth until the age of five.

Between the ages of 5–14, many people have a genetically programmed reduction in the ability to produce the enzyme lactase, resulting in only 5–15% of enzyme activity they had in the first five years. So, we obviously "grow" ***into*** this deficiency, and we're much more likely to do so based on our genetic predisposition. Only about 25% of the world's population is able to maintain a high degree of lactase activity throughout adult life. If you have your full genetic complement of lactase as an adult, you are referred to as having lactase persistence. In contrast, if you are an individual with lactase nonpersistence, your levels of lactase are less than 10% of infantile levels.

Based on genetic predisposition, it would make sense that lactase activity would vary by ethnic group. The approximate percentage of low lactase activity by ethnic group and worldwide is as follows:

White	20%
Hispanic	50%
Black	75%
Native American	90%
Dutch	0%
French	32%
Filipino	55%

(Polin RA, Ditmar MF. Pediatric Secrets (5th edition); Mosby Elsevier, Philadelphia PA, 2011.)

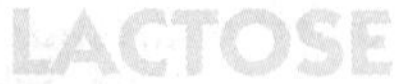

Lactose. Lactose is the naturally occurring sugar found in milk

Lactose intolerance. Many Americans have 'self-diagnosed' lactose intolerance because of the media hype surrounding this condition. Most of the individuals who are self-diagnosed actually can absorb lactose without any problem. However, as a result of their "self-diagnosis," these individuals are missing out on one of the best sources of vitamin D and calcium, as well as other essential proteins provided by milk and milk products.

New research suggests that individuals who have been definitively diagnosed with lactose intolerance may still be able to tolerate moderate amounts of this sugar. The key is to initially consume very small amounts of lactose. Start with one-half to one cup of milk with meals, and slowly increase the amount to one to two cups daily in two or three divided doses. If milk is consumed regularly, the bacteria in the large intestines can adapt and metabolize lactose. (Shaukat A, et al. Systemic review: Effective management strategies for lactose intolerance. *Annals of Internal Medicine 2010* (April); Levitt MD, et al. A commonsense approach to lactose intolerance. *Patient Care* 1997;31:185–187)

Lactose containing foods (amount of lactose).

Food	Amount of lactose
Yogurt (8 oz.)	10–15 grams
Milk (8 oz.)	10–12 grams
Ice cream (4 oz.)	4.5–5 grams
Hard cheese (1 oz)	0–1 mg

(*Environmental Nutrition,* December 1997; *Patient Care;* April 15, 1997.)

Lead. Lead poisoning is much more common in infants and children for various reasons. First, the blood-brain barrier is immature prior to the age of three, allowing lead to enter the brain more readily. Second, ingested lead has a 40% bioavailability in children, as compared to a 10% bioavailability in adults. Third, childhood behaviors associated with frequent hand-to-mouth gestures greatly increase the risk of lead ingestion. The recommended lead levels are less than 10 micrograms per deciliter (10 µg/dl). The Agency for Toxic Substances and disease registry estimates that approximately 17% of U.S. preschool children have abnormally high levels of lead, exceeding 15 µg/dl.

Serum lead levels once thought to be safe have been shown to be associated with IQ deficits, behavior disorders, slowed growth, and impaired hearing. The impairment of cognitive function begins at levels greater than 10 µg/dl, even though clinical symptoms are not apparent. Sources of exposure include lead-based paint (inner-city housing and old homes), soil and dust (near old lead-based painted houses with falling paint chips), tap water (hot tap water from old homes with lead solder on pipe connections), occupational and recreational exposures (furniture refinishing, stained glass or pottery making), airborne exposures (smelters or battery-manufacturing plants), dishware and canned foods.

Most china, porcelain, earthenware, and crystal contain varying amounts of lead used during the manufacturing process. However, if properly fired during manufacturing the dishes are not considered to be dangerous. Regulations vary from country to country. The U.S., Japan, and Great Britain have the strictest regulations on lead content. Imported food products may also be contaminated by lead used to solder cans. Foreign countries do not have to adhere to U.S. restrictions, so your canned refried beans from Mexico might be laced with lead.

One important point to remember: after years of use, lead may leach out of the china, porcelain, or crystal container. Avoid storing food or drink in these containers for long periods of time. If you desire to serve wine in a crystal decanter, this is perfectly safe and lovely. But don't *store* the wine in the decanter—either drink it all or pour it back in the original bottle. My suggestion, based on rigorous scientific research, is to drink the entire bottle.

Diets low in calcium, iron, and possibly protein increase the body's absorption and retention of lead, while a diet replete with these nutrients protects against lead build up.

Some people do wonderful things with leftovers—they throw them out.
—Anonymous

LEFTOVERS

Leftovers. Contrary to popular belief, do not allow leftovers to cool before you refrigerate them. You are just inviting bacteria to multiply if the food cools down below 140° F. The bugs will continue to multiply until food has cooled below 40° F. So, get those leftovers into the refrigerator as soon as possible, and don't worry about heating up the refrigerator with warm food! Put the leftovers in shallow containers to help the foods cool down as quickly as possible. In fact, if your freezer has a bit of room, throw the leftovers in the freezer temporarily to cool them faster. (Webb D. Nutrition myths that refuse to die continue to create confusion. *Environmental Nutrition,* September 2000.)

Leftovers—the 2/2/4 rule

- 2 hours from oven to refrigerator (refrigerate or freeze leftovers within 2 hours of cooking. Otherwise thrown them away)
- 2 inches thick to cool it quick (store food in a shallow pan at a shallow depth—about 2 inches to speed chilling)
- 4 days in the refrigerator—otherwise freeze it…use leftovers from the refrigerator within 4 days; exception: use stuffing and gravy within 2 days; reheat solid leftovers to 165° F and liquid leftovers to a rolling boil. Toss what you don't finish. (*Nutrition Action Healthletter*. March 2010)

HISTORICAL HIGHLIGHT

In the 1500s, a big kettle was often used for cooking. Every day families lit a fire and added vegetables to the pot with just a bit of meat. They would eat the stew or porridge for dinner, leaving leftovers in the pot to get cold overnight. The process would start all over again the next morning when more vegetables and small portions of meat were added. The stew could stay in the pot for days on end, spawning the rhyme, "Pease porridge hot, pease porridge cold, pease porridge in the pot, nine days old."

Legumes. The legume family includes an extensive variety of what are commonly referred to as "dried beans and peas." These include kidney beans, navy beans, pinto beans, black beans, cannellini beans, and other types of beans, as well as black-eye peas, split peas, and chick peas. Lentils and peanuts are also tossed in for good behavior. All legumes qualify as heart-healthy and colon-healthy proteins.

The B vitamin folate (folic acid), the insoluble fiber, and the top quality and quantity of protein all make legumes a food source not to be missed. Beans are also very low in sodium, unless you consume them straight out of a can. Canned beans have as much as 400 mg of sodium per half-cup. A quick and easy remedy for reducing the sodium by 40% is to rinse the canned beans under cold water before serving.

HISTORICAL HIGHLIGHT

In the mid-fourteenth century, Italians began to call glass eye disks "lentils." This was because of their resemblance in shape to the popular legume, the lentil, which is circular with biconvex surfaces. The Italian for "lentils" is lenticchie, and for more than two hundred years eyeglasses were known as "glass lentils." Lentil is the origin of our word "lens." Brilliant.

Lemons. Light up a lemon! Researchers are substituting inhaled citric or ascorbic acid derived from lemons for nicotine to facilitate smoking cessation. When inhaled in small quantities either of these acids simulates some of the respiratory tract sensations that accompany cigarette smoking. Smokers actually rated the respiratory tract sensations of a citric mist more enjoyable than puffs from low tar and nicotine cigarettes. (Rose JE. Nicotine and nonnicotine factors in cigarette addiction. *Psychopharmacology* 2006;184:274–285)

The custom of serving a slice of lemon with fish started way back in the Middle Ages. The acid of lemon juice was originally intended to dissolve a fish bone if accidentally swallowed by the diner. Today it's a delicious way to flavor the fish.

Leptin—(from the Greek "leptos," meaning thin). Leptin, the hormone of satiety, was first discovered in 1994 and was heralded as the be-all-and-end-all hormone for weight loss. Leptin is a hormone produced by fat cells in the body. Leptin signals the brain that we are full and that we can stop eating. Obviously, it doesn't seem to work in the majority of us. Genetically altered mice that lack the leptin gene become obese. Since they lack the leptin signal for fullness or satiety, it's a feeding frenzy from the get-go.

As soon as leptin was discovered weight loss experts were touting it as the beginning of the end of all of our weight loss problems. It was assumed that we could just bottle it and consume it on a daily basis and our weight problems would miraculously melt away. Unfortunately that hasn't been the case. We're still working on the weight loss issue, and leptin doesn't seem to be the quick fix that we once thought it was going to be.

Leptin levels, obesity, and C-reactive protein levels. C-reactive protein (CRP), an inflammatory protein that is especially abundant in the blood of obese individuals, inactivates leptin. Wow. Obese individuals typically produce the same amount of leptin that thin people do; however, CRP binds to leptin and prevents it from binding to its receptors. (Zhao AZ. *Nature*, April 2006).

Leptin and puberty. The leptin molecule may also be the signal for puberty. Preliminary studies have shown that when researchers inject young prepubescent female mice with leptin, the young "ladies" reach sexual maturity much earlier than their giggly prepubescent mice counterparts who only received a saline injection. This makes the leptin molecule a prime suspect as the principal initiator of puberty and links previously published data that ties the amount of fat cells in young girls to the onset of puberty. Rose E. Frisch and colleagues at the Harvard School of Public Health published the first paper showing that a critical amount of fat was necessary for puberty and continued ovulation. This landmark study was quite controversial back in 1974 when it was first published.

Over 100 studies have been published on the subject since that time. Evidence continues to build supporting the fat/leptin/puberty hypothesis in young girls. The verdict is still out on what triggers the onset of puberty in the male.

Leptin and weight loss. Let's revisit the leptin as a potential weight hormone. When weight is lost by reducing fat stores, leptin levels decline, sending a hunger signal to the brain that it's time to eat to replenish fat stores. This would obviously be to our advantage throughout evolution when food wasn't plentiful for our ancestors—especially foods such as French fries and Moon Pies. The body responded by developing a system to store an optimal

HISTORICAL HIGHLIGHT

Lettuce, as an aphrodisiac. Lettuce was considered a powerful aphrodisiac in the 9th century Egypt. Egyptian pharaohs would offer lettuce to the god of fertility—Min. The pharaohs would pray to Min and slip him a little lettuce on the side when they needed Egyptian women to conceive more soldiers for their armies.

amount of fat to draw upon in lean times. Times have changed dramatically. We have a potential for a caloric overload in today's environment that is readily accessible twenty-four hours a day, seven days a week. Drive-thru's, take outs, deliveries, sit downs, stand ups, recliners, and a never- ending supply of fat-laden, readily accessible food that leads to reward-driven eating. The result is the replenishment of fat stores without any endogenous signals.

Licorice root (Glycyrrhiza glabra or "sweet and smooth root"). Licorice root has been used for medicinal purposes and for flavoring foods for over 3,000 years. The Greeks, Egyptians, and Chinese worshipped this root. It is 50 times sweeter than sugar and is capable of masking pungent tastes in medicine. It is often used as a flavoring in cough syrups, throat lozenges, gum, candy, and tobacco. In fact, 90% of the licorice used in the United States is used to flavor tobacco products including cigarettes and chewing tobacco. Most of the "licorice" candies, including Twizzlers (the red ones), Good & Plenty, and black jelly beans in the United States are flavored with anise, not natural licorice. (Black Twizzlers contain natural licorice root extract in combination with anise oil.)

You might wonder why our candies in the U.S. contain mostly anise instead of the natural licorice root. Our Food and Drug Administration allows candy to contain up to 3% natural licorice by weight, but most contain no more than 2%, or about 0.5 gram in four twisted "ropes" of Twizzlers. In Europe, it's a different story. Black licorice, candy, and cough drops contain from 5% to 65% natural licorice.

Two or more "twists" of European black licorice per day for seven days can increase cortisol levels and result in a weight gain of one to five pounds. The main active ingredient of licorice is glycyrrhizin or glycyrrhetic acid, which has a chemical structure similar to aldosterone, the adrenal hormone responsible for sodium and water retention. This retention can lead to hypertension with headaches, vomiting, and photophobia. A syndrome resulting from the excessive intake of glycyrrhizin occurs during Halloween season. This is referred to as Halloween Hypertension, and is primarily seen in children during the week or two after Halloween. The physical assessment clue is a black tongue!

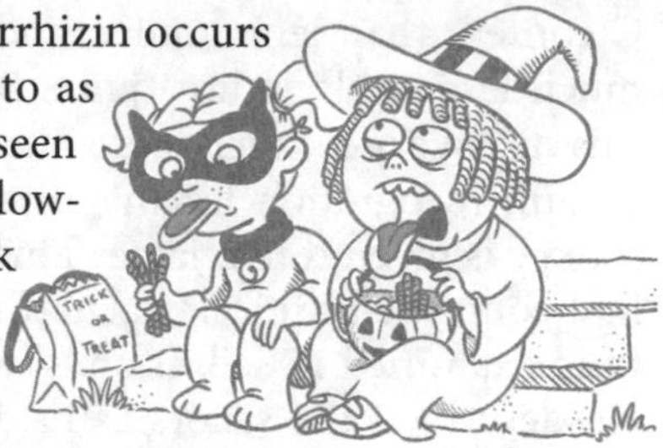

If natural licorice is taken for long periods of time, the sodium retention can result in potassium loss through the kidneys, resulting in clinically low potassium. Low potassium interferes with many physiologic functions including cardiac conduction and the result is an abnormal cardiac rhythm. Natural licorice can also potentiate potassium loss with drugs including the thiazide (hydrochlorothiazide) and loop diuretics (bumetanide/Bumex, furosemide/Lasix, ethacrynic acid/Edecrin, and torsemide/Demadex). Natural licorice in any form is not recommended for individuals with high blood pressure, heart disease, diabetes, or for pregnant or lactating women.

Why would you take natural licorice root as an alternative therapy? As a medicinal herb, licorice has been used to soothe irritated stomachs, squelch irritating coughs. Flavonoids, anti-inflammatory compounds present in licorice root, are thought to be responsible for soothing the lining of the upper GI tract and suppressing the cough reflex. Herbalists in Europe and the U.S. also use licorice root to treat stomach and duodenal ulcers and to treat adrenal insufficiency.

How much licorice should you take? Read all labels on any products before taking a slug for your cough. The recommended daily dose is 5–15 grams of the dried root made into a tea. Do not take licorice for longer than 4–6 weeks. Read the label, read the label, read the label. Did I mention that you should read the label? (Pronsky AM. *Food Medication Interactions*, 15th ed. 2008)

Lima beans. It's not often that one happens upon a delicious lima bean recipe. So, here's one to tempt the taste buds:

Sauté 1 chopped tomato and 3 diced garlic cloves in 2 Tbs. of olive oil. Add 2 cups of frozen lima beans and stir until heated through. Toss in 1 Tbs. of chopped parsley, 2 Tbs. of red wine vinegar, and salt and pepper to taste.

Limey. Limey is the American slang expression for British sailors, who regularly consumed lemons and limes and other citrus fruits to prevent scurvy on their long ocean voyages. This is somewhat of a misnomer, however, because if the truth is told, the lemon is better equipped to protect from scurvy (vitamin C deficiency) than the lime. Lime juice has lower vitamin

C content than lemon juice, and it appears that the vitamin C molecule is much less stable in lime juice. But enough of the specifics...the history of this discovery is much more interesting.

Full recognition for this discovery of the relationship of vitamin C to scurvy is given to Dr. James Lind, a British ship's surgeon credited with the first controlled clinical trial in the history of medicine. On May 20, 1747, Dr. Lind examined 12 sailors on board ship with signs and symptoms of scurvy. He described the sailors as having "putrid gums, the spots and lassitude, with the weakness of the knees." He divided the sailors into six groups, two sailors per group. One of the groups was given two oranges and one lemon per day, which he said, "They ate with greediness." By the end of six days one of the two was ready to return to duty and by the end of the trip (June 16, 1747) both sailors in the fruit group had recovered. The second sailor to recover was appointed as the nurse to the other patients. The other five groups received various combinations of other concoctions (including cider, wine, puddings, boiled biscuits with sugar, and mutton-broth) but they did not receive fresh fruit. None of the men in these other groups recovered from their scurvy.

There's no danger of my getting scurvy [while in England], as I have to consume at least two gin-and-limes every evening to keep the cold out.
—SJ Perelman (1904–1979)

Lime added to a Corona beer. Why does a bartender shove a lime wedge into the neck of the bottle of a Corona beer? Some people say that it keeps the flies out of the Corona...then why don't they shove limes down the bottle necks of all beers? Others claim that it disinfects the top of the beer bottle. Again, my point—why don't they shove lime wedges down any and all bottles of beer. And lastly, some people say that it masks the icky taste because of the clear bottle. None of the above is true.

It all started in 1981 when, reportedly on a bet with his good friend, a bartender crammed a lime wedge into the Corona bottle to see if it would start a trend. Well, now you know the rest of the story. It started a trend all right—it has been single handedly responsible for Corona beer overtaking Heineken as the best-selling imported beer in the U.S. beer market.

LISTERIA

Listeria monocytogenes. *Listeria* is an environmental foodborne pathogen that thrives in cold temperatures and can be found in water droplets on ceilings and floor drains. It is killed during pasteurization and heating, so prepared meats that are contaminated during processing and are not re-cooked are most susceptible. In addition to deli meats and other ready-to-eat meats (i.e. hot dogs, bologna), poultry products, smoked fish such as lox (smoked salmon), and refrigerated pâtés and meat spreads are perfect mediums for *Listeria.* Soft cheeses such as feta, brie, camembert, and blue-veined and Mexican-style varieties are also vulnerable to *Listeria.*

Listeriosis. Symptoms of *Listeria* infection can range from gastrointestinal symptoms with cramping, nausea, vomiting, and diarrhea to life-threatening meningitis (inflammation of the coverings of the brain). Cooking can kill bacteria, but many of the contaminated foods are not generally heated at home after possible contamination during processing. How many of you cook bologna before you slap it between two slices of white bread? Symptoms of *Listeria* can take up to two months to appear after someone has eaten contaminated food.

The latest outbreak of *Listeriosis* in cantaloupe was the most deadly food borne outbreak (30 died) in the U.S. since the1924 outbreak of typhoid in raw oysters in New York City that killed 150 people and sickened 1,500 throughout the United States.

You might be wondering how oysters became contaminated with *Listeria.* It's an interesting story. New York City was the center of the oyster trade business in the 1920s. Oysters that had been harvested were hung underwater in oyster baskets in the harbor to keep them alive before they were shipped by train on ice across the country. The problem was the location of the baskets when hung underwater for safe-keeping. Unfortunately the baskets were hung near an untreated sewage outtake pipe, and the sewage contained typhoid. Thanks to "refrigeration on ice" on the trains, the infected oysters were distributed throughout the U.S. The oysters were eaten raw when they reached their destination and a deadly outbreak ensued.

Let's get back to the 2011 cantaloupe outbreak of *Listeriosis.* The cantaloupe came from Jensen Farms near Holly, Colorado. The *Listeria* was found on the equipment in a packing facility at Jensen Farms, so the contamination occurred as the cantaloupes were being packaged for transport. *Listeria* was found on the outside rind of the cantaloupe and when consumers cut through the rind the *Listeria* was spread to the interior portion and eaten by the unsuspecting consumer. (*Centers for Disease Control,* 2011)

Lush. Dr. Thomas Lushington (1590–1661) has the distinction of having his name shortened to lush, the term fondly used for an individual who enjoys a little too much fruit of the vine. Dr. Lushington was an English chaplain known for his fondness for liquor. The term lush was actually originally used as a slang term for beer, but has evolved into the slang term for a drunkard.

Lutein. A number of studies have found a lower risk of both cataracts and advanced macular degeneration in patients who consume the highest amounts of the potent antioxidants, lutein and zeaxanthin.

Foods with the highest lutein and zeaxanthin levels include (½ cup with vegetables cooked):

Kale	11.9 mg
Spinach	10.2 mg
Swiss chard	9.6 mg
Collard greens	7.3 mg
Spinach (1 c raw)	3.7 mg
Peas, frozen	1.9 mg
Broccoli	1.2 mg
Romaine lettuce (1 c)	1.1 mg
Brussels sprouts	1.0 mg
Zucchini	1.0 mg

Other foods with lesser amounts lutein and zeaxanthin include asparagus, corn, green beans, iceberg lettuce, nectarines, and oranges. Don't forget that both lutein and zeaxanthin are also found in egg yolks—especially eggs that have been fortified. Lutein is better absorbed from eggs than from other lutein-rich foods like spinach. (Source: U.S. Department of Agriculture, 2011)

Lycopene is a red pigment known for its powerful antioxidant activity. Lycopene has twice the antioxidant properties as beta carotene. Lycopene belongs to the family of carotenoids that give vegetables and fruits their vibrant colors. This carotenoid just so happens to give tomatoes their lusciously deep red color. Other vegetables that contain lycopene include pink grapefruit, watermelon, and guava.

In order for the lycopene to exert its powerful effects tomatoes should be cooked. Cooking breaks down the cell walls in tomatoes and unleashes the effects of lycopene. By cooking the tomatoes in a little olive oil, lycopene will be absorbed even further, because it is fat-soluble.

So what are your best bets for adding lycopene to your diet? Tomato sauces top the list with twenty-three mg of lycopene per one-half cup serving. Watermelon also packs a powerful lycopene punch with 9–13 mg per cup and a half. Watermelon has 40% more lycopene than raw tomatoes. Salsa is at the bottom of the list with 3 mg per two tablespoons, and canned tomatoes sit right in the middle with 11 mg per ½ cup. (Tomatoes and lycopene: A case when fresh isn't best. *Environmental Nutrition,* March 1999; Arnold J. Watermelon packs a powerful lycopene punch. *Agricultural Research.* June 2002 (50):12–14)

Everything you have ever wanted to know about lycopene can be found at www.lycopene.com. This site is chock-full of research findings, recipes for lycopene-healthy eating, and of course, none other than the H.J. Heinz Company sponsors the site.

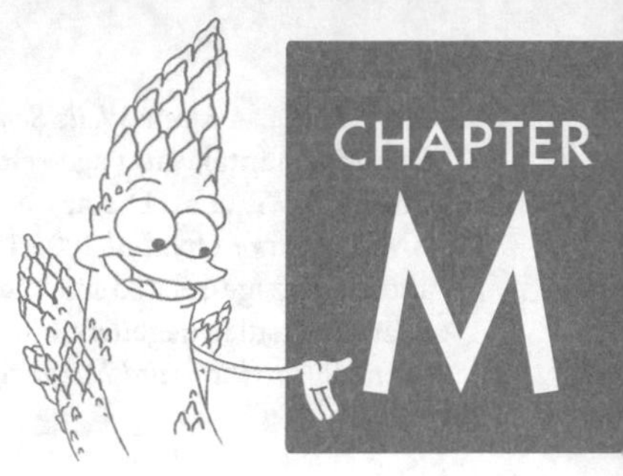

The 3-Martini lunch is the epitome of American efficiency. Where else can you get an earful, a bellyful, and a snootful at the same time?
— Gerald Ford

Macular degeneration. Age-related macular degeneration (AMD) is a common cause of impaired vision and blindness in older adults. Age-related macular degeneration is estimated to affect more than eight million individuals in the U.S. The advanced form of the disease affects more than 1.75 million individuals. AMD occurs when the cells in the central part of the retina (called the macula), degenerate, slowly resulting in blurred central vision. When the macula degenerates it is difficult for the patient to drive, read, or perform other activities that require central vision. Most macular degeneration is referred to as "dry" AMD. A rare form, "wet" AMD, occurs when abnormal blood vessels grow in the retina and lead blood and serum into the back of the eye. This can result in a sudden deterioration of vision.

How can this be prevented or delayed? Go straight to the produce counter and stock up on those "green leafys," especially spinach, kale, broccoli, and collard greens. These contain the antioxidants lutein and zeaxanthin, and may reduce the incidence of age-related macular degeneration by as much as 43%. Beta carotene is another antioxidant that has been shown to slow down the progress of AMD. Next stop—the seafood counter. Stock up on the fish that contain the highest amounts of omega-3 fatty acids. A study in the March 2000 *Archives of Ophthalmology* found that older adults who ate fish more than once a week had only half the risk of AMD as those who ate it less than once a month. Third stop—the vitamin and dietary supplement section of the grocery store. Vitamin C and vitamin E, potent antioxidants, may help reduce the risk of developing AMD and decrease the progression of the disease. Last stop—look in the B section of the dietary supplements and consider buying the herb bilberry. Preliminary studies suggest that bilberry extract may halt the progression of AMD as well as cataracts. And, lastly, you may want to make sure you get enough zinc in your diet. The mineral zinc has also been associated with a reduction in the incidence of

AMD. (*Dr. Andrew Weil's Self Healing,* March 2001; Smith W, Mitchell P, Leeder SR. Dietary fat and fish intake and age-related maculopathy. *Arch of Ophthal* 2000 (March);118:401–404; Chong EWT, et al. Dietary omega-3 fatty acid and fish intake in the primary prevention of AMD. *Arch of Ophthal* 2008;126:826–833; van Leeuwen et al. Dietary intake of antioxidants and risk of age-related macular degeneration. *JAMA* 2005;294:3101–3107; Johnson EJ. Age-related macular degeneration and antioxidant vitamins: recent findings. *Current Opinion in Clinical Nutrition and Metabolic Care* 2010;13:28–33)

ASPARAGUS TIP

Since the "wet" form of AMD is due to bleeding beneath the retina it would be prudent to have patients, friends, and family with this condition avoid any dietary supplements that predispose to bleeding. These dietary supplements include garlic, ginkgo, ginger, glucosamine, large doses of vitamin E, and greater than 3 grams of omega-3 fatty acids per day. Each of these dietary supplements inhibits platelet aggregation and predisposes the individual to bleeding.

MAD COW DISEASE

Mad cow disease. This devastating neurological deterioration is fatal in all cases—whether you are a sheep, a cow, a cannibal, or a human with non-cannibalistic preferences. In sheep the disease is referred to as scrapie (SCRAY-pee); in cows it is known as bovine spongiform encephalopathy (BSE), or as the tabloid term, "mad cow disease"; in the Fore cannibal tribe of New Guinea it is known as kuru; and in non-cannibalistic humans it is referred to as variant Creutzfeldt-Jakob disease (vCJD).

Creutzfeldt-Jakob disease (CJD) is a form of brain damage that leads to a rapid decrease in cognitive function and movement. The disorder is extremely rare, occurring in about 1 per 1 million people. It manifests between the ages of 20 and 70, but usually presents in the late 50s. The causative factor is believed to be a prion, a protein that causes normal proteins in the brain to fold abnormally. CJD is classified as either classic CJD or variant CJD. The classic types of CJD are sporadic and familial. The age of onset of the sporadic form is 65. The familial form may present earlier. The familial form is rare—most cases are sporadic. Classic CJD is *not* related to mad cow disease, however, the brain pathology is similar.

The first cases of "mad cow" disease appeared in Britain twenty-six years ago, November, 1986 to be exact. At that time it was called the "mystery brain disease" that was killing the England's dairy cows. Cows were observed to be disoriented, irritable, apprehensive, and unable to stand or walk without a staggering, unsteady gait. Since the cows were exhibiting bizarre behaviors the phrase "mad cow disease" emerged. Autopsies on the bovine (cow) brain revealed "spongy" areas, and the name bovine spongioform encephalopathy (BSE) was given to this disease in cattle. The pathologic findings in the cow's brains were similar to those seen in humans dying of CJD and in sheep dying of scrapie. (The term scrapie originates from the behavior of sheep with this illness: the disoriented sheep would stand next to a barn or fence and continually scrape their flanks against the structures until they started bleeding.)

Cattle throughout Europe were involved, but the United Kingdom was hardest hit. The disease reached a peak in 1992 with more than 37,280 new confirmed cases in cattle that year. In all, 184,500 cattle were found to be infected with BSE in over 600 herds. (CDC, Department of Health and Human Services. www.cdc.gov/ncidod/dvrd/bse/; Coghlan A. Curtain falls on mad cow disease. *New Scientist* 2011 (January 29): 6–7)

Through February 2010, BSE surveillance identified a total of 21 cases in cattle in North America: three BSE cases in the U.S. and 18 cases in Canada. Of the three cases in the U.S. one came from Canada. Of the 18 cases identified in Canada, one was imported from England.

The first confirmed human case of the "mystery brain disease" occurred in 1994 and the first death occurred in May 1995 in England. In 1996, ten additional British citizens were diagnosed with "mad cow" disease. Since their brain tissue resembled that of cows with bovine spongioform encephalopathy as well as that of humans dying of CJD, the British pathologists named it variant CJD (vCJD).

Since 1996, 170 people worldwide have died from vCJD. Other European nations with deaths from vCJD include Italy, Germany, France, Spain, Ireland, Belgium, Denmark, Luxembourg, the Netherlands, Switzerland, and Liechtenstein. The average age of death in patients with the variant form, vCJD, is 28, compared to age 70 in patients with the non-variant CJD. It appears as if the crisis is over. The number of deaths from vCJD in 2011 was in single digits.

Three cases of vCJD have been reported in the United States. Variant CJD cases are ascribed to the country of initial symptom onset, regardless of where the exposure occurred. There is strong evidence to suggest that two of the three cases in the U.S. were exposed to the BSE agent in England (onset of symptoms occurred in 2001 and 2005 while living in England) and that the third case was exposed while living in Saudi Arabia (onset of symptoms occurred in 2006).

The cause of BSE is a mutant prion.This is not a virus, parasite, bacteria, fungus, or any other type of known infectious agent. In fact, the brains of all mammals (and that includes the human mammal) contain structural proteins in the brain known as prions. An unknown trigger causes prions to undergo a structural "unfolding," causing the surrounding brain tissue to degenerate. Once the prion unfolds, the damage to neighboring tissue results in a progressive, unremitting, and rapid deterioration of mental and motor function.

The most likely trigger for vCJD is the consumption of brain or spinal cord tissue from another infected animal. The consumption of cattle infected with the mutant prion was the cause of BSE in Europe. The cattle were infected by eating rendered meat-and-bone meal protein supplements made from sheep, cows, pigs, poultry, roadkill, and any other dead animals that happened upon the rendering machine. The renderings of sheep with scrapie and the renderings of other cattle with BSE have been blamed for the outbreak of BSE. (Rendering, by the way, is the process of boiling and grinding up carcasses of dead animals—including bones, brains, spinal cords, and internal organs.)

As the outbreak unfolded, the FDA, USDA, and other regulatory agencies in the United States actually worked together (surprise) and safeguards were put into place almost immediately. First of all, as far back as 1950, long before vCJD appeared, the USDA banned the importation of sheep and goats to the U.S. Why? A flock of British sheep was reported to have scrapie and even though there was no inkling that a problem would occur in the future, the USDA decided to be proactive and ban sheep and goats from entering the US. The importation of cattle from England was banned in 1989. Fewer than 500 cows from the British Isles made it across the Atlantic Ocean in the 1980s. Only 32 of the approximate 500 cows entered the food chain. The chance that even one cow was infected was one in 10 billion. Beef exports resumed from England in 2006.

Second, the FDA has prohibited animal-feed mills from mixing meat and bone meal made from rendered cows and sheep into feed for other cows and sheep. The supplements can be fed to swine and poultry because they do not get BSE-like illnesses from food.

The third reason it will be tough for BSE to make its way into our food chain is because of the good old McDonald's fast food restaurant chain. Even though we can argue that their fries and burgers might be causing a myriad of other health problems when consumed daily, they are adamant that their hamburger sources are free of contamination. And, when McDonald's talks, everyone listens. McDonald's rules the roost when it comes to beef sales throughout the world. They mandate that any cattle used for its all-beef patties should have documentation that they have not been fed meat-and-bone meal made from rendered cows and sheep. No one wants to lose McDonald's as a customer by sneaking in a few rendered cattle.

Finally, the beef industry banned the use of stun guns to prepare cattle for slaughter. The explosive blast from the stun gun blew brain tissue throughout the carcass, causing a potential route of infection with prions from nervous system tissue. In cows with BSE, brain tissue is highly infectious.

Hmmmm, you say. If people didn't eat cow brains or spinal cords, how did they acquire this illness? Most likely from eating inexpensive beef products that contained mechanically separated meat. This type of meat is a paste produced by compressing carcasses. This paste may have contained spinal cords and was used in preparing hot dogs, sausages, and burgers. Do we use mechanically separated meat in the U.S.? Yes, but rarely. And the label on the package must state if a product contains mechanically separated beef. Unfortunately, there are no labels on hot dogs purchased from hot dog stands, or on beef sausages at your favorite breakfast establishment.

Did vegetarians acquire vCJD? Yes. Their exposure was hypothesized to be through milk or gelatin (which is made from beef). Or, vCJD may incubate for decades and the vegetarian may have eaten infected beef in the years prior to becoming a vegetarian.

Mad cow disease and kosher meat. Can eating kosher meat reduce the risk of developing mad cow disease? If you're still worried after the last discussion, the answer is yes. Eating kosher meat can virtually guarantee a mad cow disease-free meal. Why?

1) Mad cow disease occurs mainly in older cows. Cattle chosen for kosher meat are usually between 18 and 24 months. The current USDA's age limit for cows chosen for human consumption is under 30 months. In other words, cows that have the highest risk for carrying the agent responsible for Mad Cow disease are cows over the age of 30 months. In April 2009 our FDA made a final ruling barring brains and spinal cords from cattle 30 months and older in all animal feed, including pet food.
2) "Downers" cannot be used for kosher meat. What is a "downer"? Downers are cows that are sick, injured, or unable to walk. Many cows with mad cow disease appeared sick and wobbly, and were considered "downers." The person who selects the cows for kosher meat, known as a "shochet," is trained to detect any signs of illness. If present, the cow is obviously not chosen for kosher consumption. The USDA banned the use of "downers" for consumption in 2005.
3) The animal used for kosher meat is killed as quickly as possible by severing the carotid arteries with one swift stroke of the shochet's knife. Cattle for nonkosher markets have traditionally been killed by a "stun" gun that injects pressurized air into the skulls. This high pressure can theoretically scatter brain or spinal cord tissue throughout the body of the cow. As mentioned previously, the USDA has also banned this stun gun procedure.
4) And, finally, even though this has no proven benefit for reducing the transmission of mad cow disease, kosher meat is prepared by draining all of the blood from the animal. This is accomplished by soaking the meat in water, covering it with coarse kosher salt, and then washing it. This salting process may also make kosher meat safer from contamination with bacteria from the cow's bowel, including *E. Coli O157:H7* and *Salmonella.*
5) One last word for the non-kosher folks reading this blurb— certified organic meats also provide a high level of safety standards. So, either go kosher or go organic to reduce your risk of mad cow disease to practically zero. Zilch, Nada. (*Environmental Nutrition,* May 2004)

Magnesium. Magnesium is a metallic element that plays a major role in human metabolism. Sixty percent of stored magnesium is found in bone and 38% in skeletal muscle and other soft tissues. The free "ionic" form of magnesium is available in the body to move wherever it's needed, hence the term "free." Only 1% to 2% of magnesium is in the free ionic form. Research links magnesium to more than 300 enzyme systems. Magnesium is essential for the formation of the energy-producing cyclic adenosine monophosphate. Many of the conditions that magnesium supplementation benefits involve muscular or vascular tone. Decreased magnesium levels have been studied in relation to migraines, heartburn, hypertension, asthma, preterm labor, cardiac arrhythmias, diabetes, osteoporosis and constipation. Who can forget those commercials for Phillips Milk of Magnesia?

Women need 360 mg per day for ages 14 through 18, or 310 mg per day from ages 19–30, and 320 mg per day for 30 and over; men need 410 mg per day for ages 14 through 18, 400 mg for ages 19–30, and 420 mg for over 30. The upper limit from supplements **alone** should not exceed 350 mg/day. The total amount of magnesium from supplements and diet should not exceed 700 mg per day. (Dietary Guidelines for Americans 2010; http://www.cnpp.usda.gov/DGAs2010-DGACReport.htm)

So why is the average American deficient in this element? For starters, the average American doesn't consume enough magnesium to replace what he/she is losing through urine on a daily basis. The biggest reason for the under consumption is that magnesium is not found in pizza, French fries, hamburgers, and processed foods. It is, however, found in the foods that most Americans do not consume in adequate amounts. This includes leafy green vegetables, whole grains, beans, and nuts. For example, a slice of whole-wheat bread has 24 milligrams of magnesium while a slice of white bread has only 6 milligrams of magnesium. Once a whole grain has been refined and made into white flour, certain nutrients are re-introduced, but magnesium isn't one of them. It appears that in order to consume approximately 400 mg daily you will need to eat an all-around healthful diet. Go figure.

The following is a list of magnesium-containing foods—you have no excuse not to get enough magnesium in your diet, there are plenty of foods to choose from.

1 oz dry roasted almonds (24 nuts) ....86 mg
1 oz Brazil nuts, unblanched (6-8 nuts)...........107 mg
2 shredded wheat biscuits ....80 mg
1 cup of cooked spinach ....163 mg
1 medium baked potato with skin ....55 mg
1 cup plain, low-fat yogurt...................................43 mg
½ cup cooked brown rice.....................................42 mg
½ cup vegetarian baked beans.............................40 mg
½ cup canned white beans ....67 mg

1 banana..32 mg
1 cup skim milk..28 mg
3 oz. grilled salmon..28 mg
1 (1-oz slice whole-wheat bread)...............................24 mg

A good way to remember magnesium in food is to remember that foods high in fiber are usually high in magnesium. So, beans, vegetables, seeds, and nuts tend to be on all lists for magnesium-containing foods.

What are the symptoms of magnesium deficiency? Premenstrual syndrome, leg muscle cramps, coldness of the extremities, weakness, anorexia, nausea, digestive disorders, lack of coordination and confusion have all been reported with low levels of magnesium. Low levels of magnesium have also been demonstrated during migraine headaches.

Another interesting way to get a dose of magnesium is to drink hard water. Whoa, you say...yes, in fact, drinking hard water, containing magnesium, calcium, and other minerals it contains—reduces the risk of heart disease, according to new research from Finland. The harder the water in areas of Finland, the lower the incidence of heart attacks. It appears as if fluoride in the water also reduces the cardiovascular risk. (*UC Berkeley Wellness Letter,* June 2004) (*American Journal of Clinical Nutrition,* 55: 1992;1018. and *The Journal of Clinical Epidemiology,* 48: 1995;927; Sun-Edelstein C and Mauskop A. Food and Supplements in the management of migraine headaches. *Clin J of Pain.* June 2009;25(5):446–452)

Magnesium and cardiovascular benefits. Women with the highest intakes of magnesium containing foods (more than 345 mg per day) have a 34% reduced risk of sudden cardiac death compared to women who don't get enough magnesium in their diet. A study published in the February 2011 issue of *The American Journal of Clinical Nutrition* examined the magnesium intake in 88,375 healthy women, and the results were definitive. Higher intakes of magnesium were definitely associated with the lowest risks of sudden cardiac death. Magnesium deficiency can lead to dangerous cardiac arrhythmias, particularly when the heart is already compromised with chronic heart failure or an acute coronary event such as a myocardial infarction. Cardiac patients are often treated with oral or intravenous forms of magnesium to prevent these life-threatening arrhythmias.

Magnesium and diabetes. In a 2007 study of more the 85,000 women, the Harvard Nurses' Health Study, almost 43,000 men in the Harvard Health Professionals Follow-Up study, and some 40,000 women in the Iowa Women's Health Study—all suggest that people with the highest levels of magnesium in their diets have the lowest risk for developing type 2 diabetes. Magnesium is required for the secretion of insulin from the pancreas. Without enough magnesium, the pancreas will fail to secrete the needed amount of insulin to control blood glucose levels. Insulin becomes ineffective, the patient becomes less insulin-sensitive, and the trek toward the development of type 2 diabetes has begun. People with diabetes also tend to have reduced stores of magnesium and to excrete more magnesium in their urine than individuals without diabetes. (Larsson SC, Wolk A. Magnesium intake and risk of type 2 diabetes: A meta-analysis. *J Intern Med.* 2007;262:208–214)

Magnesium and hypertension. Physiologically, magnesium affects blood pressure by facilitating the endothelial resting tone and smooth-muscle reactivity.

Magnesium also exerts a mild calcium channel blockade, resulting in a vasodilatory effect, and reduces inflammation and oxidative stress. In 12 clinical trials on patients with established hypertension, magnesium supplementation demonstrated an impressive reduction in diastolic (the bottom number) blood pressure. (Beyer FR et al. Combined calcium, magnesium and potassium supplementation for the management of primary hypertension in adults. *Cochrane Database Syst.* Rev. 2006)

Magnesium and kidney disease. Eating a diet high in magnesium does not pose a health risk, but people with renal disease can receive too much if they take a multivitamin or supplement with additional magnesium. Neuromuscular toxicity is the most common complication of too much magnesium.

Magnesium and migraines. Studies have shown that there are low brain levels of magnesium during migraine attacks. Also, "migraineurs" have systemic magnesium deficiency. A small number of women who suffer from migraine headaches may be deficient in magnesium. In one of two small studies, patients who took 600 mg of magnesium a day for 12 weeks went from three attacks per month to two. That might not sound like a lot; however, if you are the one with debilitating migraine headaches, this reduction may be a lifesaver. (*Cephalgia* 16; 257, 1996; Sun-Edelstein C, Maskop A. Food and supplements in the management of migraine headaches. *Clin J of Pain* 2009 (June);25(5):446–452)

Magnesium and osteoporosis. It appears that magnesium is also important for strong bones and for the prevention of osteoporosis. Choosing a calcium supplement with magnesium may give an added boost for bone protection, but eating foods high in magnesium can be just as beneficial. (www.iom.com)

Magnesium and preterm labor. Magnesium deficiency can be an acute problem during pregnancy. Magnesium plays a role in fetal growth and development and is essential in controlling uterine muscle wall excitability. Preterm labor is thought to be related to low magnesium levels and is the most common condition treated with intravenous magnesium. (Durlach J. New data on the importance of gestational Mg deficiency. *J Am Coll Nutr.* 2004 Dec;23(6):694S–700S)

MALNUTRITION

Malnutrition in the elderly. There is no uniformly accepted definition of malnutrition in older adults. Commonly used definitions include the following:

In community-dwelling older adults:

- Involuntary weight loss (e.g., greater than or equal to 10 lb. [4 kg] over 6 months; or greater than or equal to 4% of the total body weight over 1 year)
- Abnormal body mass (e.g., BMI greater than 27; BMI less than 22)
- Hypoalbuminemia (e.g., less than or equal to 3.5 g/dl) (albumin has a half-life of 18–20 days, prealbumin has a half-life of 48 hours and may be valuable in monitoring nutritional recovery)
- Hypocholesterolemia (e.g., less than 160 mg/dl)
- Specific vitamin or micronutrient deficiencies (e.g., vitamin B12)

In hospitalized older patients:

- Dietary intake (e.g., less than 50% of estimated caloric intake)
- Hypoalbuminemia (e.g., less than 3.5 g/dl)
- Hypocholesterolemia (e.g., less than 160 mg/dl)

Nursing-home patients

- Weight loss of greater than or equal to 5% in past 30 days; greater than or equal to 10% in 180 days
- Dietary intake less than 75% of most meals

Focus on whether the following issues may be affecting nutritional status:

- Economic barriers to securing food
- Availability of sufficiently high-quality food
- Dental problems that preclude ingesting food
- Functional disability that interferes with shopping, preparing meals, or feeding
- Poor appetite
- Food preferences or cultural beliefs that interfere with adequate food intake
- Depressive symptoms
- Medical illnesses that:
    - o Interfere with digestion or absorption of food
    - o Increase nutritional requirements
    - o Require dietary restrictions

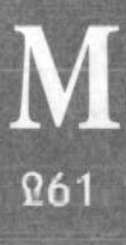

Malnutrition and nutritional supplements. Protein and energy supplements appear to have beneficial effects in elderly patients with malnutrition. Weight gain, decreased mortality, and shorter hospital stays are three major benefits. Nutritional supplements include Boost and Boost Plus (50% more calories than Boost), Ensure and Ensure Plus (50% more calories than Ensure), Carnation Instant Breakfast lactose-free and Carnation Instant Breakfast lactose-free Plus (50% more calories than Carnation Instant Breakfast lactose-free). All protein and energy supplements have 40 and 55 grams of protein per liter, as well as sodium and potassium. Boost Plus is the only nutritional supplement with fiber.

MANGO

Mango. The common mango or Indian mango originated in Southeast Asia thousands of years ago and is one of the most cultivated fruits of the tropical world. More than one third of all mangos are cultivated in India. The taste of the mango fruit has been described as a combination of nectarine, a pineapple, and an orange.

The mango is a nutritionist's dream. Rich in vitamin C (76% of the daily value), vitamin A (25% of the daily value), and potassium (257 mg), mangos also contain an ample amount of fiber (3 grams). Each mango has approximately 110 calories.

ASPARAGUS TIP

The mango peel and the sap of the mango both contain urushiol, the chemical that causes the itchy, miserable dermatitis that some people experience upon exposure to poison ivy and/or poison oak. People with a history of poison ivy or poison oak may develop a contact dermatitis when handling mangos. During mango's primary season, it is the most common source of plant dermatitis in Hawaii.

MARGARINE

Margarine. Just exactly what is margarine? Both sticks and tubs of margarine must contain 80% vegetable oil (the rest is mostly milk and water). You can call a product margarine if it's made with less vegetable oil as long as it's called reduced-fat, light, low-fat, or fat-free. Without the above descriptors, margarine with less than 80% oil must be called "vegetable oil spreads," a generic name for margarine.

Traditional stick margarines contain 100 calories per tablespoon and is the least healthful of all margarines. It's higher in fat and trans fats than tub margarine. Total fat for 1 tablespoon is 11 grams, with trans fats of 2 grams and saturated fats of 2 grams.

Traditional tub margarines have 70 calories per tablespoon, 8 total grams of fat, with 0 trans fats and 1.5 grams of saturated fats. Regular tub margarines contain 61% to 79% vegetable oil and are now labeled trans-fat-free. Companies add olive oil, yogurt, sweet cream buttermilk to entice you to buy them, but truth be told, the additions are not present in enough quantities to be of any health benefits. Not so for calcium added to margarines—most have 100 mg per tablespoon and this is helpful for a boost.

Reduced Fat/Calorie Tub Margarine (60% or less oil and 25% less fat) has 50 calories per tablespoon, 6 grams of saturated fat, 0 grams of trans fats, and

1 gram of saturated fat. Light/low-fat Tub Margarine has 40% or less oil and 50% less fat, with 5 grams of saturated fat, 0 grams of trans fats, and 1 gram of saturated fat.

How about spray products…5 sprays is the equivalent of one tablespoon and 5 calories—no fats. (*Environmental Nutrition,* April 2007)

Margarine or butter? Butter or margarine? Which one is better? Butter? Well, neither of the choices wins the contest for health food extraordinaire. They are both full of the "bad" fats—either saturated fats in butter or trans fats in margarine. Margarine might be considered the more ominous of the two, because of its trans fats. Now, having said that, not all margarines are created equal in terms of trans fat content. As a general rule of thumb, the softer the margarine, the less trans fat it contains. Margarine that comes in a tub container is better for you than stick margarine. You can also check the grocery shelves for the trans fat-free margarines or the "smart-margarines" that contain plant sterols or stanols. (See Chapter P for plant stanols and sterols)

MARTINI

Martini. The martini cocktail was invented in 1863 by a San Francisco bartender named Jerry Thomas. He purportedly named the drink after the town of Martinez upon learning that this was the destination of a departing customer.

Martinis should be shaken, not stirred. Was James Bond right after all? The shaken martini contains more microscopic shards of ice, giving it a more pleasant texture or "mouthfeel." In addition, the shaken martini helps reduce the taste of residual oil left over when vodka is made from potatoes, the base vegetable used at the time Ian Fleming wrote his James Bond books. (University of Western Ontario, *British Medical Journal* 2010; 310:1600)

MAYONNAISE

Mayonnaise, the origins. There are many popular theories on the origin of mayonnaise. Of course, the Romans and the Egyptians had their version of mayonnaise—a combination of oil and eggs they used to mask the flavor of rotten food. The *real* origin of mayonnaise is most likely in the middle of the 18th century. It is believed that the recipe was acquired from the town of Mahón in Minorca in 1756 after a victory over the British by Louis-Francois Armand du Plessis de Richelieu. Whoa. Is that one, two or three guys? The French originally dubbed it Mahonaisse and it was considered a delicacy in Europe. The Spanish called it *mahonesa.* In American it was known as mayonnaise, and it was regarded as a delicacy for only the most elegant meals. Finally, in 1921, a German immigrant and delicatessen owner, Richard Hellman, (ringing any bells?), began packing it and selling it in jars from his New York deli. He named it Hellman's Mayonnaise and it became the first mass-merchandised condiment that we all know and love on our sandwiches today.

Mayonnaise—a new use for creepy crawly head lice. Instead of slathering that mayonnaise on your next ham and cheese sandwich, consider slathering it on your child's lice infected noggin first. For patients whose pediculosis (head lice) persists despite the usual treatments, try the following:

Liberally apply plain mayonnaise (any kind) to the patient's hair, cover the scalp with a plastic bag (not their entire head!!) and expose the head to sunlight.

This method has been shown to be effective at killing lice and nits (Clinical Pearl, Cathy Clark, APRN-C, Basset, Nebraska) (*Clinician Reviews* 2006; 16(10):50).

Mayonnaise—other uses. Mothers have used mayonnaise to cool the burn of the sun, to smother blood-sucking ticks, and as a popular hair conditioner in the 1970s. So what if your head smelled like a tuna fish sandwich.

McDONALDS

McDonalds—SUPER SIZE ME. In 2003, a film-maker named Morgan Spurlock decided to eat at McDonald's for 30 days, three meals a day. Spurlock gained 24 pounds in those 30 days and named the movie SUPER SIZE ME (2004). And it wasn't just the weight—he was depressed, he had erectile dysfunction and his liver was chock full o' fat.

Wow. No sex, a fatty liver, and depression—why would you do that to yourself? Apparently his goal was to make a statement about the link between fast food, obesity, and clinical disease.

The film premiered at the Sundance Film Festival in 2004. Obviously it made an impression on someone from McDonald's. Shortly after the film was launched nationwide, McDonald's not only phased out the SUPER SIZE option from their menu they also began offering a line of healthier alternatives.

The average American will eat at McDonald's 1,811 times in his or her life. Only 4 percent of Americans say they didn't eat at a McDonald's restaurant in the previous year.

A 29-year Big Mac attack. From April 1972 to May 2001, Donald Gorske of Fond du Lac, Wisconsin downed two Big Macs every day. After finishing 18,000 Big Macs he was assured of his spot in the *Guinness Book of World Records.* By polishing off 18,000 Big Macs, the 6-foot, 178-lb prison guard has eaten the equivalent of 800 heads of lettuce, 820 onions, 1,900 whole pickles, 563 pounds of cheese, almost 100 gallons of special sauce, 14.5 head of beef cattle, 6,250,000 sesame seeds and 18,000 buns.

M&Ms. One of the biggest sellers for the Mars Company is M&Ms. The average number of M&Ms per standard package is 57, give or take one or two. Of that number, 33% are dark brown, 25% are yellow, 19% are orange,

14% are blue, and 9% are green. Since the green M&Ms have the folklore reputation of being a powerful aphrodisiac, one wonders if the Mars Company hasn't lost its libido. Each M&M has 4.2 calories.

In 1976 the Mars Company took red M&Ms off the market, responding to the mass hysteria triggered by the media, which hyped the notion that red M&Ms were made with the carcinogenic red dye number 2. This wasn't true; red dye number 2 was not used. However, the damage was done. The teeming masses became so hysterical that canceling red M&Ms was the company's only recourse. Red M&Ms have since been reintroduced to the market without the mass hysteria. Red M&Ms are colored with red dye number 3, a noncarcinogenic chemical additive.

The M&M was named after Victor Mars (the owner and founder of Mars Company) and his associate Mr. Merrie. They developed the M&Ms as a taste treat in 1941.

MEAT

Meat. If you are a typical American, you ate nearly 220 pounds of meat last year. In 2008 the world consumed about 280 million tonnes of meat. (UN Food and Agriculture Organization, 2010)

Meat-eater. Meat-eater is a slang term for a policeman or politician who accepts or extorts bribes (graft).

Meat, lean. Lean beef cuts include eye or round roast or steak (143 calories, 1 g saturated fat, 4 g of total fat), sirloin tip side steak (143 calories, 2 g of saturated fat, 4 g of total fat), top round roast and steak (178 calories, 2 g saturated fat, 5 g of total fat), bottom round roast and steak (150 calories, 2 g saturated fat, 6 g of total fat), top sirloin steak (180 calories, 3 g saturated fat, 8 g of total fat). All nutritional values are based on a 3-oz. serving of cooked beef. (Women's Nutrition Connection, April 2012)

Meat and kidneys. How does animal protein harm the kidneys? The harmful effect of animal protein on the kidneys is associated with its high content of valine and lysine, amino-acid building blocks of protein. Valine and lysine are present in much higher concentration in meat than in dairy products, and are completely absent from vegetable protein. These two amino acids contribute to edema and intraglomerular hypertension (high blood pressure within the vessels of the kidney) in the kidneys that have already been damaged, contributing to acceleration of kidney failure.

Meatless Mondays. The Meatless Monday campaign began in 2003 in an effort to reduce meat consumption in the U.S. by going one day a week without eating meat. By going meatless one day a week, the average American can reduce saturated fat intake by 15 percent. Monday was picked because studies suggest that people are more likely to stick with changes in behavior if they begin those changes on Monday.

Why don't you try substituting plant-based proteins one day a week? A perfect way to remember to do this would be to try a month of meatless Mondays. Instead of plopping a piece of chicken, fish, or meat on your plate and building a meal around it, consider some of the following options:

- Quinoa and beans (see Chapter Q)
- Whole wheat pita bread with tomato sauce, mozzarella cheese and ricotta cheese
- Spinach salad with tofu
- Yogurt with nuts and berries

Lots of choices, give it a try. Say yes to Meatless Mondays and reward yourself with 'tini' Tuesdays. That would be martini Tuesdays—see Chapter A for the benefits of alcohol.

Meat and mortality. A 2009 study by the National Cancer Institute found that people who eat the most red meat and processed meat have a higher risk of death than those eating the least. In the study the patients with the highest meat intake averaged 2.2 ounces per 1,000 calories per day. On a 2,000 calorie daily diet, that's like eating a quarter-pound hamburger per day, or nearly 2 pounds of beef and port in one week. Higher consumption of poultry and fish was associated with a lower death rate. Step away from the red meat table, folks. Perhaps a meatless Monday, Tuesday, and Wednesday would be prudent for a longer, healthier life.

Meat packers. Perhaps the most famous of all meat packers in North America was Sam Wilson of Troy, New York. His nickname was Uncle Sam Wilson and he supplied meat to the troops during the War of 1812. The beef Wilson shipped out was stamped with the initials U.S., and although he intended the U.S. as an abbreviation for the United States, it also came to be identified with Wilson himself, or Uncle Sam. Cartoonists of the time portrayed him with the white goatee, dressed in a top hat and the patriotic colors of red, white, and blue. In 1961 Congress made Uncle Sam official as the United States "mascot," so to speak.

MEDITERRANEAN DIET

Mediterranean diet. What is the Mediterranean diet? Well, if you have a history of heart disease or if you have already had a myocardial infarction (heart attack), you may want to listen up. The Mediterranean diet is rich in fruits, vegetables, whole grains, legumes, and fish, with 30% of the calories from fat but only 8% of the fat calories as saturated fat. And, you get to throw in a glass of wine along with your meal. Twelve years ago a study in the February 16, 1999, issue of the journal *Circulation,* found that patients with heart disease who followed the Mediterranean diet guidelines had a 50–70% lower risk of a second heart attack in the four years of follow-up, as compared with the patients who followed the traditional western diet of 34% fat, with 12% of the total fats as saturated fats. The authors of the study cited the omega-3 fatty acids found fish, nuts, canola oil, and flaxseed as playing a major role in cardiac protection. A 20-year follow-up from the Nurses' Health Study in 2009 found that the nurses with the greatest adherence to the Mediterranean diet had a significantly lower cardiovascular mortality rate. (Fung TT et al. Mediterranean diet and incidence of mortality from coronary artery disease and stroke in women. *Circulation* 2009;119:1093–1100)

Numerous studies over the past 10 years have reported the similar results. Do you need information on how to switch to a Mediterranean-style diet? Call your local nutritionist for a consultation or go straight to the local bookstore and purchase one of the many cookbooks that have been written on the subject.

Mediterranean diet and Alzheimer's disease. The Mediterranean diet, characterized by high intakes of fruits, vegetables, and cereals and low intakes of meat and dairy products, lowered the risk of Alzheimer's disease by 38% over a four-year period.

Seven nutrients most often reported in studies related either positively or negatively to Alzheimer's disease include saturated fatty acids, monounsaturated fatty acids, omega-3 polyunsaturated fatty acids, omega-6 polyunsaturated fatty acids, vitamin E, vitamin B12 and folate. A diet high in omega-3 and omega-6 polyunsaturated fatty acids, vitamin E, and folate, but poor in saturated fatty acids and B12, was similar and significantly correlated with the Mediterranean diet. The protective effect of folate reduces circulating homocysteine levels, vitamin E has strong antioxidant properties, and "fatty acids may be related to dementia and cognitive function through atherosclerosis, thrombosis, or inflammation via an effect on brain development and membrane functioning or via accumulation of beta-amyloid". (Gu Y, et al. Food combination and Alzheimer disease risk: a protective diet. *Arch Neurol* 2010; DOI:10.1001/archnneurol. 2010.84)

A second study published in the March 2011 issue of the *American Journal of Clinical Nutrition,* found that participants whose diets most clearly adhered to the Mediterranean diet pattern experienced slower rates of cognitive decline than those who didn't eat Mediterranean style.

Melatonin and tumor growth. Linoleic acid, the primary omega-6 fat in corn oil, has been shown to stimulate the growth of tumors in rats, but only in the ***absence*** of melatonin, the hormone produced by the pineal gland at night. During the nighttime hours when an animal produces melatonin, tumor production of a growth chemical produced from linoleic acid decreased to negligible amounts. Cancer in these rats grew at roughly one-half the rate of the tumors in rats with their melatonin-producing pineal gland removed. Providing extra melatonin as a late-afternoon supplement was important—giving it early in the daytime had no effect.

OK, so that's rats—what about humans? First of all, melatonin is a powerful anti-oxidant and helps to prevent free radical damage to healthy cells. In addition, melatonin may stimulate powerful cancer-destroying cells called natural killer cells. So, do sleep-deprived humans have a higher risk of developing certain cancers due to their lower amounts of circulating melatonin? Good question. Some research says yes—especially with occupations that work during the night. Nurses would be one of those occupations and studies have shown that the incidence of breast and colorectal cancer is slightly higher in "night-duty" nurses.

Several studies have also looked at the use of melatonin to treat cancer. Melatonin has been used alone or combined with chemotherapy, radiation therapy, hormone therapy (such as tamoxifen in breast cancer patients), or immunotherapy (interleukin-2) in a number of studies involving different types of cancer. A few of these studies have suggested that melatonin may extend survival and improve quality of life for patients with certain types of untreatable cancers such as advanced lung cancer and melanoma. This is not a panacea as other studies indicated that melatonin caused little or no response in certain types of tumors. (American Cancer Society. http://www.cancer.org/Treatment/TreatmentsandSideEffects/ComplementaryandAlternativeMedicine/PharacologicalandBiologicalTreatment/melatonin

Memory. Try this for a short-term memory boost: one large tart apple and a cup of cashew nuts blended until smooth and chilled. Spread a little on whole-wheat crackers and enjoy. Nibble on this while studying and it may help you remember what you are reading. (Alzheimer's Prevention Foundation, Dharma Singh Khalsa, MD, Tucson, AZ.)

Mercury, methyl. Methyl mercury is a heavy metal that accumulates in fatty fish. Methyl mercury excess is particularly dangerous for pregnant women, since it crosses the placenta and has the potential to cause birth defects in the developing embryo. Not all fish is created equal when it involves the amount of methyl mercury accumulation. Various fish accumulate mercury in varying amounts. A point scale is used for determining the methyl mercury toxicity of each type of fish. On a scale from 1 to 10, with one point being the least amount and 10 points being the most methyl mercury per ounce of fish.

Consuming more than 70 points per week can cause symptoms of mercury poisoning, including numbness in the extremities and diminished motor skills. The highest amounts of mercury are found in swordfish, fresh bluefin tuna, king mackerel (not Atlantic mackerel) and tilefish. Each one-ounce serving of the one of the above fish provides ten points. Note: Most servings of fish are 3 to 4 ounces—so a 4-ounce filet of swordfish would provide 40 points. One ounce of halibut is five points and canned tuna, shrimp, crab, lobster, and salmon receive two points per one-ounce serving.

If you are worried about the methyl mercury content of the fish you eat, you may want to cook it at home instead of ordering from the menu in restaurants. When researchers compared the methyl mercury content of tuna sushi sold in 54 restaurants with tuna-grade sushi sold in 15 supermarkets across three states, restaurant tuna contained up to 50% more methyl mercury than supermarket tuna. Why? Supermarket tuna sushi is usually made with yellowfin, a smaller tuna species that accumulates less methyl mercury than the larger bigeye or bluefin tuna species typically prepared in restaurants. (Michael Gochfeld, PhD, professor, Environmental and Occupational Health Sciences Institute, Rutgers University, Piscataway, NJ. December 2010)

The content of methyl mercury in fish from low amounts of methyl mercury to the highest amounts of methyl mercury (Low, Medium, High):

- Catfish/shrimp (Low)
- Salmon (Low)
- Sardines (Low)
- Pacific oysters (Low)
- Trout (Medium)
- Bluefin tuna (High)
- Flounder (Medium)
- Chilean sea bass (High)
- Swordfish (High)
- Mackerel (High)
- Tilefish (High)
- Grouper (High)
- Halibut (High)

Metabolic syndrome. A 2002 report by the National Cholesterol Education Program (NCEP) Adult Treatment Panel III (ATP III) report identified a constellation of factors that increased an individual's risk of developing cardiovascular disease and type 2 diabetes. This constellation of factors is referred to as metabolic syndrome and includes insulin resistance manifested by hyperglycemia (high blood sugar), dyslipidemia (abnormal blood lipids with high triglycerides and low HDLs), hypertension, and abdominal obesity. Somewhere in the neighborhood of 34% of adults in the U.S. have metabolic syndrome. (FYI: A slew of other organizations has thrown their two cents in and has varying definitions of the syndrome but for this book we'll use the NCEP ATPIII definition as outlined above). (Thomas J, Walker D. A practical guide to metabolic syndrome. *The CLINICAL ADVISOR* 2012:39–48)

Dietary treatment of the metabolic syndrome centers on reducing calorie intake by 500 to 1,000 calories per day and ramping up the exercise. The Mediterranean diet appears to be the best when it comes to having a positive effect on the dyslipidemia and insulin resistance. The Mediterranean diet consists of lots of green leafy vegetables, fiber, fish, olive oil, and nuts; low intake of saturated fats, trans fats, and cholesterol has proven to be effective in aiding weight loss in patients with metabolic syndrome. (Brand J. Metabolic syndrome: the complex relationship of diet to conditions of disturbed metabolism. *Functional Foods Health Dis.* 2011:2:1–12)

Microwaving vegetables. The FDA maintains that foods cooked in a microwave oven keep more of their vitamins and minerals because microwave ovens can cook more quickly and without adding water. The wave energy produced by microwave ovens causes molecules in food to rapidly realign millions and millions of times—it's this agitation that causes the food to heat up.

Keeping nutrients intact is the good news; however, some experts think that microwaving food may alter the chemical structure of the nutrients in an unhealthful manner. This chemical alteration may prevent nutrients in microwaved foods from performing the desired function in our bodies and possibly creates cell-damaging free radicals. This has certainly not been proven, so as of the printing of this book, microwaving is assumed to be a safe and effective way of heating up foods.

The first commercial microwave oven weighed 670 pounds and was almost six feet tall. You needed an electrician and a plumber to install it. Total cost? $2,000 in 1947 or about $20,000 in 2012.

Migraine headaches and food triggers. Of course, everyone with migraines may have their own "special" triggers, but the most common foods known to trigger migraines are: alcohol, especially red wine, tannins in tea, chocolate, caffeine, and foods that contain nitrates (hot dogs, deli meats, sausages, bacon, and other processed meats). Foods that contain tyramine, a compound formed in foods during the fermentation process may also trigger migraines—pork, hard cheeses, yogurt, and aged or pickled meat or fish. The food additive MSG (monosodium glutamate) has been linked to migraines and can be found, most famously, in Chinese foods. You can request "no MSG" at any Chinese restaurant today, however, MSG has also been added to canned soups, sauce and gravy mixes, soy sauce, and other prepared foods. Foods containing sulfites may also be a trigger—dried fruits such as apricots, prunes, and figs, and white wine. (Joy Bauer MS, RD, www.joybauer.com; Food and Fitness Advisor, Weill Cornell Medical College, December 2010.

MILK

Milk. Nonfat dry milk can provide a significant protein and calcium boost to foods without adding fat or cholesterol. Simply mix the powder into casseroles, creamy soups, puddings, dressings, quick breads, pancakes, cookies, or shakes. One-third of a cup of the powder contains only eighty calories, yet provides eight grams of protein and 300 mg of calcium, the same as in a cup of liquid milk.

Milk and hypertension. Drink milk and lower your blood pressure. Yes, low-fat calcium products are also part of the DASH diet (see Chapter D), but

HISTORICAL HIGHLIGHT

For more than five millennia, human beings have treated their ailments with extraordinary creativity. For example, in 2000 BC Assyrian and Babylonian doctors used a salve made of frog bile and sour milk for treating infected eyes, but this concoction was considered effective only after the patient ate a sliced onion followed by a swig of beer. Milk baths became famous in Napoleon's regimen. His sister, Pauline, maintained a herd of 400 asses for the production of enough milk to fill her daily bath.

research also shows that low-fat milk and milk products alone are also beneficial for lowering blood pressure by themselves. Dutch researchers noted that participants with the highest dairy consumption of all types were 24% less likely to develop hypertension than the group consuming the least dairy products. For low-fat dairy products, the difference in risk was 31%. Low-fat milk and milk products specifically were associated with lower hypertension risk, while no benefit was seen for cheese or high-fat dairy. (www.ajcn.org/cgi/content/abstract/89/6/1877)

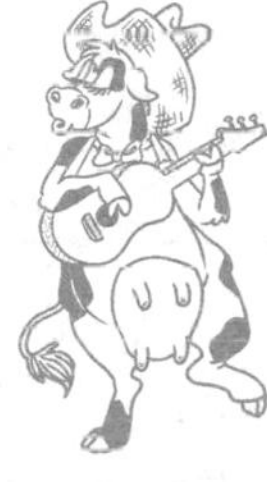

Milk production. How do you coax a cow to produce more milk? A kick in the dairy air? Not exactly. The 43rd International Science and Engineering Fair in Nashville shed some light on this dilemma. An eight-week study found that cows increased their production of milk by 6.2% if they listened to country music. Rock music only increased the output by 4.7%, and Mozart was a dismal failure—only a 1.6% increase in milk output with classical music.

Happiness is seeing your mother-in-law's picture on the back of a milk carton. —Anonymous

---

Milk as a contrast dye for abdominal CT scans. How many patients absolutely adore the taste of contrast media for CT scans of the abdomen?

ASPARAGUS TIP

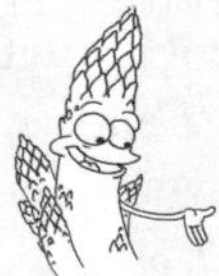

- It takes 10 pounds of milk to make one pound of cheese.
- In 1936 a quart of milk cost 12 cents.
- A glass of milk may contain minute amounts of up to 80 different antibiotics.
- In 2008 the world consumed about 700 million tons of milk.

(United Nations Food and Agriculture Organization (FAO), 2010.

None. And, in fact, most patients ABHOR the taste of VoLumen, the barium-based contrast media. Researchers at St. Luke's-Roosevelt Hospital in New York compared milk to the barium-based agent and found that milk was at least as good for contrast as the commercial agent. Well, whaddya know? And, moreover, the "dose" of milk cost a whopping $1.39 compared to the cost of VoLumen at $18 bucks a dose. (Radiological Society of North America Meeting, December 2006, Chicago)

Milk. Hold the milk for vascular benefits of black tea. In a study of 16 postmenopausal women, those who drank about two cups of black tea without milk had a greater than four-fold increase in flow-mediated vasodilation from baseline in the forearm brachial artery. However, those who drank a mix of 90% black tea with 10% skim milk had no more of an increase in vasodilation than if they had consumed two cups of hot water. It appears as if three of the milk proteins—alpha casein, beta-casein, and kappa-casein blunt nitric oxide production. Nitric oxide is the MOST potent vasodilator known to man. Other milk proteins did not interfere with nitric oxide. (Lorenz M et al. Addition of milk prevents vascular protective effects of tea. *Eur Heart J*, Advanced online publication. January 8, 2007)

I am thankful for laughter, except when milk comes out of my nose. —Woody Allen

---

MILK THISTLE

Milk Thistle. Milk thistle (silymarin) is an antioxidant that protects and nourishes liver cells, stimulating protein synthesis and cellular regeneration.

Milk thistle and chemotherapy. Andrew Weil, M.D., suggests taking milk thistle for at least two months after receiving chemotherapy. Milk thistle is a natural remedy that helps the liver to recover from toxins. He suggests the brand name Thisilyn from Nature's Way. (Weil, A. *Self Healing*. January 2001)

Milk Thistle and hepatotoxicityfrom chemotherapy in children with acute lymphoblastic leukemia (ALL). A randomized, double-blind, placebo-controlled trial of children with ALL concluded that children with hepatotoxicity from chemotherapy had significant reductions in toxicity with taking milk thistle. Further study is needed to determine the most effective doses and duration of milk thistle and its effect on hepatotoxicity and leukemia-free survival. (Ladas EL, et al. A randomized controlled double-blind, pilot study of milk thistle for treatment of hepatotoxicity in childhood acute lymphoblastic leukemia (ALL). *Cancer* 2010 (January); 116(2):506–513)

Miso. Miso is a fermented soybean paste made with salt and often with rice or barley. The lighter varieties tend to be milder; the darker colors are more flavorful. So, if you are looking to add a bit of soy to your diet, try a cup of miso soup.

Molasses. What is this stuff, anyway? Molasses is a concentrated byproduct of refining sugar cane into table sugar. Unlike sugar or artificial sweeteners, molasses is a source of minerals your body needs including manganese, magnesium, iron, copper, calcium and potassium. Amounts vary widely by brand, so check the label if you're buying molasses for a specific mineral content. Each tablespoonful of molasses contains about 50 calories.

HISTORICAL HIGHLIGHT

The Great Molasses Flood of 1919. On January 15, 1919 a gigantic steel vat exploded in Boston, spewing 2.3 million gallons of molten molasses. Thirty-foot waves of the sticky stuff flowed through the streets, catching men, women, children, horses, and other live animals in its flow. Horses were stuck in the muck, cars, people, and houses were smashed to pieces as the molasses flowed at speeds of up to 35 miles per hour. In fact the flood killed 21 people and injured another 150.

Molecules with characteristic flavors—for all you chemists out there...
Linalool (tea)
Benzaldehyde (almond)
A-sinensal (mandarin, orange)
(+) nootkatone (grapefruit)
1-p-menthene-8-thiol (grapefruit)
2-trans-6-cis-nonadienal (cucumber)
4-phenyl-2butanone (raspberries)

Monosodium Glutamate (MSG). MSG is a flavor enhancer frequently used in Asian cuisine. Foods containing MSG can also be misleading as MSG on a food label is also known as *calcium caseinate, sodium caseinate, autolyzed yeast,* or *hydrolyzed protein.*

Moonshine and lead poisoning. Yep, moonshine continues to be distilled in car radiators in the hills of Georgia, Tennessee, Ohio, and "Kaintucky." Dr. Brent Morgan of the Georgia Poison Center was concerned about a clustering of patients that had been treated at an Atlanta Hospital emergency room for lead poisoning symptoms such as seizures, abdominal pain, and anemia. All of the patients had been imbibing homemade moonshine that was contaminated with lead from making and storing the moonshine in old car radiators. Dr. Brent surveyed 531 people and found that almost 10 percent reported drinking home-distilled alcohol in the past five years; more than one-fourth of the group downed some homemade hooch in the previous week. Clearly this continues to be a problem, so Practitioners, beware! Remember, too, that the anemia of lead poisoning mimics the anemia of iron deficiency, so order the basophil stippling test to pick up lead poisoning. (*Annals of Emergency Surgery.* September 2003)

MULTIVITAMINS

Multivitamins. Multivitamins are the most common dietary supplement used by adults in the U.S. According to a national nutrition survey, 30% of Americans take multivitamins and minerals regularly, downing 1 to 14 pills per day, at a cost that can hit $75.00 per month.

A recent study from the *Archives of Internal Medicine* (2011) tracked approximately 38,000 women from Iowa between the ages of 55 and 69 for 19 years. Those who regularly took multivitamins had a 6% higher risk of dying within that period of time. Whoa. Before you toss your multivitamins please note that this study does not provide compelling evidence that multivitamins are detrimental to your health. First of all, the risk of dying was very small. Secondly, the study couldn't prove that taking a multivitamin caused the higher risk of dying, because researchers didn't randomly assign women to take either a supplement or a placebo. Something else about the vitamin takers might explain their higher risk of dying. (*Arch. Intern. Med.* 171;1625, 2011)

Over time the focus of vitamin supplements has shifted from treatment of deficiency to prevention of chronic disease. However, current science doesn't support the use of multivitamins to treat any chronic disease. There's little, if any, evidence that people who take multivitamins live any longer nor are they less likely to get heart disease, have a stroke or develop cancer. Performances on memory and cognitive function are no better with multivitamin use either. People taking multivitamins are just as likely to develop a cold or other infection, stay sick just as long and miss planned activities as those taking a placebo.

The original power of vitamin supplements was to augment what was lacking in the diet—and, this remains their appropriate role in diet and disease today. If you eat a well-balanced diet you will be getting all of the nutrients you need—you won't need a multivitamin.

1940—the debut of the "One-a-Day" multivitamin.

Multivitamins. Questions and Answers—the scoop.

Q. Should you buy generic multivitamins, or should you fork out the big bucks for the expensive brands?

A. Generic multivitamins are usually just as effective as the more expensive brands, so unless you just enjoy being a "name dropper" and paying more money to have a brand name on the shelf, buy the less expensive stuff.

In fact, a Consumer Report study showed that Costco brands were top of the line when it comes to multivitamins.

Q. Some of the multivitamins say they contain sugar and starch additives. Should I shun those in favor of multivitamins that don't have those "fillers"?

A. No. Don't shun the sugar and starch additives as they help with the absorption of the contents of the multivitamins. They are not just "fillers." However, do ignore the hype about special features such as "extended release," "time-release," etc. There is no optimal time to absorb nutrients. Therefore, having vitamins available throughout the day is of little value.

To improve absorbability, take your supplement with food. "Chelated" vitamins supposedly offer superior absorption. However, a chelated nutrient breaks down as soon as it hits the acid-rich stomach, and is absorbed just like other nutrients. Do not take vitamins with coffee, since the acid in the coffee can cancel out some of the nutrients.

Q. Should you buy the natural form or the synthetic form of vitamins?

A. Folic acid and vitamin B12 are better absorbed as supplements. The natural form of folic acid, folate, is not absorbed well from foods (even from good sources like spinach, orange juice, and beans), making supplements a good idea. Besides a multivitamin providing plenty of folic acid (at least 400 micrograms or 0.4 mg), the U.S government also now mandates that all "enriched" grains contain folic acid. The same is true for B12. A B12 supplement is better absorbed than foods containing B12.

Q. How many vitamins and minerals should be included in a "multivitamin?"

A. Look for at least 20. Several "key" nutrients fall short in the American diet and should be included *for sure* in a multivitamin. These include vitamin D (especially if you are over 50 and trying to protect your bones), B12, folate, calcium, copper, iron, magnesium, selenium, and zinc.

Q. What does the DV mean on the label of the multivitamin?

A. Nutritionists have traditionally used the RDA (Recommended Daily Allowance) to provide information on the amount of vitamin or mineral needed daily in order to prevent a nutritional deficiency. The DV (Daily Value) is a variation on that theme and a recent name change to take the place of RDA. These amounts are calculated with an added margin for protection, so anything more than 100% is not necessary except in strict vegetarians, individuals on restricted weight loss diets, or the elderly.

The amounts listed on the side of multivitamin bottles are generally not therapeutic doses of vitamins. The doses are considered to be enough of a dose to prevent any complications from vitamin E deficiency.

Q. Should I buy a vitamin that has a USP designation on it?

A. YES. The USP on the label indicates that a supplement meets five quality standards set by the United States Pharmacopoeia for vitamin, mineral, botanical, and herbal supplements: 1) disintegration, 2) dissolution, 3) potency, 4) purity, and 5) expiration date. Don't be impressed with a label that only advertises "laboratory-tested" or "quality-assured." This means little without the USP label.

Q. What does fat-soluble vs. water-soluble mean?

A. Vitamins A, D, E, and K are fat-soluble vitamins, which means that they attach to lipids in the blood. To reap the necessary benefits of fat-soluble vitamins, you need to have some fat in your diet. The body can store excess amounts of fat-soluble vitamins.

The B vitamins and vitamin C are water-soluble, which means they dissolve in water. Most are not stored in the body, and excess vitamins are excreted via the kidneys. For example, the body can only retain 500 mg of vitamin C at one time. The kidneys will immediately excrete a dose greater 500 mg. So, your toilet will reap the benefits of a 1,000 mg dose of vitamin C; you will not.

Vitamins A, D, C, B6, and niacin may be toxic if taken in large amounts. The recommended safe limit for vitamin A is 10,000 IU or 25 mg per day; for vitamin D, 800 IU per day; for vitamin C, 1,000 mg per day; for B6, 200 mg per day; and for niacin (niacinamide, nicotinic acid, nicotinamide or B3), 500 mg for regular niacin, 250 mg for slow-release niacin, and 1,500 mg for nicotinamide.

Q. Why does my urine turn bright yellow after taking a multivitamin or vitamin B complex?

A. The riboflavin (B2) from the multivitamin is the culprit.

Q. Are there specific multivitamins for the over-50 crowd?

A. Yes. Look for a multivitamin that has more B12, is higher in vitamin C and E and calcium, and has *no* or very low iron. Check out Centrum Silver, even though it is quite low in calcium. It is high in B12 and does not have any iron. One A Day 50 Plus is similar to Centrum Silver, but is higher in vitamins C and E. It is also low in calcium. Flip over to the V chapter for some new information on vitamin E. If you don't feel like flipping over at this moment, suffice it to say that you don't want much vitamin E at all in a multivitamin. The synthetic form is less active than the natural form and vitamin E supplements have not been found to offer any conclusive protection against disease in large clinical trials. If anything, vitamin E supplements have deleterious effects.

When purchasing a multivitamin, men and postmenopausal females should choose one without iron. If you can't find one without iron, purchase a multivitamin with no more than 10 mg or take a multivitamin with 18 mg iron every other day. Why? Preliminary evidence shows that iron may oxidize LDL-cholesterol in the arteries and increase the risk of heart disease. Men with high iron levels have a higher risk of heart disease than men with low levels of serum iron. Postmenopausal women have stopped losing

ASPARAGUS TIP

Just remember that most health experts advocate getting nutrients from foods—however, that doesn't mean a well-balanced multivitamin/mineral is a bad idea. It primarily provides insurance against scurvy, beriberi, and other nutritional deficiencies. The studies on vitamin B complex, soy, fish oil, and others found that the prevention benefits were from food, not a vitamin pill.

iron via menstruation and therefore will also accumulate iron. Note: The DV (Daily Value) for iron is 18 mg for premenopausal women (in order to replace the amount lost with menstruation), but 0 mg for all men and postmenopausal women.

On the subject of wild mushrooms, it is easy to tell who is an expert and who is not: the expert is the one who is still alive. —Donel Hanahan

---

Mushrooms. The six most popular mushroom varieties include white button, crimini, portabella, maitake, shiitake, and enoki. All of the mushroom varieties are rich in total dietary fibers, including those linked to cholesterol-lowering and heart health. White button mushrooms are the most popular variety in the U.S. but each mushroom variety has its own unique nutritional profile. Portabella mushrooms and crimini mushrooms contain beta glucans—sugar molecules that are only partially digestible and are considered prebiotic, meaning they promote the growth of healthful bacteria in the colon.

Mushrooms are rich in antioxidants such as polyphenols. Most of the nutrients are fully retained after mushrooms are cooked, which makes them ideal for soups and stews, sautéed for appetizers; or grilled as a substitute or accompaniment for meat.

Shiitake and maitake are medicinal mushrooms used to boost the immune system. Mushrooms may be especially beneficial in the treatment of cancer, and research studies are ongoing for their direct anti-cancer activity as well as their immune-enhancing response in cancer patients.

Mushrooms are also the only vegetable source of vitamin D. Mushrooms also come in extracts containing shiitake, maitake, reishi, zhu ling, and others. Check out Fungi Perfecti at 1-800-780-9126 or www.fungi.com for more information on mushrooms.

A dietary change that could make a huge difference in weight loss is to swap your meat for mushrooms. Instead of ground beef for tacos and burritos, use chopped mushrooms. Use a portabella mushroom instead of a

ASPARAGUS TIP

Do not rush out and buy a frilly picnic basket and start hunting for mushrooms on your own. Check out the story of Nicholas Evans, author, *The Horse Whisperer.* In a nutshell, or a mushroom cap, as it were, his entire family was poisoned in September 2008 after hunting and consuming deadly webcap mushrooms on his brother's estate in the Scottish Highlands. The entire family was critically ill and Nicholas needed a kidney transplant, which his daughter willingly donated.

burger. Trade three ounces of lean ground turkey for a half-cup of chopped Portabella mushroom once a week and save 7,280 calories per year.

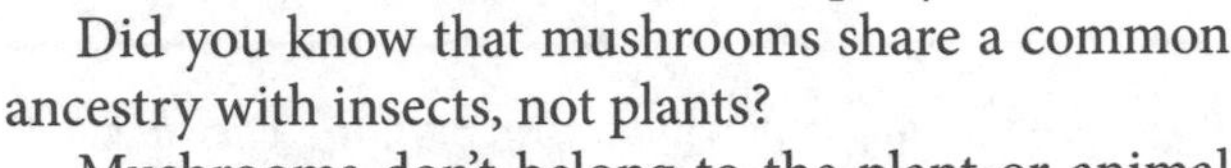

Did you know that mushrooms share a common ancestry with insects, not plants?

Mushrooms don't belong to the plant or animal kingdom. They are classified in the kingdom of fungi.

A single mushroom can produce as many as 40 million spores in an hour.

Mustard. Mustard is the third most common popular American condiment. Romans made "mustumardens," or "burning must" by combining "must" (unfermented grape juice) with seeds of the "Sinapishirta" plant. Why am I telling you this? Because we often think, mistakenly, that mustard is made from the mustard plant.

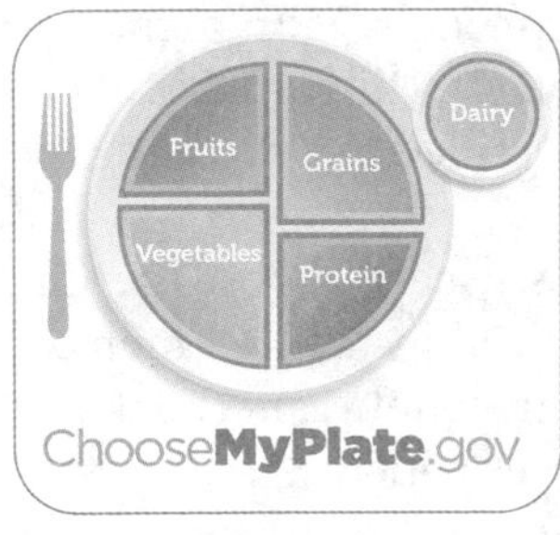

MyPlate. No, that's not spelled wrong. MyPlate is the new "food pyramid." So, what's up? The food pyramid is history and the new government recommendation is a plate graphic divided into four wedges. One half of the plate is for fruits and vegetables—and filling that half with any mixture of the two is generally fine. In other words you don't have to "count" the number of fruits and vegetables—just fill half of the plate with a variety of the two. The other half of the plate is divided between protein and grains—with the grain wedge slightly larger than the protein wedge. Hanging off the plate icon is a small circle that adds a place for dairy—anything from a glass of skim or low-fat milk to a cup of yogurt. So, if you would like to know more about the 2 million dollar project paid for by the Department of Agriculture, log on to ChooseMyPlate.gov.

CHAPTER N

Avoid fruits and nuts. You are what you eat.

—Jim Davis

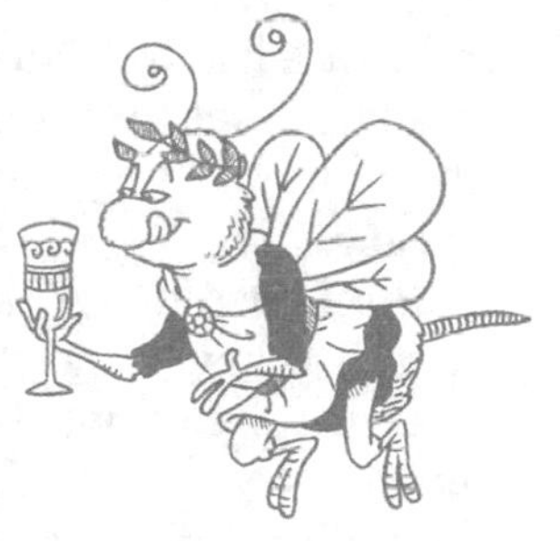

Nectar—the "divine drink of the Gods." The word nectar is derived from the Greek *nek,* for "death," and *tar,* for the verb "to overcome," signifying its immortal nature. Nectar is a sugary fluid secreted by plants, especially within flowers to encourage pollination by insects and other animals. It is collected by bees to make honey. To make a single pound of honey it takes 80,000 bees and about 2 million flights between the plants and the hive.

Nitrosamines. Nitrites give cured meats like hot dogs, ham, bologna, sausage, and bacon their characteristic pink color and sharp flavor. Beef manufacturers use the nitrites as a preservative and to prevent bacterial food-borne infections. Nitrate, made up of nitrogen and oxygen, occurs naturally in the diet. Six percent of the nitrates that we consume comes from meat products, 21 percent comes from nitrogen-contaminated drinking water, and 70% comes from vegetables grown in the soil. When added to meat, nitrates break down into nitrites. Nitrates can also be converted to nitrites in the stomach, especially if the pH of gastric fluid is high. And these nitrites can react with food proteins to form cancer-causing compounds known as nitrosamines. These compounds can also be created in meats cured with nitrite, especially when frying is the selected method of cooking.

On the other hand, nitrates found in plant foods may actually be beneficial for heart health. The DASH diet is very high in nitrate-based plant foods and the benefits of the DASH diet have been proven over and over again. Apparently the body processes plant nitrates differently than those found in meats. (*Environmental Nutrition,* May 2010)

Noroviruses. Also known as the Norwalk virus family, the noroviruses have been documented in foodborne outbreaks involving a variety of foods, including fruits, salads, eggs, clams, shellfish, chicken and bakery items. Shellfish and salad ingredients are the foods most often implicated in Norwalk outbreaks. Ingestion of raw or insufficiently steamed clams and oysters poses a high risk. Water is also a common source of outbreaks and may include water from municipal supplies, well water, recreational lakes, swimming pools, and water stored aboard cruise ships. In fact, nothing in the world returns a cruise ship to port faster than a norovirus outbreak on board.

Infection with the noroviruses causes a self-limiting gastroenteritis characterized by nausea, vomiting, and diarrhea (diarrhea and vomiting are also known as "shuking"—the hybridization of two words used by average Americans to describe bodily functions), and abdominal pain. Headache and low-grade fever may occur. The incubation period is 24 to 72 hours.

Nuts. *"Sometimes I feel like a nut"*...and if you do, you should go ahead and have a handful. Nuts have been food staples for thousands of years. Nut bread was a staple for one of the great pharaohs; walnuts were used as a remedy for headaches, and newlyweds were pelted with almonds as a fertility blessing.

The numerous varieties of nuts include walnuts, almonds, peanuts, pistachios, hazelnuts, Brazil nuts, cashews, macadamias, chestnuts, and pecans. A serving size of nuts is one ounce (¼ cup), and various nuts have varying nutritional values. Each type of nut contains a different mix of nutrients, fats and protective antioxidants. Nuts contain L-arginine, the precursor to nitric oxide, and a potent vasodilator. Nuts are also packed with protein, fiber, B vitamins, magnesium, calcium, copper, zinc, selenium, phosphorus, and potassium. Almonds and walnuts are also great sources of vitamin E.

HISTORICAL HIGHLIGHT

Origin of the macadamia nut. John MacAdam, M.D., was a Scottish physician who relocated to Australia circa 1855 to teach and practice medicine. He befriended a botanist after his move, a gentleman by the name of Ferdinand von Mueller. Von Mueller was exploring the outback of Australia one fine day in 1857 when he happened upon what he thought was an entirely new species of tree that produced a fascinating nut. He was intrigued by his find and reviewed the world's botanical literature to determine whether or not this tree existed in the world of botany at the time. He determined that it was a new species, and he named the nut of the tree after his physician and friend, John MacAdam.

The lowest fat and lowest calorie nut is the chestnut, which just happens to be roasting on an open fire at Christmas. The highest fat and highest calorie nut is the macadamia nut.

Nuts and cardiovascular disease protection. What is the relationship of nut consumption and heart disease? Let's look back to the Nurses' Health Study of 86,016 healthy nurses aged 34–59 at study entry in 1980. As of 1990, 1,255 coronary artery events had occurred. After adjusting for the usual risk factors for coronary artery disease, women who ate more than five ounces of nuts per week had a 35% lower risk of coronary artery disease compared with those who never ate nuts or who consumed less than one ounce per month. The results were the same when the diet was adjusted for all the usual dietary variables—dietary fats, fiber, vegetables, and fruit. The results continued to be the same when the subgroups were stratified by smoking, high cholesterol, alcohol consumption, use of multivitamins including vitamin E supplementation, body mass index and exercise.

Another study of 31,000 individuals found that those who ate nuts more than five times a week lowered their risk of heart disease by more than 50%. Those who ate nuts one to four times per week cut their risk by 27%. A pooled analysis of four U.S. studies found that the highest intake group of nut consumption had about a 35% reduced risk of coronary artery disease incidence. The study by Albert, et al. reported that an inverse association between nut consumption and total coronary artery disease death was due primarily to a reduction in sudden cardiac death. Compared with men who rarely or never consumed nuts, those who consumed nuts two or more times per week had a 47% reduced risk of sudden cardiac death.

Sounds as if nuts might be the be-all and end-all for coronary artery disease, eh? Why is this? Although nuts are high in fat, each nut contains a different percentage of saturated fats, polyunsaturated fats, and monounsaturated fats. All nuts should lower your LDL-cholesterol if you eat them instead of meat, butter, or other saturated fats. But only nuts that have at least twice as much polyunsaturated fat as saturated fat lower LDL if you eat them instead of pasta, bread, or other carbohydrates. The nuts that have at least twice as much polyunsaturated fats as saturated fats are pistachios, walnuts, pecans, almonds, peanuts, and hazelnuts. The nuts that *don't* fit this picture are macadamia nuts, cashews, and Brazil nuts. (Albert CM, et al. Nut consumption and decreased risk of sudden cardiac death in the Physician's Health Study. *Arch Intern Med.* 2002;162:1382–1387; Hu F, et al. Frequent nut consumption and risk of coronary artery disease in women: Prospective Cohort Study. *British Medical Journal* 1998 November 18;317:1332–33. Tunstall-Pedro H. "Nuts to you [...and you, and you]: Eating nuts may be beneficial—though it is unclear why. *British Medical Journal* 1998 November 14;317; *Nutrition Action Healthletter,* October 2009)

Nuts not only protect your heart, but a study in the 1999 *Journal of Neurology* found that a diet high in the monosaturated fats contained in nuts can also help protect against age-related memory loss and declining cognitive function.

So let's look at a few nuts…

…..Almonds—my favorite, contain flavonoids that prevent the oxidation of LDL-cholesterol. If you can't oxidize LDL-cholesterol, you can't pack your coronary arteries with it. Almonds are also a great source of vitamin E, and, here's a show stopper—in a study comparing weight loss of participants, almonds were as helpful as complex carbs for dropping the pounds. Almonds also contain around 80 mg of calcium in a handful of nuts (20–25 nuts), so even though you wouldn't want to get your entire recommended daily calcium (1000 mg) from nuts, a handful is helpful. And, we're not done with the benefits of almonds yet. One serving of almonds contains one-fourth of the recommended daily amount of magnesium which, in conjunction with calcium and potassium, helps control the relaxation of blood vessels. Hence, a blood pressure lowering effect is observed.

…..Brazil nuts—a big bold yummy nut containing a big bolus of selenium. Just two Brazil nuts contain 155 mcg of selenium and the recommended daily amount of selenium is only 55 mcg. So, no more than 2 Brazil nuts a day as an overdose of selenium over time can cause problems. Brazil nuts are also high in vitamin E. The Selenium and Vitamin E Cancer Prevention Trial found that men getting selenium and vitamin E, alone or in combination, reduced their risk of prostate cancer by 60 percent. Selenium gives the immune system a boost and vitamin E is a potent antioxidant—a winning combo in a great nut. Brazil nuts are also high in calories—so the 2 nut rule is a good one. Each nut is 100 calories. NOTE: If you are taking a multivitamin that has more than 50% of the daily value of selenium, just eat one Brazil nut a day. Don't forget that Brazil nuts do not protect the heart.

A note on this nut: Brazil, the country, got its name from the nut, not the other way around.

…..Macadamia nuts—17 out of the 21 grams of fat found in an ounce of Macadamia nuts are the monosaturated type of fat. This lowers the harmful level of LDL-cholesterol without lowering the beneficial effects of the good HDL-cholesterol. Macadamia nuts also have anti-oxidant and anti-inflammatory properties.

…..Peanuts—okay, okay, if you want to get picky, peanuts are actually a type of legume and not a true nut. Peanuts contain a hefty amount of folate (34 µg per ounce), a B vitamin that lowers the level of homocysteine, an amino acid that damages arteries and contributes to the deposition of fat in the arteries. Peanuts are also high in L-arginine, the precursor to nitric oxide, the potent vasodilator that improves blood flow to all body parts.

…..Pecans—the pecan is a nut chock full of antioxidants. These nuts have been shown to keep the eyes in tip top shape and help protect from cataracts and macular degeneration. The National Eye Institute's Age-Related Eye Diseases Study reported that patients with macular degeneration who had adequate intakes of antioxidants were 29% less likely to experience disease progression than those who got lower levels.

.....Pistachios—A 2007 study conducted by Penn State University found that pistachios lower blood pressure. Men who added 1.5 ounces of shelled pistachios to their daily diets had drops in systolic pressure of 4.8 points. (Presented at the April 30, 2007 Experimental Biology Meeting, Washington DC, West SG, lead investigator). Pistachios have also been shown to lower plasma lipids by as much as 25%. They can also significantly reduce the glycemic index of foods when a handful of pistachios is tossed back with a high glycemic food such as a baked white potato or bowl of white rice. (*Environmental Nutrition,* June 2008)

One daily serving of pistachios (~45 nuts) can lower LDL-cholesterol by 9%, seven times more than expected based on the nuts' fatty acid content. Compounds such as fiber and phytosterols found in pistachios may contribute to the benefits. (*The Am J of Clinical Nutrition,* 2008 October)

ASPARAGUS TIP

Why are some pistachios dyed red? Pistachios were first mass-marketed in the U.S. in the 1930s during the Great Depression. At that time they were placed in vending machines mixed with the bland cashew nut and the pallid peanut. Some ingenious pistachio seller decided that he would dye them red to make them stand out in the crowd. It worked and pistachios became a hit.

.....Walnuts have a special claim to fame. They are the only nut that contains alpha linolenic acid (ALA) a polyunsaturated fat that is converted to omega 3 fatty acids in the body. So, apart from fish and flaxseed, walnuts are considered one of the best sources for omega-3 fatty acids. So, we all know the positive benefits of omega-3s, and if you don't, flip over to Chapter O immediately. But to give you a preview—omega-3s lower LDL-cholesterol, lower triglycerides, increase HDL cholesterol, inhibit clotting factors, and reduce arterial inflammation. The omega-3s have also been shown to help maintain healthy levels of serotonin in the brain. Serotonin in the brain keeps you happy. So put a smile on your face and reach for the bowl of walnuts...have a nice, big handful. (see Chapter W for more on walnuts.)

What's a handful (approximately 1 ounce)? (*Nutrition Action Newsletter,* November 2005)

- 8–11 halves of walnuts (175 calories)
- 30 large/60 small Roasted peanuts (160 calories)
- 45 shelled pistachios (165 calories)
- 20–24 whole almonds (170 calories)
- 18–20 halves of pecans
- 18–20 hazelnuts (Filberts)

- 150–157 pine nuts
- 10–12 Macadamia nuts
- 16–18 cashews
- 6–8 Brazil nuts

Nuts—salted? Roasted or Raw? Salted nuts usually have between 100–300 mg of sodium per 1 ounce serving. If you want to skip the sodium, buy nuts that say "raw" or "unsalted." If you need a bit of the salty taste to satisfy your own cravings, buy nuts that have "50% less salt" or "lightly salted" on the label. As far as roasted nuts are concerned, you'll see "dry" roasted or "oil-roasted" nuts. It doesn't matter which one you choose—roasted nuts are no higher in calories or saturated fats.

Nutritionist. Need a nutritional advisor in your area? Visit www.eatright.org and click "Find a Registered Dietician."

Oysters are supposed to enhance your sexual performance, but they don't work for me. Maybe I put them on too soon.

—Gary Shandling.

Oat bran. Why is it that when a label states that two tablespoons of oat bran are good for your bowels, that you will automatically assume that three times that much must be even better for you? This was the case with a 75-year-old man who arrived at the emergency room one evening with bloating and severe abdominal pain. During his yearly physical exam the week before, his physician had recommended that he increase his intake of fiber and that two tablespoons of oat bran would be a great way to start his day. The physician also recommended that each tablespoon of oat bran be accompanied by an eight-ounce glass of water. The older man decided that six tablespoons would be much better for his bowels than two. He forgot that water was to accompany the increase in fiber intake, and in less than one week he arrived at the emergency room with the clinical signs of intestinal obstruction.

As a general rule in the world of emergency medicine, when an older patient arrives at the emergency room with intestinal obstruction, one of the first thoughts is that the obstruction is due to cancer of the colon. So the gentleman was whisked up to the operating room to remove the 'blockage,' most likely caused by a malignancy.

Much to the dismay of the surgeon, the 'blockage' was a two-foot long column of oat bran obstructing the sigmoid colon. Upon removal of the oat bran, the bowels were free to move again. Too much oat bran, without the benefit of the water, overwhelmed the ability of the intestines to move, and hence the blockage.

Does anyone need to hear the moral of this story?

Obesity and the average American. The average American consumes 64 pounds of fat and oils each year and 65 pounds of sugar. Is it any wonder why the average American is larger than the average American? In fact, being larger than the average American reduces longevity depending on the actual amount of extra weight carried around. For every 7% above the ideal weight, the life span is reduced by one year. Individuals weighing more than 100 pounds above their ideal weight find themselves fully 50% more likely to die in any given year than their thinner colleagues, friends, family, and peers. When all of the risks are added together, the risk of dying from obesity in a given year is one in 200,000. (Flegal KM et al. Prevalence and trends in obesity among U.S. adults, 1999–2008. *JAMA* 2010;303(3):235–241)

Let's compare that to other risks of dying within a given year:

One in 1 to 10 million risk of dying from a lightning strike

One in 1 to 10 million risk of dying from cancer by eating a charbroiled steak once a week

One in 1 million is the point below which the FDA deems any risk of cancer from a food additive to be too small to be of a concern over a lifetime

One in 1 million chance of drowning in a bathtub

One in 100,000 extra risk of cancer from eating a peanut butter sandwich every day

(Up to Your Armpits in Alligators? How to Sort Out What Risks Are Worth Worrying About. John and Sean Paling, 1997)

Obesity in the U.S. Mississippi has held the title of the most obese state since 2004. Approximately 32.5% of the Mississippians are obese, *but watch your back, Mississippians!* Alabama is on target to steal your crown and is closing in fast with a 31.2% obesity rate. West Virginia comes in a very close third, with 31.1% obesity, and Tennessee is fourth with a rate of 30.2%. Mirror, mirror, on the wall, who's the leanest of them all? Colorado! Only 18.9% of the mountain-high folks weigh in as obese, and Massachusetts is the number 2 most lean state with 21.2% considered obese. (CDC; http://www.cdc.gov/obesity/data/trends.html#State)

The 10 most obese U.S cities? Memphis, TN (34%), Birmingham, AL (31.3%), San Antonio, TX (31.1%), Riverside/San Bernardino, CA (30.8%), Detroit, MI (30.4%), Jacksonville, FL (29.8%), Nashville, TN 28.8%), Oklahoma City, OK (27.5%), Kansas City, MO (26.9%), San Diego, CA (26.7%).

The baby boomers are contributing mightily to this obesity problem, so Medicare beware. Obesity's associated costs add $93 billion to the nation's debt annually. Each year 112,000 people die from obesity-related causes, and the condition is responsible for an increased risk of chronic conditions such as diabetes, cancer, dementia, hypertension, sleep apnea, and heart disease—just to name a few. Over one-fourth of the American population is obese—26.1% according to the latest report released in September 2009 by the Centers for Disease Control.

Some numbers of interest:

- In 1950 the average dress size was 8
- In 2002 the average dress size was 14
- In 1971 approximately 14.4% of Americans were described as "clinically obese"
- In 2002 the percentage of clinically obese Americans jumped to 30.9%
- In 1971 each person in the U.S. consumed 1497 pounds of food per year
- In 2000 each person in the U.S. consumed 1775 pounds of food per year (an additional 278 pounds per person per year)
- The good news: we're eating more vegetables
- The bad news: one-third of the vegetables are fries, chips and iceberg lettuce

On the parental side, statistics are not much better. According to a recent national study, only 42% of mothers of children in grades one through four exercised at all, and only 48% of the fathers. One in four adults is obese, and nearly half of adults are overweight. It is estimated that 12% of all U.S. deaths could have been prevented with even moderate physical activity. Approximately 60% of adults don't get enough physical activity to benefit their health.

Obesity in childhood. A Kaiser Family Foundation study found that, on average, kids now spend nearly four hours a day watching TV or videos, one hour and 44 minutes listening to music, and at least one hour using the computer. Some of these activities overlap, but they are all obviously sedentary.

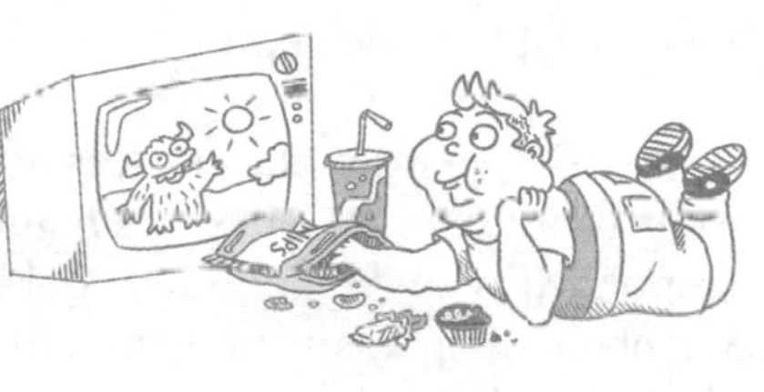

The same Kaiser Family Foundation study found that nearly 75 percent of all ads aimed at young children and teenagers were hawking candy, snacks, sugary cereals, or fast foods. Children ages 2–7 see an average of 12 food ads per day, or about 4, 400 per year. Teens view about 6,000 food ads per year.

Only 50% of our children engage in regular physical activity. One of every four boys and girls engages in no exertional activity at all. Contrasted with a decade ago, today's typical child is five pounds fatter. One in five children is obese. Running a mile takes children one full minute longer than it did a decade ago.

Obesity and cancer. Is fat tissue a risk for cancer? Evidence continues to mount concerning the relationship between obesity and certain types of cancer. In terms of breast cancer, there's no question that gaining weight after menopause raises the risk. Endometrial cancer is also strongly associated with obesity. Eighty-five percent of all women who develop cancer of the endometrium are overweight. Epidemiological studies have also provided convincing evidence that obesity increases the risk for cancers of the esophagus, colon, pancreas, and kidney. The magnitude of the increase in risk varies between cancer sites. (Key TJ, Spencer EA, Reeves GK. Symposium 1: Overnutrition: consequences and solutions. Obesity and cancer risk. *Proceedings of the Nutrition Society.* 2010; 69:86–90)

Obesity and depression. In a study from the *American Journal of Public Health,* obesity was correlated with a 37% higher risk of depression in women and a 37% lower risk of depression in men. Similarly, a 10-unit increase in body mass index (BMI) was associated with a 22% increase in thoughts of suicide and suicide attempts in women, but a 26% and 55% decrease, respectively, in men. Underweight men had a marked increase in depression (25%), thoughts of suicide (81%), and suicide attempts (77%). Once again, which came first? Do extremes in BMI lead to depression or does depression lead to extremes in BMI? The implications are obvious in terms of screening gender for risk factors for depression and suicide. (*American Journal of Public Health* [February]: 90(2): 2000; Wit L, et al. Depression and obesity: A meta-analysis of community-based studies. Psychiatry Research. 2010; 178(2):230—235; Luppino FS, et al. Overweight, obesity, and depression. *Archives of General Psychiatry.* 2010; (67):220–229).

Obesity and gasoline. Obese individuals burn about nine gallons more fuel per year in their cars than normal-weight people because of the drag of their weight on the engine.

Obesity, gender differences and favorite foods. When asked to name their favorite foods, obese men answered "steak and roasts." Obese women responded with "doughnuts, cookies and cakes." The second favorite meal for obese men was ice cream and frozen desserts, however, obese women chose bread, rolls, and crackers. Third on the list for men was chicken and turkey, and the women preferred ice cream and frozen desserts as their third choice

Obesity and men—the perils of being portly. In a survey of 1,981 men aged 51–88, 24% reported moderate to severe erectile dysfunction (ED). The men with ED were more likely to be older, have hypertension, and weigh more than their study counterparts. Men with waistlines measuring 42 inches were found to be twice as likely to suffer from ED compared to men whose waistlines measured 32 inches. Men who were sedentary were also twice as likely to suffer from ED as men who exercised at least 30 minutes per day. Guys, listen up. Get off that couch, pick up those weights, and hit the gym runnin'.

Let me put it this way. According to my girth, I should be a ninety-foot redwood. —Erma Bombeck

Obesity and viruses. Do viruses cause obesity? The year was 1990. The place was Bombay, India. The scene was a veterinarian discussing a serendipitous observation with a nutritionist. During the discussion, the veterinarian commented that he had made the observation concerning a lethal viral infection in chickens and their tendency to gain a significant amount of weight prior to their demise. Within a 3-week period from the time they acquired the viral infection to the time of death, the chickens gained 60–75% more fat than the chickens that were not infected. In chickens, the virus appeared to alter metabolism such that, even with the same food and exercise, infected birds gained more weight than uninfected ones.

The nutritionist, Nikhil Dhurander, found the correlation fascinating enough to continue the research and to look for a human corollary. He moved to Madison, Wisconsin, to continue his research. The human counterpart to the chicken virus was found to be Adenovirus-36 (AD-36). After six years of research, he reported his findings to the North American Association for the Study of Obesity.

Dhurander found that obese patients (15% of 150 patients weighing 250 pounds or more) had antibodies to the virus, compared to the control group who did not have any antibodies and who were lean. Lab animals injected with AD-36 gained enough weight to be classified as clinically obese. A paradoxical characteristic of the virus is that it appears to cause low cholesterol and triglycerides along with obesity. This is good. Obese individuals with AD-36 antibodies also had lower cholesterol and triglycerides than other obese individuals.

Does this mean that antiviral drugs can be used to reduce weight, or even better, to prevent weight gain? Wouldn't that be the answer to all of our obesity problems? The answer is a resounding "no." Researchers state that the large majority of obese Americans gain their weight the "old-fashioned" way: too many calories and too little exercise. (*ADVANCE for Nurse Practitioners*, November 1997; Atkinson RL, Dhurandhar NV, Allison DB, et al. Human adenovirus-36 is associated with increased body weight and paradoxical reduction of serum lipids. *Int J Obes* (Lond). 2005; 29(3):281–286)

Smoking is responsible for 400,000 deaths per year...obesity for 300,000 deaths per year. Whom should our government sue for obesity deaths? —Anonymous

Obese moms, dyslipidemia, and neural tube defects. Two studies have demonstrated a link between obesity (pre-pregnant weight) and the risk of neural tube defects. One study noted a twofold risk increase among women with a body mass index (BMI) greater than 29. This finding was independent of other known causes of neural tube defects including folic acid deficiency, type 1 diabetes, use of diet pills, and even previous pregnancy affected by neural tube defects. The second study confirms these findings. Since as many as 10% of women may be obese prior to conception, these findings are important. (Shaw GM, et al. Risk of neural tube defect-affected pregnancies among obese women. *JAMA* 1996; 275(14):1093–1096)

Obesity and breakfast. A new study shows that the more often adolescents eat breakfast; the less likely they are to be overweight. There was a direct relationship between body mass index and eating breakfast—the more often they had breakfast, the lower their BMI. Interestingly, breakfast eaters consumed greater amounts of carbohydrates and fiber, but consumed fewer calories from fat and exercised more. Consumption of fiber-rich foods may improve glucose and insulin levels, making people feel satisfied and less likely to eat later in the day. (Dr. Mark Pereira, University of Minnesota, March 2007)

At the start of the study, consistent breakfast eaters had a BMI of 21.7; intermittent eaters 22.5; never had breakfast—23.4. Over the next five years the BMI increased in exactly the same pattern even after controlling for age, sex, race, socioeconomic status, smoking and concerns about diet and weight.

Obstruction due to dried fruit. Abdominal surgery was performed on an older woman with the clinical diagnosis of obstruction. Once again, since the woman was elderly, it was presumed that the obstruction was due to a malignancy blocking the bowel. However, once the surgeon arrived at the designated area, he found a complete undigested apricot blocking the lumen of the intestine. He was perplexed, naturally, and asked the daughter if she might be able to explain the finding. The woman's daughter said that she had given her mom some dried fruit several days before. Could it be that the dried fruit absorbed water and expanded into the mass that blocked the bowel?

As an experiment, the surgeon soaked some dried apricots in water for twenty-four hours. Over that period of time the dried apricots absorbed enough water that they enlarged to the size of a fresh whole apricot, about the size of a golf ball. He speculated that the older woman did not chew the dried apricot adequately and most likely swallowed it in its entirety.

Oils. Olive oil contains about 85% monounsaturated fatty acids, mainly oleic acid, and about 15% saturated fatty acids, mainly palmitic acid. In contrast, soybean oil has only about 8% saturated fat, and has a lot more essential fatty acids—both omega-6 (mainly linoleic acid) and omega-3 (mainly alpha-linoleic acid, ALA). Canola oil also has quite a bit of ALA and much more omega-6 than olive oil, though somewhat less than soybean oil. Fish oil, of course, contains at least 50% eicosapentaenoic acid (EPA) and docosahexanoic acid (DHA—the omega-3 fatty acids that are good for the brain and the heart.

OLESTRA

Olestra. Oh no, oh no, olestra. What is olestra? Olestra is a calorie-free fat substitute that is licensed by Proctor and Gamble under the trade name of Olean. It is Procter and Gamble's way of saying you can eat more *fat-free* potato chips and not worry about the calories—WOW! No-guilt chips. Fabulous. But is it? Frito-Lay has licensed olestra for its Doritos, Lay's, and Ruffles potato chips. It depletes the body of carotenoids (antioxidant compounds that have been shown to reduce the risk of cancer and coronary artery disease) as well as vitamins A, D, E, and K. Eating chips with olestra does help cut the fat intake, which in turn, does reduce caloric intake. Unfortunately, most people make up for the missing calories by boosting their intake of other high caloric foods and any calorie savings is lost. But, if you eat snack food with olestra/Olean, don't forget to read the small print. Two of the dreaded side effects of olestra include severe abdominal cramping and "anal leakage." Anal leakage is Frito-Lay's way of saying: diarrhea-that-is-almost-impossible-to-reach-the-toilet-in-time-with.

OLIVES

Olives. In order to cut costs, American Airlines eliminated one olive from each salad in their first class meal service. They saved $40,000 per year with this cost-cutting stroke of genius. Apparently it wasn't enough.

OLIVE OIL

Olive oil (extra virgin). The biggest health benefit of olive oil is that nearly three-quarters of its fat content is monosaturated fat, which lowers LDL-cholesterol (the bad guy) while leaving the good cholesterol, HDL, undisturbed. This makes it a perfect fat to use to protect the heart. Olive oil also contains polyphenols which are antioxidants. Extra-virgin olive oil is the *least* processed form of olive oil, so it provides the most nutrients. Virgin olive oil is next and "light" olive oil has the exact same amount of calories as virgin and extra-virgin, but it has gone through more processing, so it has a lighter color and milder flavor. It's a popular choice for baking.

"YUCK, I can't stand the taste of olive oil…" Yeah? That's because you're too *cheap* to buy the good stuff. Spend a little extra on the extra-virgin olive oil. Olive oil should have a little "bite" to it when you use it as dipping oil for your breads or for making sauces, and as a component of oil and vinegar salad dressings. The more expensive olive oils are much more flavorful.

Ah yes, but it 'tis a fat, albeit a "healthy" fat—the monounsaturated type of fat. Note that it contains about 120 calories per tablespoon, so it isn't considered a "skinny" fat.

Which oils are best for your health? Oils low in saturated fat but high in monosaturated fat are considered to be the best for health's sake. Below is a chart you can use to check percentages of saturated fat (the bad fat) and monosaturated fat (if there is a good fat, this would be the one).

Content	**Saturated fat**	**Monosaturated fat**
Canola	6%	62%
Grapeseed	7%	79%
Safflower	9%	12%
Sunflower	11%	20%
Peanut	13%	49%
Corn	13%	25%
Olive	14%	77%
Soybean	15%	24%
Vegetable shortening	26%	43%
Butter	54%	30%

(Source: USDA Nutrient Database: www.nal.usda.gov/fnic/cgi-bin;nut_search.pl)

Does cooking with olive oil destroy the health benefits? Some nutritionists and health professionals, including Dr. Oz, state that it's a waste to cook with extra virgin olive oil because the heat dissipates some of the flavor and destroys some of the antioxidants that make extra-virgin olive oil special. While that's true, it doesn't destroy all of the health benefits. (Krasner D. The Flavors of Live Oil: A Tasting Guide and Cookbook, Simon & Schuster, 2011).

OMEGA-3

Omega-3 fatty acids. Can you say seafood? "Seafood, seafood, and seafood." Okay, okay, okay. Seafood is rich in omega-3 fatty acid. Which seafood? All seafood? Mrs. Paul's fish sticks? Fried Mississippi catfish? No, not exactly. The types of fish that contain the greatest amounts of fatty acids also tend to have high fat contents. When choosing a fish for omega-3 content, choose a fish with the most omega-3 fatty acids for the least amount of fat. The fish containing the most omega-3 fatty acids, more than 1,000 mg

HISTORICAL HIGHLIGHT

On March 35, 1935, two physicians from St. Mary's Medical School in London announced that they had successfully treated pneumonia by emulsifying olive oil and injecting it into the veins of the patients. The high temperatures in the patients with pneumonia returned to normal within twenty-four hours after the oil injections and within three weeks the patients had recovered from pneumonia. Olive oil injections were also used in patients with septicemia and acute rheumatism. The physicians hypothesized that the olive oil absorbed the pneumonia and other toxins circulating in the blood.

Fast forward to 2011. Was this really such a wacky concept? Not really. Using oil to neutralize and/or sop up bacterial toxins was actually based on scientific knowledge of neutralizing foreign substances—similar to what the immune system does. (*Science News*, November 5, 2011)

per 3½ oz. serving, include anchovies, Atlantic halibut, herring, mackerel, salmon (Atlantic chinook, coho, king, pink, sockeye), sardines, shark, trout (rainbow, lake), and tuna (albacore, bluefin). Fish weighing from 500 to 900 milligrams include Pacific halibut, rockfish, salmon, smelt, squid, striped sea bass, swordfish, turbot, tuna (yellowfin), and whitefish. Krill, tiny shrimp-like crustaceans also contain omega-3 fatty acids.

OK, so you are a vegetarian, vegan, allergic to seafood, or just plain don't like seafood. You also have options. Non-marine based omega-3 fatty acids are found in walnuts, green leafy vegetables, canola oil, soybean oil, flax oil, algae oil, ground flaxseeds and tofu. The omega-3 fatty acid in the non-marine based foods is alpha-linolenic acid. It has to be converted into omega-3 fatty acids once consumed.

The two major marine-based omega-3 fatty acids are docosahexanoic acid (DHA) and eicosapentanoic acid (EPA). Well, you have no doubt heard about the omega-3s in the news, so just what the heck are omega-3 fatty acids? Omega-3 fatty acids are polyunsaturated essential fatty acids found primarily in fish and fish oils. The term "essential" means that we "essentially" need them to live. Unfortunately, this is one of those "essential" things that we do not make ourselves, so we have to obtain them from another source. In this case, the source would be the fish we eat, the flaxseed we grind, or the walnuts we use in our Waldorf salad. (Does anybody eat "Waldorf" salad anymore?)

Omega-3s first attracted major scientific attention in 1979 when researchers studied native Greenlanders whose diets consisted mainly of cold-water fish. The risk of heart disease in this population was 50% lower than that of adults in the U.S. who were devouring T-bones and NY strip steaks and few, if any, cold-water fish.

Numerous studies have since confirmed the cardioprotective benefits of omega-3 fatty acids. One mechanism of action appears to involve a positive effect on the lipoprotein profile, with an increase in the "good cholesterol" or high-density lipoproteins, as well as a reduction in triglycerides. Another mechanism of action is that omega-3s are converted to a compound similar to prostacyclin, a naturally occurring vasodilator that also inhibits platelets.

In a meta-analysis of 12 randomized trials that involved almost 33,000 patients, investigators evaluated the effects of fish oil supplements on cardiac arrhythmias and mortality. The findings were positive:

...among all patients, fish oil significantly lowered the risk for death from cardiac causes (by 20%); however, it did not lower the risk for all-cause death.

...among patients with known coronary artery disease, fish oil significantly lowered risk for sudden cardiac death (by 26%) and for death from cardiac causes (by 20%).

The above results do not support recommending fish oil to patients without CAD, at least for the prevention of CAD. Omega-3s have numerous other benefits so everyone would benefit from a couple of servings two to three times per week. Read on for the myriad of other benefits of omega-3 fatty acids.

(Alice H. Lichtestein, DSc, director of Cardiovascular Nutrition Laboratory, Tufts Jean Mayer Human Nutrition Research Center on Aging, Boston MA, 2007; León H et al. Effect of fish oil on arrhythmias and mortality: Systematic review. *BMJ* 2008 Dec 23; 338:a2931).

Is there absolutely NO END to the benefits of eating fish containing omega-3 fatty acids? Let's get with the program folks...face it, don't make a face about it. EAT SALMON. EAT FLOUNDER. EAT COD. EAT SARDINES. "But I might be exposed to too much mercury and PCBs and dioxin," she whines. Stop whining and chow down.

A search of the medical literature, supplemented by reviews of references and direct investigator contacts, identified reports evaluating intake of fish or fish oil and cardiovascular risk, effects of methyl mercury and fish oil on early neurodevelopment, risks of methyl mercury for cardiovascular and neurologic outcomes in adults and health risks of dioxin, and PCBs in fish. An interesting note on PCBs, for those of you worried about your intake of PCBs and possible cancer risk: 91% of the PCBs in the American diet come from beef, chicken, pork, dairy products, vegetables, and eggs. Ok, so you're still worried about the risk of cancer and PCBs in fish because you are a fish "af*fish*ionado"... relax. Using data from the Environmental Protection Agency, researchers from the Harvard School of Public Health have this to say: The PCB intake from eating farmed salmon twice a week for 70 years would cause an extra 6 cases of cancer per 100,000 people, while eating wild salmon would cause an extra 2 cases. Yet eating either farmed or wild salmon twice a week for 70 years would prevent at least 7,000 deaths from heart disease. Hello? Is anyone listening out there? Clearly, the benefits of fish and cardiovascular disease far outweigh the risks of cancer from the PCB content of fish.

After all of the research and number crunching the recommendations are as follows:

1) As noted above, omega-3s stabilize heart rhythms and prevent cardiac arrhythmias.
2) In addition, omega-3 fatty acids have a beneficial effect on the lipid profile—lowering total cholesterol and increasing HDLs and reducing LDLs.
3) Omega-3 fatty acids are also anti-inflammatory, and, since inflammation is currently the biggest buzzword in the world of cardiovascular disease, anything that has an anti-inflammatory effect is beneficial.
4) Women of childbearing age and nursing mothers should consume two to four 3-ounce seafood servings per week (up to 12 ounces per week), especially the fish with highest concentrations of EPA and DHA. Everyone should limit their intake of older fish because they have had more time to accumulate mercury. These include the large predatory varieties like shark, swordfish, king mackerel, and tilefish, the species with the highest levels of mercury because they eat smaller contaminated fish. Chilean sea bass, rockfish, grouper, bluefish, and bluefin tuna also contain worrisome amounts of mercury.
5) The best sources for omega-3 rich seafood low in contaminants are salmon (wild and farmed), mackerel (but not king mackerel, which is high in mercury), mussels, oysters, anchovies, rainbow trout, herring, and sardines. Canned white (albacore) tuna has three times the omega-3 fatty acids of light tuna, but it also contains three times the mercury. Nursing women and children under 12 should limit white tuna intake to 6 ounces or less per week. The mercury levels in white tuna are thought to pose little risk to the adult nervous system.

The following is a list of the fish with their levels of omega-3 fatty acids and their relative amounts of mercury and PCBs. The relative amount of omega-3 (in milligrams, or mg) compared to the amount of mercury and PCBs (in micrograms, or mcg) is listed in the parentheses after the fish. For example, H/H/L is high in omega-3s and high in mercury and low in PCBs vs. H/L/L which is high in omega-3s, low in mercury, and low in PCBs. Cut this chart out of this fascinating book (or make a copy of it) and slap it on the front of your refrigerator for future reference. (P.S. A note on milligrams vs. micrograms. It's hard to compare the two because micrograms are one thousand times smaller than milligrams—think comparing grapefruit to raisins in terms of size/amounts.)

- Salmon (H/L/L) (wild or farmed) (farmed salmon has the highest omega-3s with 4500 mg per 2 servings; wild salmon has 1900 mg per

2 servings; negligible mercury; 50 mcg PCBs for farmed salmon; wild salmon has negligible PCBs and negligible mercury)

- Sardines (H/L/M) (2 servings = 1800 mg of omega-3s; 100 mcg PCBs)
- Trout (H/L/L) (2 servings = 1700 mg of omega 3s; negligible mercury and PCBs)
- Canned or fresh tuna (H/H/H) (white tuna has 1500 mg of omega-3s per 2 servings; light tuna has 500 mg of omega-3s per serving) (white tuna has 75 mcg of mercury per 2 servings, vs. light tuna with 25–50 mcg of mercury per 2 servings; white tuna has over 200 mcg of PCBs per 2 servings—this level of PCBs is above the "action level" given by the FDA; light tuna has 125 mcg of PCBs, below the "action level" given by the FDA)
- Tilefish (H/H) (2 servings = 1750 mg of omega-3s; 225 mcg of mercury)
- Swordfish (H/H) (2 servings of swordfish has 1500 mg of omega-3 fatty acids, BUT it also has 200 mcg of mercury, which is the upper limit of the recommended mercury limit for pregnant or lactating women and children)
- Mussels (H/L/L) (2 servings = 1500 mg of omega-3s; 50 mcg of mercury; negligible PCBs)
- Shark (H/H/L) (2 servings = 1200 mg of omega-3s and 200 mcg of mercury)
- Halibut (H/M) (2 servings = 1000 mg of omega-3s and 50 mcg of mercury)
- Shrimp/scallops/crab (M/L/L)(300 mg omega-3s, negligible mercury and PCBs)
- Pacific oysters (H/L) (4 ounces of Pacific oysters = 1550 mg omega-3s)
- Flounder (M/M)
- Chilean sea bass (M/H)
- Mackerel (not KING mackerel) (M/H)
- Grouper (L/H)

(*Harvard Heart Letter,* February 2007) {Mozaffarian D, Rimm EB. Fish intake, contaminants, and human health: evaluating the risks and the benefits. *JAMA* 2006; 296:1885-1899; Institute of Medicine; Seafood Choices: Balancing Benefits and Risks; www.iom.edu (click on "Reports"); www.oceansalive.com; www.seafoodchoices.com; www.ewg.org/issues/mercury; www.nrdc.org/health/effects/mercury/guide.asp; www.gotmercury.org}

Omega-3 recommendations. Although the FDA does not regulate supplements, it has recommended safe limits of 3,000 milligrams (mg) per day for omega-3 fatty acids from fish and supplements combined, and 2,000 mg per day from supplements alone. Supplements may increase the risk for bleeding, especially if the patient is on anticoagulant drugs such as warfarin (Coumadin), dabigatran (Pradax/Pradaxa), and rivaroxaban (Xarelto).

Don't forget that dietary supplements are not approved for safety or effectiveness by any of the approval groups such as the FDA and USDA. A recent review by the independent organization known as ConsumerLab.com found only 17 of the 24 omega-3 supplements tested passed their tests for purity, freshness, and correct dosage of omega-3 listed on the packaging. Buyer beware, once again. (*Environmental Nutrition.* February 2011)

Omega-3s and bipolar disease. In a May 1999 *Archives of General Psychiatry,* patients with bipolar disease received either omega-3 fish oil or olive oil (as placebo) along with their standard medications, including lithium and Depakote. After four months, 65% of the omega-3 recipients improved compared to only 19% of the olive oil group. Subsequent studies have also confirmed the findings.

Omega-3 fatty acids—bumping up the amount in foods. How, might you ask? Changing the diets of pigs, cows, chickens, and other farm animals may just be the answer. Eggs from chickens allowed to forage for part of their food average four times the omega-3 fatty acids found in factory-produced eggs. Just feeding chickens flaxseed can bump up the omega-3 fatty acid content of the chicken eggs. Feeding the nutritious weed purslane to animals can also bump up the omega-3s. Purslane is higher in omega-3s than any other vegetable. In addition to improving the quality of meat, purslane feed could produce healthier butter and eggs. And eggs, unlike fish, are plentiful, cheap and free of pollutants. Hmmm…just a thought. But, there's also genetic engineering—omega-3s can also be spliced and diced into foods. This, of course, would be the alternative if chicken farmers are loathe to allow those pesky chickens out of their cages to pick and peck for food a few hours a day. (*Science News,* May 27, 2006)

Omega-3s and Type 1 diabetes. Researchers in Colorado tested 1770 children with a genetic risk for developing type 1 diabetes. The researchers assessed their dietary intake of omega-3 fatty acids and measured islet cell autoantibodies as markers for developing the disease. They started measuring islet cell autoantibodies annually and found that at a mean age of 6.2 years, 58 children had developed islet autoimmunity (positive for at least 1 or 3 specific autoantibodies). After adjusting for known variables, the intake of total omega-3 fatty acid was inversely associated with the risk for islet autoimmunity. When two or more antibodies were used as an endpoint, the inverse association between omega-3 intake and islet autoimmunity was even stronger. These findings suggest that dietary intake of omega-3 fatty acids after age 1 year reduces the risk prior to age six. How long the protective effect lasts is unknown. Recommending a diet rich in omega-3 fatty acids early in life for children at risk for type 1 diabetes mellitus seems reasonable at this time. (Norris JM, et al. Omega-3 polyunsaturated fatty acid intake and islet cell autoimmunity in children at increased risk for type 1 diabetes. *JAMA* 2007 Sep 26; 298:1420)

Omega-3s and the heart. Is there no end to the benefits of fish oil and the heart? Patients with chronic heart failure taking fish oil have a small, but statistically significant reduction in death rate compared to patients in either a placebo or a statin drug. Fish oil is packed with omega-3 fatty acids, which not only increase HDLs, the good cholesterol, but also decrease inflammation throughout the arteries. The benefits of omega 3 fatty acids and the prevention heart disease are controversial to say the least. Some cardiologists swear by them, other cardiologists are underwhelmed by the literature, and some don't use omega-3s at all. All of that being said read the results of the Health Impact Study below.

ASPARAGUS TIP

If all men and women over age 65 took 1,800 mg of omega-3 fatty acids daily, coronary heart disease would be reduced to the extent that about 374,000 hospitalizations could be avoided over five years. (The Health Impact Study IV commissioned by the Dietary Supplement Education Alliance September, 2009)

Obviously more research is necessary. But, before you toss your bottle of fish oil capsules, read on—omega-3s have numerous benefits throughout the body.

Omega-3s and cancer prevention. Omega-3 fatty acids may play a role in preventing certain cancers, as well as enhancing traditional cancer therapies. New evidence suggests that omega-3 fatty acids may also slow the rate of metastatic disease. Women whose diets consist mainly of fish (Asian women for example) exhibit a relatively low incidence of breast cancer. Clinical studies have demonstrated that fish oils inhibit mammary tumor growth in the laboratory, not only preventing the tumor from growing in the first place, but also reducing tumor size in existing breast cancers.

Omega-3s and macular degeneration. Eating marine-based omega 3 fatty acids at least once a week compared with less than once a week was associated with a reduction of developing severe neovascular macular degeneration by half. Studies also found that a high dietary intake of omega-3 fatty acids was associated with a 38% reduction in the risk of late macular degeneration. Fish intake at least twice a week was associated with a reduced risk of both early and late macular degeneration. (Augood C, et al. Oily fish consumption, dietary docosahexaenoic acid and eicoapentanoic acid intakes, and associations with neovascular age-related macular degeneration. *Am J Clin Nutr* 2008; 88:390—406; Chong EWT, et al. Dietary omega-3 fatty acid and fish intake in the primary prevention of age-related macular degeneration. *Arch Ophthalmol* 2008; 126:826—833)

Omega-3s and rheumatoid arthritis. Omega-3 fatty acids inhibit the production of leukotrienes, inflammatory mediators produced in various tissues including the joints. This has implications for individuals with chronic inflammatory pain syndromes such as rheumatoid arthritis.

A report on the use of complementary medicine for arthritis published in February 2009 by the UK-based Arthritis Research Campaign, showed that 62 percent (13 out of 21) of complementary treatments were shown to have little or no effect, scoring only one out of five on the effectiveness scale. These included feverfew, flaxseed oil, homeopathic remedies, selenium, and the antioxidant vitamins A, C, and E. By contrast, fish oil containing omega-3 fatty acids scored ***five out of five*** on the effectiveness scale.

Researchers from the University of Washington and the Fred Hutchinson Cancer Research Center examined the diets of 324 women who later developed rheumatoid arthritis. The study also followed 1,245 women who remained free of rheumatoid arthritis and served as the control group. The women who ate at least one to two servings of baked or broiled fish each week were 22% less likely to develop rheumatoid arthritis, compared with those who ate fewer servings of fish.

Omega-3s and sockeye salmon. Just one serving of sockeye salmon has 27 times the amount of omega-3 fatty acids as a piece of sole. Alaskan natives whose chief form of protein is salmon have less than one-third of the heart attack rate of U.S. Caucasians, even though twice as many of the Alaskan natives smoke cigarettes. Omega-3 fatty acids have anti-inflammatory properties, anti-platelet properties, and anti-arrhythmic properties. Broil it, grill it, pan-fry or poach it. To get the richest flavor from a salmon fillet, begin cooking with the skin side up. There is a layer of fat just beneath the skin, and by starting with the skin side up when you grill or broil fillets, the fat will trickle down into the flesh of the fish, adding flavor and moisture.

Omega-3 fish oil supplements. Fish oil capsules are one of the most popular nutritional supplements. But do you really get all of the health benefits from these capsules? YES, but make sure you get a combined amount of EPAs and DHAs of 500 to 1000 mg/day. Choose wisely as all fish oil supplements vary widely in the amount of actual fish oil they contain.

ONIONS

Onions. Why do raw onions bring a tear to your eye? Slicing an onion damages the cell walls, releasing enzymes and sulfur-containing amino acids that trigger a chemical reaction when coming in contact with each other. These volatile sulfur-containing compounds irritate the eyes and stimulate the tear glands. The irritating chemicals just happen to be water-soluble, and the flowing tears help dissolve them. Two helpful hints to reduce the tearing that accompanies raw onion cutting: Hold the onion under cold water while cutting it and/or chill the onion before peeling it.

Onions most likely possess these tearing compounds as a sort of chemical survival system that keeps predators away. It must have worked—onions and other members of the lily family have survived for thousands of years.

In Bluff, Utah, the law forbids barbers from eating onions between 7 a.m. and 7 p.m.

HISTORICAL HIGHLIGHT

For more than five millennia, human beings have treated their ailments with extraordinary creativity. For example, in 2000 BC, Assyrian and Babylonian doctors used a salve made of frog bile and sour milk for treating infected eyes, but this concoction was considered effective only after the patient took a swig of beer chased by a slice of onion.

The round shape of the onion signified eternity to the Egyptians. The Egyptians would place their right hand on an onion when taking an oath.

Oranges. Say yes to oranges! An orange is every bit as nutritional as an apple. In fact, it might even bypass the apple if you look at the Overall Nutritional Quality Index of an orange vs. an apple. But we're splitting hairs here, really. Not into apples? Grab an orange.

Oranges are native to Asia but they arrived in Europe via the trade routes in the 15th century. Christopher Columbus brought orange seeds to the Caribbean on his second voyage and by the 16th century orange trees were blossoming in Florida. Spanish missionaries took oranges to California in the 18th century.

The peak season for navel oranges, my favorite, is January through March. Valencias, the most popular orange for orange juice, are available February through October, peaking in the summer months.

Oranges' best known nutritional benefit is their overabundance of vitamin C. If fact, one orange contains 130% of the daily value—more than you actually need per day. Vitamin C wasn't isolated in the laboratory until 1907, but its power to prevent scurvy was known centuries earlier. Even the scientific name for vitamin C—"ascorbic acid"—derives from the Latin for "no scurvy." (For more on vitamin C, please go to chapter V)

Besides vitamin C, oranges contain an abundance of lesser-known antioxidants, including more than 179 phytonutrients and 60 flavonoids. Of particular interest are compounds called limonoids, which scientists are currently studying for cholesterol-lowering benefits.

Oranges contain carotenoids, phytochemicals that gives them their distinct and beautiful color. Beta-cryptoxanthin, the orange color phytochemical, may also provide some protection against lung cancer. Another carotenoid in oranges, zeaxanthin, may help reduce the risk of rheumatoid arthritis—by as much as 52% in one study. (EPIC-Norfolk study, 1999)

One orange provides 12.5% of the daily value of dietary fiber—most of which is lost when you squeeze it into a glass. A cup of orange juice only contains a half a gram of dietary fiber, the whole medium orange contains three grams of fiber. If you've avoided oranges because you are avoiding carbohydrates, think again: Most fruits contain quality carbs that release their energy slowly. Oranges have a glycemic index (GI) of 44. The lower the glycemic index the slower the rise in glucose after a meal and the slower the release of insulin.

And, we're not done yet. Oranges contain folate (9.9% of the daily value), potassium (6.8% of the daily value), thiamin (7.3% of the daily value), vitamin A (5.4% of the daily value), and calcium (5.2%) of the daily value. All of that for only 80 calories for a whole medium orange! WOW.

There is no word that rhymes with orange.

Organic foods. Just what is an "organic food"? Americans pay more than $6 billion per year for these foods, so what are you getting when it says "USDA Organic" on the label? Organic foods are supposed to be grown without herbicides, pesticides, synthetic fertilizers, sewage sludge (ick), hormones, artificial additives, chemicals, or any other "unnatural" substance or preservative. However, until recently, many unscrupulous food growers would slap "organic" on the label and consumers had little assurance that this is what they were getting.

Finally the USDA released a set of standards for labeling organic foods in 2002. The rules divide organic products into four categories with products that are advertised as "100% organic" at the top of the list. These products must contain only organic ingredients, excluding water and salt. The next category must contain 95% organic ingredients, once again excluding water and salt. Any of the remaining 5% must be non-agricultural products on an approved list, or non-organically produced products that are not available commercially in organic form. The above categories can proudly display the new USDA organic seal that most likely took 10 years to develop and another 10 for the government officials to agree on.

The remaining two categories are the "also rans." The first food products in this category can carry the label that says they are "Products made with organic ingredients" as long as they contain at least 70 to 90% organic ingredients. The last category can list specific organic ingredients on the package, but cannot have "organic" on the label if they have less than 70% organic ingredients.

ASPARAGUS TIP

Fungus and molds on foods cause health risks, and they are more common on organic crops that don't use fungicides to kill them. A mold that grows on corn and peanuts produces the carcinogen alflatoxin, and can cause an entire crop to be rejected.

Are organic foods more nutritious and delicious than non-organic foods? A very simple answer to this one—No. (Dangour AD, et al. Nutritional quality of organic foods: A systematic review. *Am J Clin Nutr* 2009 Sep; 90:680)

Do organic foods cost more than non-organic foods? A very simple answer to this one—Yes, by about 50% in supermarkets and natural food stores. Organic foods are more expensive to grow and harvest. If you choose not to pay the additional 50% for overhead, make sure that you wash your pesticide-grown produce with soap and water or acidic vegetable washes or diluted vinegar and water.

Health nuts are going to feel stupid someday, lying in hospitals dying of nothing. —Redd Foxx

---

Orthorexia nervosa. Do you spend more than three hours per day thinking about healthy food? Do you care more about the virtue of what you eat than the pleasure you receive from eating it? Have you found that as the quality of your diet has increased, the quality of your life has correspondingly diminished? Do you keep getting stricter with yourself? Do you sacrifice experiences you once enjoyed to eat the food you believe is right? Do you feel an increased sense of self-esteem when you are eating healthy food and look down on others who don't? Does your diet socially isolate you? When you are eating the way you are supposed to, do you feel a peaceful sense of self-control? Do you plan your food for tomorrow today? Do you feel guilt or self-loathing when you stray from your diet?

If you have answered "yes" to one or two of these questions you may have a mild case of orthorexia, an obsession with eating healthfully that becomes so strong it leads to progressively rigid dieting that eliminates crucial food groups and nutrients. If you have said "yes" to four or more questions this means that you are in a bit of trouble concerning your unhealthy obsession with food, and if you answer "yes" to all of the questions, you are out of control and definitely need the services of a trained psychiatric professional.

Orthorexia nervosa is an obsession with the quality of food, not the quantity of food (anorexia nervosa). Healthy eating becomes a disease in its own right. Individuals lose sight of their obsessive behavior, believing that by managing their diets they can ward off illness and live happily ever after.

Orthorexia is not present at birth. This condition gradually develops over time as the obsession with diet and eating properly occupies a greater part of the day. An orthorexic will lose all pleasure at a dinner party if she eats a piece of cooked broccoli instead of eating broccoli raw. She will berate herself tirelessly if she eats a spoonful of ice cream. Interested in reading more about this horrifying condition? (Health Food Junkies: Overcoming the Obsession with Healthful Eating by Dr. Steven Bratman, Broadway Books, 2004)

I will not eat oysters. I want my food dead. Not sick, not wounded, dead. —Woody Allen.

OYSTERS

Oyster alert. If you like oysters, make sure you cook them well before eating them. Raw oysters are a delicacy of the past, unless you want to play Russian roulette with your health. Even oysters harvested from regularly monitored beds can make you sick if you don't cook them through and through. A 13-state outbreak of food poisoning in 1998 was traced to raw or undercooked oysters from Galveston Bay, Texas. This outbreak followed a summer of record-breaking heat which most likely spawned a population explosion of the bacteria *Vibrio parahemolyticus.* Despite monitoring of water quality and bacteria levels at the harvesting sites, more than 400 people in 13 states reported becoming ill with diarrhea, cramping, nausea, headaches, and vomiting within 24 hours of exposure to the infected oysters.

Another *Vibrio* species that contaminates raw oysters is *Vibrio vulnificus.* This bacterium is also commonly found in waters where oysters are cultivated such as the Gulf of Mexico The hotter the month the higher the concentrations of the bacteria. However, the old wives' tale that says it's safe to eat oysters in any month that has an "r" in it is not true. While fresh oysters are highest in bacteria in the summer months of May, June, July, and August, they can also be deadly in the other eight months as well. (FDA, "The danger of eating contaminated raw oysters: *Vibrio vulnificus* health education kit." Updated October 2009. http://www.fda.gov/Food/ResourcesForYou/HealthEducators/ucm085368.htm

So, it would behoove all avid oyster eaters to cook them before eating them, and walk right by the raw oyster bar. If you are cooking your own oysters (or clams), make sure they are cooked to an internal temperature of 140° F. It's rather tough to use a thermometer with oysters, so just make sure that you cook them another 4 to 6 minutes after the shells have opened.

ASPARAGUS TIP

True? Adding lime juice or hot sauce to raw oysters can kill the bacteria. Not true.

Oysters and the Doctrine of Signatures. As mentioned in the Chapter D, the Doctrine of Signatures is based on the concept that for every part of the human body there is a corresponding part in the world of nature. The ancient physician-priests used this doctrine as the basis for their medical therapies.

The oyster has long been held in high esteem as an aphrodisiac. Oysters were believed to boost libido, elevate testosterone levels, and increase sperm counts. Is there any truth to this claim? A platter of raw oysters somehow doesn't trigger lascivious thoughts in the average American, but if you look a little closer with the Doctrine of Signatures in mind, the oyster resembles a human testicle—in size, in shape, and in color.

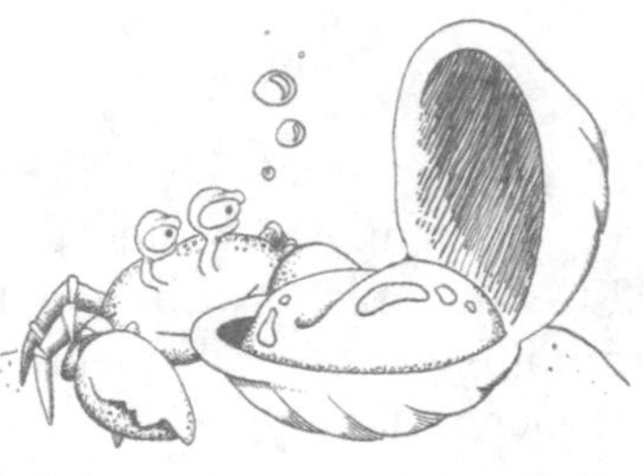

Combine the physical appearance of the oyster with the fact that oysters are nature's most concentrated source of zinc. Batches of oysters can vary in their amounts of zinc, and that variation can be anywhere from 28 mg/100 g sample in an April batch to 55 mg/100g sample compared to other natural medicinal plants used to correct male factor infertility which range from 2.09 mg/100 g sample to 6.2 mg/100 gram sample. Zinc contributes to the production of the testosterone and sperm. Normal males with zinc deficiency fail to produce enough testicular testosterone, resulting in erectile dysfuntion and low sperm count. Eat your oysters! (Modupe O, et al. Determination of the concentrations of zinc and vitamin C in oysters and some medicinal plants used to correct male factor infertility. *Journal of Natural Products* 2009;2: 89–97)

CHAPTER P

I had left home (like all Jewish girls) in order to eat pork and take birth control pills. When I first shared an intimate evening with my husband, I was swept away by the passion (so dormant inside myself) of a long and tortured existence. The physical cravings I had tried so hard to deny, finally and ultimately sated…but enough about the pork.

—Roseanne Arnold

Packer, Alfred (1842–1907). Alfred Packer's claim to fame is that in 1873 he led a party of amateur prospectors through the San Juan Mountains during one of the worst snowstorms of the century. He returned alone, saying that his companions abandoned him. Months afterwards, search parties found the bodies of the missing men, most of which had been stripped of their flesh and cannibalized. Packer was tried, found guilty of murder, and sentenced to 40 years of hard labor. As the judge was issuing his sentence he said, "Packer, you depraved Republican son of a bitch, there were only five Democrats in Hinsdale County, and you ate them all!"

Pain management and foods/supplements. Can certain foods actually reduce pain and inflammation? Yes. These foods are discussed in various sections of the book but for the sake of convenience here's the list:

…..Coffee has been shown to reduce muscle pain during and after exercise. It's the caffeine. Caffeine is added to many drugs for its synergistic effects on pain management.

…..Curcumin is an anti-inflammatory spice found in curry. Give it a try for osteoarthritis.

…..Ginger has been shown to reduce the pain of too much exercise. ☺ Yes, there is such a condition as "too much exercise."

…..Glucosamine and chondroitin, supplements that are usually packaged together, have demonstrated positive benefits in some people some of the time for some arthritis pain. In other words, sometimes it might help, but give it a three month trial before pooh-poohing it.

…..Green tea has been shown to reduce inflammation and the pain of arthritis.

.....Olive oil contains oleocanthal, a compound similar to prostaglandin-inhibiting properties of ibuprofen.

.....Omega-3 fatty acids are used to ease arthritis pain—have similar action and effectiveness as ibuprofen.

.....Pomegranate and cherries can be added to the ginger statement. Both are linked with reducing musculoskeletal pain after a round of heavy exercise.

.....Red grapes or wine. I prefer the wine. But either will do as both contain resveratrol and resveratrol has been shown to reduce inflammatory pain.

.....SAMe (S-adenosylmethionine) supplements appear to be as effective as anti-inflammatory drugs such as ibuprofen and celecoxib for the relief of arthritis pain.

Pancreas. It takes 45 minutes from production to final secretion for digestive enzymes from the pancreas to enter the small intestine.

Parkinsonism from dietary sources. The island of Guam and the island of Guadeloupe in the Caribbean have something in common—an unusually high rate of Parkinsonism. It appears as if some of their traditional foods and teas might be the culprit. On the island of Guadeloupe there is an unusually high incidence among the natives who consume a lot of pawpaws, custard apples, and herbal teas made from leaves, seeds, or bark. These contain "actively insecticidal" neurotoxic alkaloids with presumed sedative and aphrodisiac properties. Parkinsonism has also been reported from Guam (known as the "Guam Syndrome") and has been attributed to a slow toxin found in their traditional food. A high prevalence of Parkinsonism has also been reported among Afro-Caribbean and Indian immigrants in England, many of whom continue to eat their own ethnic food. (*Lancet* 354:281, 1999)

Parsley. There's actually no current research to support the claim that chewing a sprig or two of parsley freshens one's breath. However, research from 60 years ago suggested that chlorophyll does have a breath deodorizing effect. Parsley contains chlorophyll so the natural progression would be that parsley could help freshen a case of nasty halitosis. Not willing to eat fresh parsley for presumed fresh breath? There are pills on the market today that contain chlorophyll or chlorophyllin, but some contain only small amounts of the active compound. Research suggests you need 100—300 mg a day to be effective. (*Environmental Nutrition.* April, 2008)

And, as an extra-added benefit, parsley contains an antioxidant punch with flavonoids and may have some anti-inflammatory properties. Certainly a sprig of parsley won't hurt you, and it provides three vitamins–A, C, and K.

If a parsley farmer is sued, can they garnish his wages? —George Carlin

---

Pâté. Pâté is 120 calories and nearly 4 grams of saturated fat per ounce, but it also provides almost 30% of the daily intake of Vitamin A.

Peas, frozen as an ice pack. Use an unopened bag of frozen peas as a substitute for an ice pack. This bag can readily mold itself to the shape of the body part to which it is applied. If the ice pack or bag of peas is applied over an injured part within five minutes, before any swelling takes place, you may reduce the risk of bruising and reduce edema (swelling).

Peanuts. The peanut was believed to be discovered by Spanish and Portuguese explorers in Peru around 2000 B.C. They distributed the peanut around the world. It most likely reached the U.S. via the slave trade from East Africa but it may have also made its way up from South America through Central America and Mexico. When peanuts were first cultivated in the United States, they were used for livestock feed to fatten pigs, turkeys and chickens. However, after the Civil War, they gained economic importance thanks to one of the most distinguished African Americans of the nineteenth century—George Washington Carver of the Tuskegee Institute. And today? Peanuts contribute more than $4 billion to the U.S. economy each year.

HISTORICAL HIGHLIGHT

After the Civil War the South's economy was in a tailspin. The cotton crops were being destroyed by the boll weevil and by over-planting. George Washington Carver showed that the neglected peanut, soybean, and sweet potato could produce hundreds of trade goods and replace soil minerals depleted by cotton. Carver spent most of his life studying the various uses of the peanut, and as a result he is credited with single-handedly revolutionizing the South's post-war economy.

The number one peanut producing state today is Georgia, followed by Texas, Alabama, and North Carolina. Former President Jimmy Carter is the most famous peanut farmer in this day and age. Little Jimmy first sold boiled peanuts on the streets of Plains, Georgia when he was just knee-high to a grasshopper, translated in "Georgia speak" as five years old. After his presidency, he moved back to Plains to run the family farm and peanut business. Of course, one of his greatest contributions to mankind is not the peanut. Jimmy Carter is an extraordinary humanitarian and has led humanitarian efforts all over the world on behalf of poor and indigent populations.

The average age of peanut allergy onset in the U.S. for babies born before 2000 was 24 months; the average age of peanut allergy onset in babies born after 2000 is 18 months.

Peanut allergies—some interesting new findings. The rise in peanut allergies has been astronomical and of course, explanations have NOT been forthcoming. However, a few hypotheses have been proposed and most of them related allergies to genes and a genetic predisposition. But, that really doesn't make any sense because genes don't change as rapidly as the rise in peanut allergies. Another hypothesis having nothing to do with genes seems to stand out amongst all others. A 2003 study by allergist Gideon Lack of King's College of London found that preschool children who were allergic to peanuts were much more likely as infants to have been treated with skin lotion containing peanut oil than were children who didn't have the allergy. The researchers hypothesized that exposure to peanut protein through the skin laid the foundation for an aberrant immune reaction that resulted in allergy.

A second finding by the same researcher found that early exposure to peanuts via the diet decreases a child's risk of developing a peanut allergy later in life. This of course, flies in the face of the usual recommendations given to parents by pediatricians. The new study suggests that early exposure to peanuts, in the form of eating peanut butter, might induce tolerance and head off the aberrant immune response that underlies an allergic reaction. (*Journal of Allergy and Clinical Immunology,* November 2008)

Peanut butter and allergies. BEWARE! Peanut butter has become one of the most popular "convenience" foods for children. What's better than a peanut butter and jelly sandwich? Delicious, convenient, and inexpensive. So, what's the problem? As peanut butter becomes more and more popular, the risk of peanut allergy increases in direct proportion to its use. Peanut allergy is not only the fastest growing allergy in the United States, it also causes more life-threatening anaphylactic reactions than all other food allergies combined. Increased consumption of peanuts is partially responsible; however; the number of peanut-containing products is also on the rise.

In fact, new research from Food Beat, Inc. shows that total peanut mentions on top restaurant chain menus have grown 142 percent, from 74 mentions in 2000 to 179 in the second have of 2006.

HISTORICAL HIGHLIGHT

In 1890, A St. Louis physician who wanted to make a high-protein diet supplement for his elderly patients first discovered this gummy yummy spread. Actually he was given credit, but George Washington Carver also noted that when peanuts were ground into a paste, peanuts were delicious and filling. Carver, an agricultural chemist, actually figured out 300 different uses for the peanut.

Peanut butter facts: A sandwich-size 3-tablespoon serving of peanut butter contains 13.5 grams of protein—about the same amount found in 2 large eggs or a 12-ounce glass of milk. Three tablespoons also contains 4 grams of fiber—about as much as a couple of slices of whole wheat bread. The downside: 3 tablespoons of peanut butter equals 300 calories. Ouch. The upside: peanut butter will remove bubble gum from hair.

Question: Why does peanut butter stick to the roof of your mouth?
Answer: The high concentration of protein gives it an incredible ability to absorb and hold moisture—in other words, it sops up your saliva.

Peanut butter and trans fats. Trans fat levels in both traditional commercially prepared and natural peanut butters are undetectable, according to a study by the U.S. Department of Agriculture/Agricultural Research Service. In other words, research indicates that you could eat 146 two-tablespoon servings of peanut butter (the equivalent of 97 three-tablespoon peanut butter sandwiches) without consuming even 0.5 grams of trans fat—the Food and Drug Administration threshold for trans fat to be listed on a product label. (National Peanut Board, May 2007)

Peanut butter pearls.

* Americans consume 700 million pounds of peanut butter per year.
* The average American will consume nearly four pounds of peanut butter per year.
* The average child will eat 1,500 peanut butter sandwiches by high school graduation
* Ernest Hemingway wrote most of his works on a diet of peanut butter sandwiches.
* It takes 720 peanuts to make one pound of peanut butter, and 540 peanuts to make a 12-ounce jar of peanut butter.
* Four of the top 10 candy bars manufactured in the USA contain peanuts or peanut butter.
* Arachibutyrophobia (a-racki-beu-tee-ro phobia) the clinical name for the irrational fear that peanut butter may stick to the roof of your mouth.
* The amount of peanut butter consumed in one year could wrap the earth in a ribbon of 19-ounce peanut butter jars one and one-third times.
* Women and children prefer creamy, while most men opt for chunky.
* Peanut butter is consumed in 89 percent of U.S. households.
* The average number of peanuts in a box of Cracker Jack is 27.
* The Proctor and Gamble plant that makes Jif brand peanut butter produces 250,000 jars every day.

http://www.nationalpeanutboard.org/classroomfunfacts.php

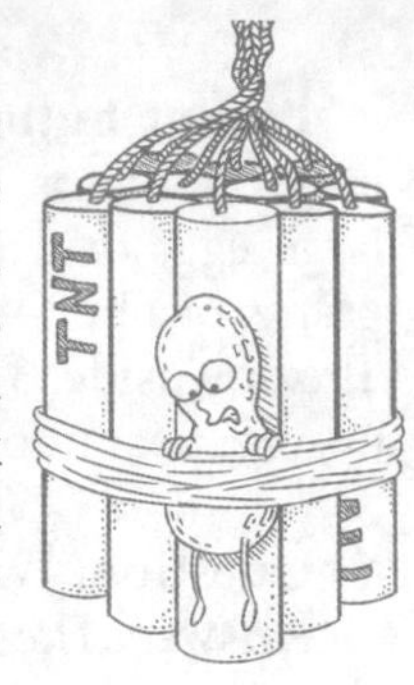

Peanuts as a component of dynamite. Peanuts are one of the ingredients used to make dynamite? Dynamite is made from nitroglycerine. Nitroglycerine is made from glycerol. Glycerol is made from peanut oil. Peanut oil is made from peanuts. You might not want to hang around dynamite if you're allergic to peanuts. Actually, I can think of numerous reasons you might not want to hang around dynamite that have nothing to do with peanuts. (www.fun-facts.com)

Peanut butter and *Salmonella*. A huge *Salmonella* outbreak in peanut butter occurred in March, 2009 in the U.S. The source of the contamination was traced to the Peanut Corporation of America's plant in Blakely, Georgia. This plant supplied wholesale peanut butter to institutions such as schools and nursing homes, and peanut paste to retail food manufacturers for use as an ingredient in ice cream, cookies, candy, and other foods. This one outbreak of *Salmonella* cost peanut producers one *billion* dollars.

How do you kill *Salmonella* in peanuts? It's called the "kill step" and it requires heating the dry roasted peanuts to an excess of 300° F for more than 15 minutes.

PEPSI

Pepsi. When Pepsi Cola was launched in China in the 1970s, the company's marketers opted to play it safe with their award-winning slogan "Come alive with Pepsi." Predictably, however, it did not translate as intended, so the product was introduced to a quarter of the world's population with the line, "Pepsi brings your ancestors back from the grave."

Coca-cola tried the same thing for the first time in the 1920s, unaware that its famous brand name translated literally as "Bite the wax tadpole." It was quickly changed to something roughly translated as "happiness in the mouth."

Pepsi Cola and "All Shook Up." Have you ever heard of Otis Blackwell? I didn't think so. Well, he was one of the most prolific songwriters of the mid-twentieth century, writing songs for Jerry Lee Lewis ("Great Balls of Fire"), and Elvis Presley ("Don't Be Cruel" and "Return to Sender"). One afternoon Otis told his agent that he could write a song about anything. His agent, drinking a Pepsi Cola at the time, started shaking the bottle and said, "Write a song about this."

The result? "All Shook Up." Elvis Presley recorded the tune and it not only topped the charts in 1957, it also became the best selling single of that year.

Persimmons. Pucker up, we're talking about persimmons. The botanical name is *Diospyros,* Greek for "food from the gods." Perhaps that's why persimmons are used in Japan for hangovers. Native Americans introduced the persimmon to Jamestown settlers to sustain them through the cold, cruel New England winters.

What are the benefits of this fall fruit? Who knows? Not a lot of research has been conducted on the persimmon but we do know that persimmons are high in fiber and have antioxidant properties. One medium persimmon has 118 calories, 6 grams of fiber (24% of the Daily Value), vitamin A–2,733 mg (100% of the Daily Value), vitamin C–13 mg (22% of the Daily Value), Copper–0.2 mg (9% of the Daily Value), Manganese–0.6 mg (30% of the Daily Value), Potassium–270 mg (8% of the Daily Value).

PESTICIDES

Pesky pesticides. The benefits of eating fruits and vegetables as a part of your daily diet far outweigh the potential cancer risks from any pesticide residues that are found in the produce you consume. This reassuring data comes from a panel of experts that reviewed over 50 studies and the risks of pesticides. One caveat—high levels of exposure, such as levels that some farm workers are exposed to, can pose a substantial risk. The group estimated that all sources of synthetic chemicals, including pesticides, are responsible for 2% of all cancer deaths. Compared to tobacco, which accounts for 30% of cancer deaths, pesticides and friends are a minimal risk.

This is certainly not a carte blanche for eating as many pesticides as you can fit into your diet. It is still important to wash those fruits and vegetables and to reduce exposure to a minimum or buy organic. (*Cancer,* November 15, 1997)

Pesticides—high risk fruits and vegetables. Apples have the highest pesticide residue when compared to all fruits and vegetables. The U.S. Department of Agriculture found that ninety-eight percent of apples tested positive for residue, even though most samples were washed and peeled before testing. The other fruits and vegetables most likely to contain pesticides include celery, strawberries, peaches, spinach, imported nectarines, and imported grapes. The good news is that all pesticide levels were within the recommended limits. (*USDA,* 2011)

Pesticides—the dirty dozen, in order, worst to best.

1. Apples
2. Celery
3. Strawberries
4. Peaches
5. Spinach
6. Nectarines (imported)
7. Grapes (imported)
8. Sweet bell peppers (imported)
9. Potatoes
10. Blueberries (domestic)
11. Lettuce
12. Kale/collard greens

(*Environmental Working Group,* April 2012)

Pesticides, the "clean 15."

1. Onions
2. Sweet corn
3. Pineapples
4. Avocado
5. Asparagus
6. Sweet peas
7. Mangoes
8. Eggplant
9. Cantaloupe (domestic)
10. Kiwi
11. Cabbage
12. Watermelon
13. Sweet potatoes
14. Grapefruit
15. Mushroom

(*Environmental Working Group,* April 2012)

Phosphorus-containing foods. The recommended daily allowance for phosphorus is 1000 mg. A normal serum phosphorus level is 3.5 to 5.5 mg/dl. Phosphorus is more easily absorbed from meat products, and you can only absorb half of the phosphorus contained in plant foods.

The kidney plays a major role in eliminating phosphorus. When kidney function is impaired, elevated serum levels of phosphorus can leech calcium out of the bone. This leads to osteomalacia, or soft, weak bones. Patients with kidney failure need to be extremely careful about the amount of phosphorus they eat and a registered dietician can teach them about phosphorus-containing foods.

The top 10 phosphorus-containing foods are as follows:

1. Bran (oat and rice)
2. Pumpkin, squash, and watermelon seeds
3. Sunflower seeds
4. Toasted wheat germ
5. Cheese
6. Sesame seeds and tahini (sesame butter)
7. Nuts (Brazil and pine nuts)
8. Roasted soy beans (edamame)
9. Flax seeds
10. Bacon

Other phosphorus containing foods: dairy products including custard, milk, cream soups, cottage cheese, ice cream, pudding, and yogurt; meats including carp, beef liver, fish roe, oysters, crayfish, chicken liver, organ meats, sardines; vegetables such as dried beans and peas, baked beans, chick peas, kidney beans, lima beans, pork n' beans, soy beans, black beans, garbanzo beans, lentils, northern beans, split peas; beverages including ale, beer, cocoa, chocolate drinks, dark colas, drinks made with milk and canned iced teas; other foods including bran cereals, caramels, brewer's yeast, nuts, wheat germ, and whole grain products. Good grief…is there any food that doesn't contain phosphorus?

Patients with kidney failure need to understand how to substitute high phosphorus foods with low phosphorus foods. For example, 8-ounces of nondairy creamer or 4 ounces of milk has less phosphorus than an 8-ounce glass of milk; 1-ounce of cream cheese can be substituted for 1-ounce of hard cheese; a ½ cup of sherbet or 1 popsicle is a great substitution for ½ cup of ice cream; 12 ounces of Ginger Ale or lemon soda is a better choice than a 12-ounce can of regular cola; a ½ cup of mixed vegetables or green beans is a can be substituted for ½ cup of lima or pinto beans.

Drugs that lower phosphorus levels include:

..... Antacids containing aluminum, calcium, or magnesium can interfere with phosphorus in the GI tract.

.....Anticonvulsants such as phenobarbital and carbamazepine (Tegretol).

.....Corticosteroids increase the excretion of phosphorus in urine.

.....Insulin in high doses may lower phosphorus absorption.

.....ACE inhibitors may lower levels of phosphorus.

.....Cyclosporine

.....Cardiac glycosides (Digoxin or Lanoxin)

.....Heparins

.....NSAIDS (non-steroidal ani-inflammatory drugs)

Phytochemicals. "Phyto" is the prefix for plant. Phytochemicals are actually toxins in plants used to ward off predators, mostly insects. When animals and humans eat plants, the phytochemicals from the plants induce enzyme systems that may allow us to detoxify foreign proteins, including carcinogens.

Carotenoids, polyphenols, and isoflavones are just a few of the many types of phytochemicals that have been spotlighted for their health benefits. Phytochemicals first came into the spotlight in the 1980s with sulforaphane, a phytochemical found in broccoli and other cruciferous vegetables that has cancer-fighting properties.

The following are four major types of phytochemicals found in various fruits and vegetables:

.....Carotenoids–alpha-carotene, beta-carotene, lutein, lycopene, zeaxanthin. Carotenoids are found in red, orange, and green fruits and veggies.

.....Polyphenols–flavonoids: flavonols, flavones, isoflavones, catechins, flavnones, anthocyanins. Flavonoids are found in tea (especially green tea), onions, soy foods, wine, and some fruits and vegetables; non-flavonoids: ellagic acid. Non-flavonoids are found in strawberries, raspberries, blueberries, and cranberries.

.....Plant sterols–sitosterol, stigmasterol, campesterol, sitostanol; plant sterols are found in vegetable oils.

.....Sulfur compounds–indoles, thiols, allicin; all types of onions, garlic, leeks.

There's something a bit absurd about taking phytochemicals in a pill when eating vegetables and fruit that are well-prepared and well-presented is one of life's joys, not one of life's miseries. You can't capture it by just popping pills. —John D. Potter, Professor of Epidemiology, University of Washington School of Public Health and Community Medicine, Head of Cancer Research at the Fred Hutchinson Cancer Research Center in Seattle, WA.

Pica. Pica is a bizarre eating disorder that has been recognized since the days of Aristotle and Socrates. The term "pica" was first coined, however, by the French physician Ambroise Paré in the sixteenth century. Pica is derived from the Latin word for "magpie," a bird known for its voracious and indiscriminate appetite for edible and inedible substances.

The actual definition of pica is "the chronic, compulsive eating of nonfoods such as earth, ashes, chalk, and lead-paint chips." The definition may also include a "false or craving appetite" or "deliberate ingestion of a bizarre selection of food." Persons suffering from pica display a persistent and compulsive need to eat non-nutritive substances such as clay, dirt, leaves, cornstarch, laundry starch, baking soda, chalk, buttons, ice, paper, dried paint, plaster, cigarette butts, burnt matches, ashes, sand, soap, toothpaste, oyster shells, or even broken crockery.

Names for various types of pica are composed of the Greek word for the ingested substance and the suffix from the Greek word "phagein," meaning "to eat." The most common pica as well as the most researched is geophagia, or the eating of earthy substances, especially clay. Other types include the ingestion of ice or ice water (pagophagia); laundry starch (amylophagia); hair (trichophagia); gravel, stones, or pebbles (lithophagia); lead paint (plumbophagia); leaves, grass, or other plants (foliophagia); unusual amounts of lettuce (lectophagia); tomatoes (tomatophagia); peanuts (gooberphagia), raw potatoes (geomelophagia), and feces (coprophagia).

As a rule, the populations most prone to pica are children under the age of six, pregnant women, persons with mental illness, and individuals who have mental disability. Pica has also been reported in breast-feeding females and individuals with seizure disorders. It may also run in families. Most likely the familial trait is environmental and not carried as a genetic trait.

As mentioned above, eating earth substances such as clay or dirt is known as geophagia. African American females in the Southeastern portion of the United States have been known to practice pica with red clay. Some, who have migrated north, have arranged to have their clay mailed from the South to continue the practice. In addition, southern grocery stores have stocked red clay for human consumption. This form of pica can result in an iron-deficiency anemia. It is thought that eating clay causes iron deficiency by binding iron in the gut and subsequently inhibiting its absorption. Some clay has been found to decrease iron absorption by 25%. Starch eating has also been associated with iron deficiency.

Pica is a serious eating disorder that can require hospitalization and medical or surgical intervention. For example, patients can be hospitalized for the treatment of phosphorus intoxication from match head consumption. Trichophagia (the ingestion of hair) is found most often in children. It is especially associated with the habit of girls chewing on long hair. Trichophagia can result in substantial amounts of hair being digested and forming "hair balls" that can obstruct the gastrointestinal tract. These "hair ball" obstructions may require surgical removal.

The cause(s) and prevalence of pica are unknown. Estimates range from 10% to 30% in kids from ages 2–6. As a rule kids who engage in pica consume things within the proximity of their grasp. These tend to be relatively harmless items such as cloth, dirt, leaves, sand, rocks, and pebbles.

HISTORICAL HIGHLIGHT

Vincent van Gogh may have suffered from pica. Van Gogh's unnatural craving involved liqueur called absinthe, which contains the chemical thujone. Thujone, a toxin in the central nervous system, is distilled from plants such as wormwood. Not only did he crave the thujone-laced absinthe, but he was also known to crave substances such as camphor. Camphor contains chemicals known as terpenes, which are also toxic to the central nervous system. He also nibbled on his paints, which contained terpene. Letters from van Gogh to various colleagues substantiated his terpene pica. One fellow artist had to restrain van Gogh from swilling turpentine one evening.

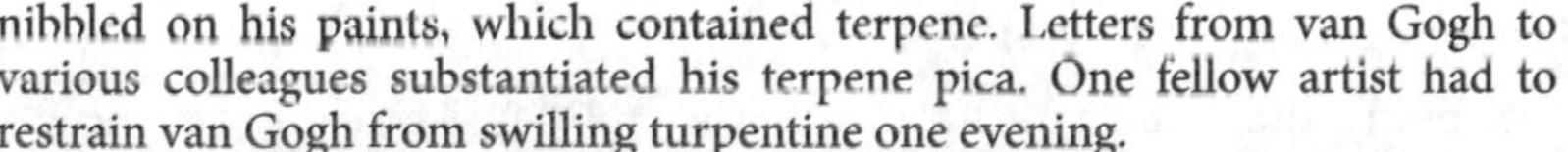

Both terpene and thujone can trigger generalized seizures when ingested in large amounts. Van Gogh had at least four documented generalized seizures during the last eighteen months of his life. The accumulation of the toxins in the central nervous system was no doubt responsible for the seizures.

As far as his missing piece of ear—did Gaugin chop it off in a fencing duel or did Van Gogh chop it off himself? The controversy continues…

ASPARAGUS TIP

The medical world uses a type of clay as a drug. Kaolinite is the common type of clay used in medicines and the primary ingredient in the commercially marketed antidiarrheal drug known as Kaopectate. Clay is also used medicinally in third-world countries where hookworm is a common parasitic infection. This intestinal parasite causes gastric distress that is alleviated with clay. Clay is also used in third world countries to relieve diarrhea, heartburn, and intestinal gas.

Theories abound as to the causes, but include nutritional, physiological, psychological, and cultural. The most common suspected factors are emotional disturbances and malnutrition resulting from a dietary deficiency.

Nutritional theory suggests that appetite-regulating brain enzymes, altered by an iron, zinc or other mineral deficiency, lead to specific cravings. However, the craved items generally do not supply the lacking minerals, so this theory has been rather difficult to prove.

The physiologic theory notes that eating clay or dirt has been used to relieve nausea, control vomiting, increase salivation, remove toxins, and to alter odor and taste perception.

In terms of psychological theories, pica has been explained as a behavioral response to stress, a habit disorder, or a manifestation of an oral fixation.

And, lastly, pica has been explained as a cultural feature in certain religious rites, folk medicine, and/or magical beliefs. For example, earth taken from a shrine or holy burial site is eaten for religious purposes or to swear oaths. (Hunter BT, Consumer's Research Magazine, 9/1/97 and the Cambridge World History of Food, 2000.)

PICK-A-pie

Pie—just a sliver, please. How about a calorie count for each pie?
Chocolate French Silk pie has 504 calories per slice
Pecan pie has 401 calories per slice
Cherry pie has 389 calories per slice
Apple pie has 328 calories per slice
Lemon Meringue pie has 290 calories per slice
Pumpkin pie has 253 calories per slice
(*Cooking Ligh*t December 2010)

How many slices did you have over the holidays? Speaking of holidays, the average weight gain is only about one pound. That's the good news. The bad news is that the pound is usually not lost over the following year. The worst news: Add 20 Thanksgiving thru Christmas holidays and you have a 20-pound weight gain in 20 years. Duh. Happy Holidays.

Pickles. What is a pickle? A pickle is a pickled cucumber. Pickling is a process by which vegetables are steeped in a preservative, usually brine or vinegar. Just about anything can be pickled, including green tomatoes, green beans, cauliflower, carrots, bologna, peppers (as in Peter Piper picked a peck of pickled peppers), pig's feet, beets, onions, eggs, and, the most popular, the cucumber. Pickling has been a popular preservative throughout history, especially before the days of refrigeration and canning. Pickle lovers of yesteryear include Julius Caesar, Napoleon, and Thomas Jefferson. Pickle lovers of today include Barb Bancroft, especially Heinz 57 Processed Dill Pickles.

If you love the sour or dill variety of pickles, you will overdose on sodium. One 5-oz dill pickle has only 24 calories but packs a walloping 1,730 mg of sodium. Ouch. The recommended daily allowance of sodium is only 2,300 mg, so you have almost used up your daily allotment with the one pickle. Enjoy it. So you like the sweet pickles you say? These are definitely lower in salt, but the calories can be as high as 150 in one large sweet pickle. So, pickles, like everything else in life, should be consumed in moderation. Small quantities of thinly sliced pickle chips are fine as an occasional condiment or as a treat right out of the jar.

A cucumber should be well-sliced, dressed with pepper and vinegar, and then thrown out. —Samuel Jackson

---

According to Pickle Packers International, the crunch of a perfect pickle should be audible from 10 paces. And who, pray tell, organized a group called the Pickle Packers International? Actually there were so many people working in pickling factories in New York City's Lower East Side in the late 1800s that they formed a trade organization known as the Pickle Packers International in 1893.

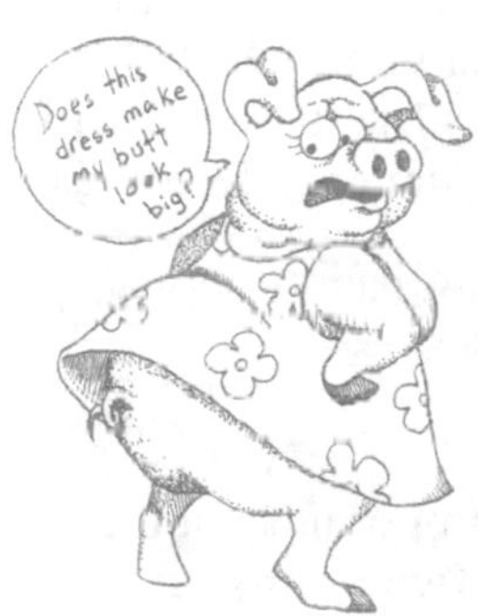

Pigs and "pigging out." Do pigs pig out? No, only humans pig out. Pigs produce a hormone known as cholecystokinin (CCK), which transmits a message from pork bellies to the pork brains that says, "Stop eating, you pig." Since pigs listen to this hormone signal, they do not overeat. Humans have the same signal; however, we typically ignore the message. Humans have other signals that tell us to stop eating, we're full, but we tend to ignore those as well. See chapter L and Leptin.

Pints and Quarts. We order beer in the U.S. by the bottle or by the glass. In jolly Olde England, ale is ordered in pints or quarts. If a customer was over-served and became a bit unruly, the bartender would holler at them to mind their pints and quarts, or their "Ps and Qs."

Piranhas. How fast do they eat? A school of piranhas, which inhabit the freshwater rivers of South America, can chew a 400-pound hog to the bone in less than 10 minutes.

Pizza pearls. Pizza, when eaten correctly, forces the diner's lips into a smile. ☺

...Ninety-three percent of Americans eat pizza at least once a month.

...Every second in the U.S. Americans eat 350 slices of pizza. And we wonder why we're having weight problems.

...Each man, woman, and child consumes an average of 23 pounds of pizza pie every year.

...Almost 70% of all Super Bowl viewers eat pizza on Super Bowl Sunday.

...Naples, Italy is the home of the traditional Neapolitan pizza pie. They "borrowed" the idea of using bread as a blank slate for all sorts of toppings from the Greeks, but they were the first to add tomatoes to the mix.

...Cheese was added to pizza in 1889 to honor the Queen Margherita, who happened to be visiting Italy at the time. The famous pizza maker, known as a *pizzaiolo,* Raffaele Esposito, created three pizzas to honor Queen Margherita and she chose her favorite from the three. She strongly preferred the pizza pie containing the colors of the Italian flag—red (tomato), green (basil), and white (mozzarella). And now you know the rest of the story—how pizza Margherita was named.

...The first licensed pizza parlor in the U.S. was Lombardi's in New York City. It opened its doors in 1905 in lower Manhattan.

...Chicago first introduced the deep dish pizza in 1943 at Pizzeria Uno.

...In 1934 there were 500 pizzerias in the U.S. By 1956 there were 20,000 pizzerias.

...In 1953, Dean Martin crooned "That's Amore!" with the famous line... "When the moon hits the sky like a big pizza pie, that's amore!"

...In 1960, Tom and James Monaghan purchased a pizza parlor in Ypsilanti, Michigan called Dominick's. They changed the name to Domino's, offered free pizza delivery, and the rest is history.

(Miller H. How a Neapolitan street food became the most successful immigrant of all. *American Heritage,* April/May 2006; 31–38).

Plant stanols and sterols. These heart-healthy compounds found in plants block cholesterol absorption in the intestines. Two grams of plant sterols or stanols daily can lower LDL-cholesterol by as much as 5 to 15% within a few weeks. Fruits and vegetables are always a great source, but you would be eating them all day, every day to get the necessary 2 grams per day. Fortified margarines such as Benecol and Take Control and fortified orange juice are available and packed with stanols/sterols. There are also supplements out there on the shelves. ConsumerLab.com reviewed and approved seven out of eight plant sterol ester supplements.

Pomegranate. Humans long ago figured out that certain plants have contraceptive powers. The pomegranate played a central role in both Greek myth and Greek birth-control efforts. According to one myth, Persephone, the daughter of the fertility goddess Demeter, was told to eat nothing during a visit to the underworld Hades, but she disobeyed and ate the pomegranate. As punishment, the gods sentenced her to spend part of the year in Hades, and for this reason, Earth experiences the barren season of winter until Persephone returns each spring. The Greeks used the pomegranate as a contraceptive, and studies have shown that it contains a plant estrogen that acts like the chemicals found in modern synthetic oral contraceptives. Pomegranates have also been used to predict fertility. The Turkish bride throws a pomegranate on the ground and the number of seeds that spill out predict how many children she will have. Yikes. It contains hundreds of seeds! The pomegranate is also referred to as "seeded apple." Historically the pomegranate was considered good for a toothache because, based on the Doctrine of Signatures (See Chapter D), when the fruit's peel was pulled away the seeds and pith resembled rows of teeth between the lips.

Pomegranates are a source of polyphenols and other anti-oxidants. One glitch: To get the full benefits of this magnanimous fruit, you would have to eat it virtually by the pound—consuming two and a half whole pomegranates per day. Hence, pomegranate juice is the way to go. Pomegranate juice is thought to have three times the antioxidants of tea and wine. A study from the *American Journal of Clinical Nutrition,* May 2000, measured the effect of pomegranate juice on various measures of atherogenesis. Pomegranate juice consumption decreased LDL susceptibility to oxidation and increased an enzyme that helps HDL protect against LDL deposition in the artery walls. Bottom line: Pomegranate juice has potent anti-atherogenic effects in healthy humans. (Aviram M et al. Pomegranate juice consumption reduces oxidative stress, atherogenic modifications to LDL, and platelet aggregation: studies in humans and in atherosclerotic apolipoprotein E-deficient mice. *Am J Clin Nutri* 2000 May; 71(5):1062–1076).

POPCORN

Popcorn. Constipated? Bad gums? Lousy teeth? Eat one to two quarts of popcorn per day for a safe, inexpensive remedy for all of the above. Americans are the largest per capita consumers of popcorn in the world. Over ten *billion* quarts of popcorn are consumed per year, grossing over one *billion* dollars for the popcorn industry.

Popcorn and the movie industry. In the 1950s, the movie popcorn was a 3-cup box with 174 calories. Today's small bag of popcorn at the movies can provide anywhere from 470 calories to 630 with 37 to 50 grams of fat—of which 29 to 34 grams is saturated. The big supersize barrel you get today is 21 cups of popcorn (buttered) and weighs in at 1,700 calories with 1500 mg of sodium. The small bag has around 500 mg of sodium.

Popcorn and polyphenols. So the above section was the bad news about popcorn. Here's the good news. Popcorn is *full* of healthy polyphenols. Polyphenols act as antioxidants, which help protect the body from the damaging effects of free radicals. Traditionally fruits and vegetables held the top spot as free radial "busters," but truth be told, research presented at the annual American Chemical Society in March 2012 showed that popcorn contains approximately 300 mg of polyphenols per serving, while fruits contain an average of 160 mg per serving. Popcorn is also a great source of fiber, making your bowels happy. It is also a completely unprocessed whole grain. And popcorn can be beneficial for weight loss because you get a large volume of food that fills you up for a small number of calories.

The catch? Choosing healthy popcorn that has flavor and doesn't taste like the box it came in. Look for packages that contain no trans fats or are labeled "light" or "94% fat free." Read the ingredients label and choose popcorns with as few ingredients as possible—basically popcorn, oil, and salt. Avoid any brand that has diacetyl in it—it's a chemical flavoring that has been associated with lung disease.

Poppy seeds and urine testing. Can a poppy seed coated bagel for breakfast prevent you from getting that new job you are applying for? Maybe seven or eight years ago the answer was yes, but not in today's urine-testing world. Let me explain. Poppy seeds are derived from poppy plants. Really. Heroin is also derived from the same source. Eating a couple of large bagels topped with an abundance of poppy seeds can register as a positive urine test for opiates. That was the bad news. Now, the good news. This must have been such a frequent occurrence for government job testing that the U.S. Government changed the threshold for opiates in the workplace setting. The old number, 300 nanograms per ml, was easily surpassed by a couple of poppy seed-coated bagels or muffins. The new number, 2000 nanograms per ml, is more likely to indicate some type of opiate use—from heroin to morphine to codeine in cough syrup. One would have to consume at least a *dozen and a half* poppy seed-coated bread products to register close to the 2000 nanogram level.

PORK

Pork—the other white meat. Pork is packed with all of the essential amino acids one needs, and it provides plenty of high-quality protein for a nutritious and delicious diet. Pork is a good source of B vitamins and also provides a bit of heme iron to keep red blood cells healthy and happy. One broiled lean pork chop has 8 grams of fat (2.6 grams of saturated fat), 92 mg of cholesterol, and 0.7 mg of iron.

Commercially-grown pigs in the U.S. are no longer a source of the parasite *Trichinella spiralis.* This was a concern many years ago when the recommendation was to cook the pork chops or pork roast to an internal tempera-

ASPARAGUS TIP

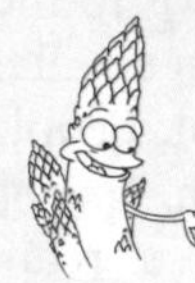

The only major source of *Trichinella spiralis* that comes to mind right now is polar bear meat. If you find yourself in a situation with polar bear meat as a choice on the menu you may want to opt for the Arctic char or the Chinook salmon.

ture of 160-170° F to kill the parasite. If the pork appeared pink in the middle it was not cooked thoroughly! As of 2011, the USDA says that a little pink in your pork is now acceptable. The latest recommendation is that pork needs to be cooked only to an internal temperature of 145° F.

Pork—organic pork vs. antibiotic-treated pork. Traces of *Salmonella* were found in 39% of pigs raised in the standard indoor pens and routinely given antibiotics, but in 54% of the organic pigs raised without drugs. The organic pigs also contained *Toxoplasma* and *Trichinella.* Are you sure you want to eat organic pork? If you do, make sure you cook it to an internal temperature of 145 degrees F. (*Foodborne Pathogens and Disease* 2008 (5); 199)

PORTIONS

Portion Distortion. How is a portion defined compared to a serving? A "portion" is the amount of food you choose to eat (or a restaurant or food packager thinks you should eat)—and a "serving" is used to describe the recommended amount of food. For example, one "serving" of meat or poultry is the size of a deck of cards. But most U.S. meals consist of 8 ounces of meat—a portion that is nearly 3 times the serving size recommended. When eating out at many of the "family-style" restaurants a portion of pasta is usually 480% bigger than the recommended serving size. Ouch. Steaks are usually 224% bigger, bagels 195% bigger, and muffin portions 333% bigger. Ouch, ouch, and a bigger ouch.

What does a serving "look" like? How can we teach patients how to estimate serving size? See Serving Size in Chapter S.

Portions of yesteryear vs. portions today. A cheeseburger in 1987 had 330 calories, today's cheeseburger averages 590 calories. The side order of fries in 1987 was 2.4 ounces and 210 calories, today's fries weigh in at 6.9 ounces and 610 calories. The blueberry muffin of yesteryear was 1.5 ounces and 210 calories, but today that same blueberry muffin is 5 ounces and 500 calories. The old, traditional cup of coffee was 8 ounces, add a bit of milk and sugar and the calorie count was 45. Today's 16 ounce coffee with milk and mocha syrup weighs in at 350 calories. Bagels have grown from three inches in diameter, 140 calories, to six inches and 350 calories—and that's before you add the cream cheese. This is just a wake-up call as to why that dang scale seems to be malfunctioning in recent years.

Portion control and smaller serving dishes. Researchers have found that using smaller bowls, smaller plates, smaller cups, and yes, even smaller utensils reduces the amount of food consumed at any given meal. People perceive that they are eating more when served on a smaller dish. In one study, subjects using a 34-ounce bowl ate an average of 31% more ice cream (137 more calories) than those scooping into a bowl half that size. (Wansink B, van Ittersum K, Painter J. Ice cream illusions: Bowls, spoons, and self-served portion sizes. *Am J of Prevent Med.* 2006;31)

POTASSIUM

Potassium. Remember that potassium plays a major role in many physiologic functions including nerve conduction, muscle contraction, the flow of fluid and minerals into and out of cells, cardiac conduction, and blood pressure regulation. Suffice it to say, potassium is an essential electrolyte but it basically "gets no respect." Its cousin, sodium, seems to get all of the glory. Hrumpf. Let's change that thinking by starting to increase your potassium intake.

What are the highest potassium-containing foods? And don't tell me bananas! How about potatoes as number one?

Food	Potassium
One medium baked potato with the skin	926 mg
Four ounces of baked halibut	654 mg
One-half of an avocado	604 mg
½ cup of raisins	543 mg
½ cantaloupe	502 mg
1 cup coconut water	480 mg
½ cup of cooked acorn squash	448 mg
½ cup of cooked spinach	419 mg
1 cup of nonfat milk	408 mg
½ cup of cooked lentils	365 mg
2/3 cup of red beans	340 mg
6 ounces of orange juice	354 mg
1 medium orange	300 mg
1/2 of a medium banana	242 mg

Can you get your potassium from foods instead of potassium supplements? It depends on how much you need and whether you are trying to prevent or treat potassium loss.

Potassium from foods usually works for prevention. Patients on a thiazide or loop diuretics need about 20 to 40 mEq extra each day. Potassium-rich foods compare to potassium supplements in the following ways:

A potato with skin or a cup of spinach provides over 20 mEq.

A cup of kidney or navy beans provides 18 mEq.

A cup of orange juice or yogurt contains 14 mEq.

An average-size banana contains 12 mEq.

Potassium from potassium supplements such as Micro-K and Klor-Con usually work better to treat hypokalemia (low potassium) than food containing potassium. (*Prescriber's Letter*, September 2008)

Potassium and prescription drugs. As noted in Chapter A, the ACE inhibitors are the number one drugs that increase potassium. Other drugs to be aware of that also have potassium-retaining properties include spironolactone (Aldactone), eplerenone (Inspra), trimethoprim-sulfamethoxazole (Bactrim, Septra), triamterene (Dyrenium), amiloride (Midamor), and the birth control pill Yaz.

Potassium and blood pressure. Don't forget about the DASH diet from Chapter D. Lower the sodium containing foods, increase the potassium containing foods, and increase the low-fat calcium containing foods to lower your blood pressure. This is the perfect recipe for lowering blood pressure.

How does potassium lower blood pressure? Potassium is exchanged for sodium in the distal tubule of the kidneys, resulting in increased sodium excretion. Potassium is also a vasodilator, lowering blood pressure. (U.S. Department of Health and Human Services, National Heart Lung and Blood Institute, National Institutes of Health. Your Guide to Lowering Your Blood Pressure with DASH. NIH Publication No. 06-4082, Revised April 2006)

Potassium in the urine—marker for a healthy diet? Is there a way to tell if we're eating a healthy diet—besides lying about it? Actually, in the future your health care provider may just ask you to empty your bladder into a cup. His/her trusty assistant will take the specimen to the in-office laboratory and check it for potassium levels and voilà! The higher the level of potassium in the urine, the more likely that the patient is following a balanced diet that meets current federal guidelines. In other words, eat "lotsafruitsa" veggies, and fiber for a potassium-packed diet. Patients with the highest levels of potassium also tend to have the lowest blood pressures, the lowest heart rates, and are less likely to be overweight than those with the lowest potassium in their urine. Stay tuned. This urine test may be coming to a toilet near you. (American Society of Nephrology National Conference, Fall 2006; Dr. Andrew Mente, Prosserman Center for Health Research, Toronto, Canada)

POTATOES

Potatoes (white). The potato is now the fourth most important world food crop, surpassed only by wheat, rice, and maize (corn). Potatoes are inexpensive, nutritious, and a good source of carbohydrates and proteins, while containing minimal amounts of fat. One small potato boiled in its skin provides 16 mg of vitamin C. Potatoes are also a great source of B vitamins (thiamine—B1, pyridoxine—B6, folate, and niacin—B3) and are a gold mine of potassium, phosphorus, and other trace elements. Potatoes provide five grams of fiber if you eat the skin of a large potato. Potatoes are also high in antioxidants.

Potatoes are members of the nightshade family Solanaceae plants that produce neurotoxins (nerve poisons) known as glycoalkaloids. The glycoalkaloid in potatoes is known as solanine, a neurotoxin made in the green parts of the plant: the leaves, the stem, and any green spots on the skin. Solanine interferes with acetylcholinesterase, a neurotransmitter that enables neurons to communicate with one another.

Potatoes exposed to light produce solanine more quickly and in higher amounts than potatoes stored in the dark, but all potatoes produce some solanine all of the time. To prevent greening of potatoes, store then in a dark, cool place that is well ventilated. Solanine persists in the potato even after it is cooked. It is estimated that an adult might have to eat about 3 pounds of potatoes or 2.4 pounds of potato skins at one sitting to experience the first gastrointestinal or neurological signs of solanine poisoning. It is estimated that it would take 1.5 pounds of potatoes or 1.4 pounds of potato skins to cause symptoms in a child. The U.S. government has mandated that potatoes cannot contain more than 200 ppm (parts per million) of solanine per potato. Most potatoes on the grocery shelf contain 100 ppm, however; to be on the safe side, don't buy potatoes with green spots on the skin or potatoes that have sprouts growing out of the skin.

Don't peel potatoes too far ahead of time, as they will lose some vitamin C to the air and water. In addition, when you cut into a potato the cell walls release polyphenoloxidase, an enzyme that hastens the oxidation of phenols, creating the brownish compounds that darken a fresh-cut potato. To slow down the reaction, soak the peeled sliced fresh potatoes in ice water.

Which potato should be chosen for various potato preparations? Russet potatoes are best for baking and mashing; round red potatoes are the best sautéed; yellow-fleshed potatoes such as Yukon Jack have a dense creamy texture; purple and blue potatoes have a slightly nutty flavor.

Microwaved potatoes or baked in a traditional oven? Microwaving retains slightly more nutrients because of a quicker cooking time than in the traditional oven. Microwaving takes about seven minutes for one medium potato. You'll save nutrients by baking or boiling potatoes in their skins. A potato boiled without its skin loses 8% more potassium, 20% more vitamin C and 5% more B6 than a potato with the skin left on. Bringing the water to a boil before adding the potatoes preserves even more vitamin C.

Potato tips and chips:

- An ordinary, unruffled potato chip is 55/100 of an inch thick.
- One 15-ounce bag of potato chips = 1 cup of oil.
- A one-ounce bag of chips has about 150 calories.
- Potato chips were invented by a chef in Louisiana in 1865.
- One medium movie popcorn (eleven cups) with "butter topping" is the equivalent of eating eight potatoes: 910 calories and 71 grams of fat.
- Each year, McDonald's alone uses 3.2 billion pounds of potatoes.
- Americans eat an average of 2.7 pounds of potatoes per week.

- One in every five potatoes grown in the U.S. ends up as French fries.
- Potato starch is used as an adhesive in stamps and as an absorbing agent in disposable diapers.
- John Dillinger reportedly carved a potato in the shape of a revolver, turned it black with iodine, and used it to escape from jail.
- The Incas measured time by how long it took a potato to cook.

Potato chips: the number one American snack food. A total of 3,468 billion pounds of potatoes are used to make potato chips each year. Another way to put it: 11% of the total United States potato crop becomes potato chips.

Potomania—drinking excessive amounts of water. All you hear today is drink more water, eight to twelve glasses of water a day, increase your water intake to five to eight glasses per day, etc. Well, yes, water has numerous benefits and all of us should probably consider increasing our intake of water, but, let's not go overboard. Patients with potomania drink copious amounts of water for absolutely no reason whatsoever, wreaking havoc with the kidneys and electrolyte balance. The most common "potomaniac" is the chronic, excessive beer drinker—the guy/gal who drinks beer after beer after beer after beer. Beer is a hypotonic solution consisting almost exclusively of water. In the usual course of events, when an individual consumes large amounts of beer, a state of inebriation occurs and they are too drunk to continue drinking beer. But chronic beer drinkers are capable of drinking copious amounts of beer without passing out. The other group at high risk for potomania is the new wave of "starvation" dieters that think if they fill up on water all day and all night they won't be hungry and will lose weight. Most of these starvation diets push the water but provide only 400 calories a day in packets of protein, salt, minerals and vitamins. Be aware of these crash diets that require extraordinary amounts of water as part of the program. (*Lancet* 2002; 359:942)

Pretzels. Pretzels are the second most popular snack food after potato chips in the U.S. The earliest story of the origin of the pretzel comes from the medieval German monk who took a scrap of bread dough, rolled it into a strip, and folded it into the shape of a child's arms folded in prayer. The monks offered these pretiola (Latin for "little bribe") to children who memorized the Scripture verses and prayers. The first pretzel factory in the U.S. was in Lititz, Pennsylvania in 1861. In 1935, the Reading Pretzel Company introduced an automatic pretzel-twisting machine that sped up the process of pretzel making considerably. Today pretzels are eaten in many shapes and sizes—hard, soft, large, small, sweet, salty.

Pringles. How about the following for a new use of the round Pringles container? Frederic J. Baur, the deceased designer of the Pringles potato chip can, recently passed away and his will mandated that his cremated remains were to be poured into one of his tubular potato chip cans and buried in the family plot.

PROBIOTICS

Probiotics. Probiotics are the naturally occurring friendly gut bacteria that assist in food and nutrient assimilation, inhibit harmful bacteria, boost immune system function, and repopulate healthy gut flora after antibiotic therapy. And that's not all—these friendly functioning gut bacteria also manufacture many vitamins in the gut, help digest lactose, contribute to cholesterol and triglyceride metabolism, and assist in hormone metabolism. Important? You bet. The two major friendly strains are *Lactobacillus,* populating the small intestine, and *Bifidobacterium*, populating the large intestine. The two strains work together to boost gut flora and maintain gut health.

So, do foods we eat influence our natural healthy gut bacteria? Yes...and you can imagine the foods that decrease the friendly bacteria. Sugar, fried foods, white flour, and caffeine are among the dietary bad guys. Taking probiotic supplements do not compensate for a lousy diet, but they can help repopulate the diminished gut flora induced by those foods.

Psychological stress can also exacerbate intestinal inflammation, wiping out the friendly gut bacteria and weakening the immune system. Probiotics can reduce inflammation, enhance the immune system, and buffer the GI effects of stress.

Another interesting connection with probiotics is the brain-gut connection in patients with irritable bowel syndrome (IBS). Serotonin deficiency has been observed in patients with IBS. Probiotics containing *B. infantis* have been shown to be helpful in boosting serotonin in the gut and may provide the missing link in the treatment of IBS.

These products have long been popular as alternative therapies in the holistic health communities. However, mainstream medicine was reluctant to embrace the world of probiotics until research supported their clinical usefulness. Well, the proof is in the probiotics as they say, and research abounds as to the clinical benefits.

When the pathogenic bacteria predominate various gastrointestinal symptoms such as bloating, gas, diarrhea, constipation, and inflammation (colitis) may occur. Commercial probiotics, taken as a pill, powder, or in liquid forms, will help fortify the intestinal tract with beneficial organisms and help restore the proper balance of healthy bacteria. Probiotics contain live microorganisms that enhance healthy microbial growth in the intestines.

Patients can take probiotics as supplements (Lactinex, etc,), or get them from yogurt and other fermented dairy products. Choose a brand of yogurt that contains "live and active cultures" such as Dannon, Yoplait, or Colombo. One of the best yogurts available in the U.S. is Stonyfield Farm Yogurt. This brand of yogurt contains six "live and active" microorganisms, which help maintain the healthy bacteria in the gastrointestinal tract and may even stimulate the immune system as an additional bonus. Most other yogurts contain only two "live and active" cultures. The "live and active" culture that appears to be most effective in colonizing the GI tract and preventing diarrhea is *Lactobacillus GG,* found in the dietary supplement Culturelle. It appears to be more effective than *Lactobacillus acidophilus,* found in Dannon, Yoplait, and Colombo yogurts.

Just what are the benefits? Improved lactose digestion for starters, and a reduced risk of intestinal infection with the likes of *Salmonella, Shigella, Listeria, E. coli,* and *Campylobacter jejuni.* In addition, the risk of *H. pylori* is reduced by 18%.

Numerous studies have demonstrated the benefits of using probiotics for the prevention of antibiotic-associated diarrhea, acute diarrheal illness (gastroenteritis), and inflammatory bowel disease. The most commonly studied probiotics are the lactic acid producing *Lactobacillus GG* and the yeast, *Saccharomyces boulardii.* (Pick M. Gut flora on a crusade for good. *ADVANCE for NPs and PAs.* March 2012; Floch MH, et al. Recommendations for probiotic use. *J Clin Gastroenterol.* 2006;40(3):275–278; Balfour SR. Bacteria in Crohn's disease: mechanisms of inflammation and therapeutic implications. *J Clin Gastroenterol.* 2007;41(Supp 1): 537–543; Environmental Nutrition, "Best designed functional foods," June 2000; *Environmental Nutrition,* 2010)

Probiotics and antibiotic-associated diarrhea. Antibiotic-associated diarrhea occurs in approximately 25% of patients receiving antibiotics. Antibiotics that can wreak havoc with the intestinal microflora include the cephalosporins, tetracyclines, trimethoprim/sulfamethoxasole, fluoroquinolones, macrolides, penicillins, sulfonamides, and isoniazid. Doron, et al. pooled 25 randomized controlled trials of probiotics for the prevention of antibiotic-associated diarrhea and found that more than half of the trials demonstrated significant efficacy of the probiotic. In particular, the lactic-acid producing *Lactobacillus GG,* and the yeast, *Saccharomyces boulardii,* and mixtures of the two were effective. A review by Jones also found the same effects of probiotics on antibiotic-associated diarrhea. Some proponents of probiotics recommend taking them for two to three weeks during and after a course of antibiotics. Give supplements during and after a course of antibiotics if clinical judgment warrants it. Taking eight ounces of yogurt twice daily at least two hours after the antibiotic and continue for several days after the antibiotic therapy is finished helps to prevent antibiotic-associated diarrhea. Another option is to take Culturelle, 1–2 capsules, each day. (Doron SI, et al. Probiotics for prevention of antibiotic-associated diarrhea. *Journal of Clinical Gastroenterology.* 2008;42:S58–63; Jones K. Probiotics: preventing antibiotic-associated diarrhea. *J Spec Pediatr Nurs.* 2010;15(2):160–162; Hulisz D. Probiotics for antibiotic-associated diarrhea. Medscape Pharmacists, *Medscape Today.* 7/25/2011; Williams NT. Probiotics. *Am J Health-Syst Pharm.* 2010;67:449–458)

Probiotics and inflammatory bowel disease. Probiotic intake has been associated with significant anti-inflammatory effects in patients with inflammatory bowel disease. Probiotics increase regulatory T cells and decrease circulating inflammatory proteins including tumor necrosis factor-alpha and interleukin-12. No changes were reported in the placebo group.The probiotics used in this particular study were *Lactobacillus rhamnosus GR-1* and *Lactobacillus reuteri RC-14*. Results were reported after 30 days. Baroja ML, et al. Anti-inflammatory effects of probiotic yogurt in inflammatory bowel disease patients. (*Clinical & Experimental Immunology.* 2010;149(3):460–479)

Probiotics, alleriges, and sepsis. Rare cases of probiotic-related bacteremia and fungemia have been reported. Because probiotics contain live microorganisms, patients who are immunocompromised, have severe underlying comorbidities, are critically ill, or have short bowel syndrome may be more susceptible to probiotic sepsis and should not receive them. Patients with lactose intolerance should not take probiotics containing *Lactobacillus* species, and patients with yeast allergies should not take *Saccharomyces boulardiispecies.* (Williams NT. Probiotics. *Am J Health-Syst Pharm.* 2010;67:449–458)

Probiotics and ventilator-associated pneumonia. Ventilator-associated pneumonia (VAP) occurs in 9% to 27% of patients receiving mechanical ventilation in the ICU (intensive care unit). The pathogenesis of VAP involves colonization of the upper respiratory tract (including the oropharynx, back of the throat, and digestive tract) and subsequent aspiration (inhalation into the lungs) of the contaminated secretions.

Researchers conducted a double-blind trial among 146 adult patients who were receiving mechanical ventilation and who were likely to require it for at least 3 days. The 146 patients received two capsules of *Lactobacillum rhamnosus GG* or a placebo twice daily. The contents of one capsule were mixed with saline and applied as a slurry to the back of the throat. The contents of the second capsule were given through a nasogastric tube directly into the gastrointestinal tract. The result? Fifty patients developed ventilator-associated pneumonia. Of these, 17 patients received the probiotics and 33 received the placebo. A second bonus in the probiotic patients was a reduction in the development of a severe type of diarrhea known as *Clostridium difficile.* The third bonus was the cost: a whopping $2.13 daily for the probiotic group. (Morrow LE et al. Probiotic prophylaxis of ventilator-associated pneumonia: A blinded, randomized, controlled trial. *Am J Respir Crit Care Med* 2010 Oct 15;182:1058)

Prosciutto. Prosciutto is an Italian ham that is salted and air-dried but not smoked. Prosciutto is often sliced paper-thin and has a sweet tang. It also has 660 mg of sodium per slice, three times the amount of sodium in bacon (but bacon has nearly four times the saturated fat).

Prostate cancer and chili peppers. Chili peppers contain the spicy chemical capsaicin, which may have the power to destroy cancer cells. When researchers gave capsaicin to mice with prostate cancer, it shrank their tumors to one-fifth their original size. Of course the prostate shrank—you not only would have to have a cast-iron stomach to consume the amount of capsaicin the scientists gave the mice but the amount of "burn" on the way out most likely fried the prostate so that it shriveled to the size of a sesame seed. The weekly dose per mouse was the equivalent of about 600 jalepeños.

> "He should be so lucky." NBC correspondent, Andrea Mitchell, responding to an erroneous closed-caption news report that her husband, Federal Reserve chairman Alan Greenspan, had been hospitalized "with an enlarged ***prostitute***." (He had undergone prostate surgery for an enlarged prostate.)

PROTEIN

Protein. The Recommended Dietary Allowance for protein is 0.36 grams per pound of body weight or 0.8 grams of protein per kg of body weight daily. No calculator? That works out to about 45 grams of protein if you weigh 125 pounds (62.5 kg), 55 grams if you weigh 150 pounds (68 kg), and 65 grams if you weigh 175 pounds (87.5 kg). A better way to figure it out is to aim for an amount of protein that's equal to half your weight in pounds. This is slightly higher than the RDA mentioned above, but a little extra protein goes a long way to keeping muscles strong and the immune system healthy. In fact, some research shows that 1.0 or 1.1 grams of protein per kg seems to be associated with slower muscle wasting in the elderly.

Protein should account for 10–35% of the total calories for adults older than 18 years of age. Proteins can come from animal sources (of course), as well as beans, and nuts, and tofu, and grains and cereals. See the list below for some suggestions for plant proteins.

PLANT-BASED PROTEINS

Food	serving size	protein (grams per serving)
Tofu (firm)	4 ounces	18
Soy nuts	¼ cup	17
Veggie burger	1 patty	13
Lentils	½ cup	9
Black beans	½ cup	8
Peanut butter	2 tbsp	8
Kidney beans	½ cup	7
Walnuts	¼ cup	7
Soy milk	1 cup	7

Chickpeas	½ cup	6
Almonds	¼ cup	6
Pumpkin seeds	¼ cup	5
Spinach, cooked	1 cup	5
Broccoli, cooked	1 cup	5

(*Food and Fitness Advisor,* September 2009; *Nutrition Action Newsletter,* April 2011; USDA Nutrient Database for Standard Reference)

A quick comparison of protein sources with animal proteins—4 ounces of chicken packs a walloping 35 grams of protein, beef and pork pack in at 30 grams of protein per 4 ounces, ground beef with 20% fat is 29 grams of protein and canned tuna is 14 grams of fat. Plain Greek yogurt, 6 ounces, provides 16 grams of protein, cottage cheese 14 grams and plain ol' milk is only 8 grams of protein.

Protein intake and osteoporosis. Each gram of protein consumed increases calcium excretion by 1 to 1.5 mg. If a woman consumes 65 grams of protein per day, which is the typical amount for the average American woman, she would lose an extra 15 to 23 mg of calcium per day. Over time, this amount of calcium loss adds up and increases the risk for osteoporosis.

Proton Pump inhibitors (PPIs) and meals. Proton pump inhibitors are prescribed for the clinical condition known as gastroesophageal reflux disease or GERD. These drugs inhibit the active pump on the luminal surface of the gastric parietal cell that pumps acid into the lumen of the stomach. The majority of the symptoms of GERD are caused by acid as it refluxes into the lower third of the esophagus. Is there a specific time of day that these drugs should be taken in order to get the greatest benefit? Yes, these drugs work the best when acid secretion is being triggered by a meal. Patients should take their PPI on an empty stomach, 30 to 60 minutes prior to meals. It's best if the drug is on board before the acid pump is activated, so PPIs should be taken before the first meal of the day.

You know you're old when 'getting a little action' means
your prune juice is working. –Anonymous

Prunes. News Flash from the California Prune Board: As of the fall of 2000, prunes officially changed their name to *dried plums.* The California Prune Board petitioned the Food and Drug administration for a name change, and the petition was approved in June. The reason given for the name change: To attract a more youthful market. Thus far there is no evi-

ASPARAGUS TIP

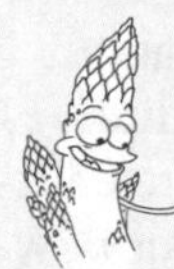

Sixty-seven percent of the dietary protein in the U.S. diet comes from animal sources, compared to a worldwide average of approximately 30 percent. The average American adult male consumes almost 70% more protein everyday than he/she needs. For women it's about 25% more than needed.

dence that the name change has pulled the proverbial wool over the eyes of the "youthful" market.

But, speaking of dried plums, aka prunes…a study in the September 28, 2011 issue of the *British Journal of Nutrition,* found that dried plums suppress bone resorption (breakdown), thus aiding in fracture prevention and osteoporosis. A 12-month study comparing a group of women taking 100 grams (10 dried plums) daily with a group consuming 100 grams of dried apples showed a markedly higher bone mineral density in the ulna of the forearm and spine in the dried plum group compared to the dried apple group. Nursing homes, listen up!! All of the Power Punch that you are serving might not only help the bowels but also may protect those old frail bones as well!

Prunes and the bowel. Prunes and prune juice have long been revered by the elderly for their ability to stimulate the bowels. What is it about constipation and the elderly? It seems as if everyone over 75 is constipated. There must be a gene that turns on at 75 that says… *"You're going to be constipated…Happy 75th Birthday…"* And there must be a gene that turns on and says…*"you're going to eat prunes every day for the rest of your life…"* AND there must be a gene that turns on at that exact same time and says… *"You're gonna talk about it all day…"*

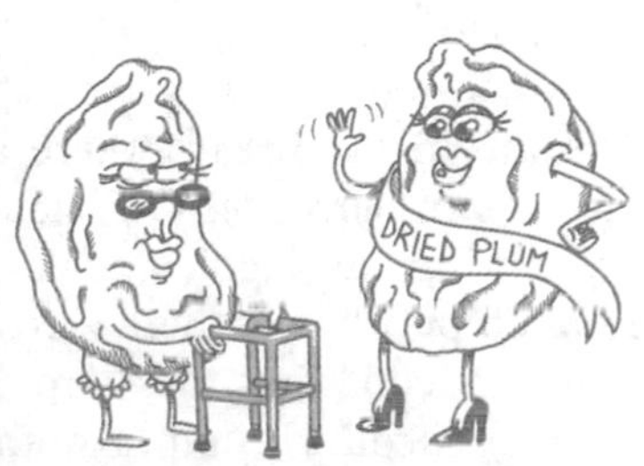

What's in a prune that makes it such an effective laxative? It's certainly not the fiber, even though prunes have a high fiber content. Prune juice has very little fiber but it's just as effective as prunes as a laxative. So, then, if it's not just the fiber, what is it? Apparently it is a derivative of the chemical isatin, which is related to another natural substance, bisacodyl, the active ingredient in some over-the-counter laxatives. Biscodyl is a contact laxative that induces the secretion of fluid in the bowel and stimulates peristalsis. Once peristalsis starts, the last stop is the toilet.

Prunes vs. psyllium for constipation. Very few clinical trials have evaluated prunes as compared to other treatments for constipation. A recent trial, supported by the California Dried Plum Board, provides some comparative efficacy evidence.

Forty adults with chronic constipation were studied in a randomized crossover trial. Treatment periods lasted three weeks, separated by a one-week washout period. One treatment period used prunes 50 g (about 6 prunes) twice daily with meals; the other treatment period used psyllium 11 g twice daily with eight ounces of water. Prunes were found to be more effective than psyllium using measures of number of complete spontaneous bowel movements (3.4 vs. 2.8 per week) or stool consistency. Improvement in global constipation symptoms was reported by 70% with prunes and by 55% with psyllium, but this difference was not statistically significant. There were no significant differences in side effects. (*Aliment Pharmacol Ther.* 2001; 33:822–828)

Prune profile. Dried prunes are called dried plums. One-fourth cup of prunes contains 32% of the daily value of vitamin K, 12.3% of the daily value of fiber, and 9% of the daily potassium, and only 104 calories. Prunes are also high in iron, folate, and vitamin C. Dried prunes have everything that fresh prunes have, with the unwanted addition of high sodium. Dried prunes are called dried plums.

Psyllium. Psyllium is the active ingredient of the over-the-counter laxative *Metamucil,* used by a myriad of average Americans for bowel-moving purposes.

Pumpernickel bread. There are many explanations for the origins of the word pumpernickel. One states that the name was coined by Napoleon's troops during the Napoleonic Wars. His men complained that although they were often poorly fed, there was always enough bread for Napoleon's favorite horse, Nicoll. Thus the word "pumpernickel" was coined—pain (bread) pour (for) Nicoll. Hmmm. Another explanation is that the word is derived from the combination of two German words—"pumpern" which means flatulence, and "nickel" which is derived from the name of a goblin or devil. Put the two together and you have bread that basically means "devil's fart." Hmmmmm….add a little sauerkraut and corned beef and your cadre of close friends will be severely depleted of their gas in no time. One last explanation is that nickel is an abbreviation of the Christian name Nikolaus (often used in Germany to designate a halfwit). Since pumpernickel is made with leaven and coarsely crushed pure rye bread, the other name could mean "a coarse bread suitable for a halfwit."

We live in an age where pizza gets to your home before the police. —Jeff Mander

---

I've been married so long I'm on my third bottle of Tabasco sauce.

—Susan Vass

QUERCETIN

Quercetin supplements. Quercetin (pronounced "kwair-sit-in") is an anti-oxidative flavonoid widely distributed in the plant kingdom. It is found in small amounts in onions, spices, apples, grapes, green tea, potatoes, and red wine.

Let's chat about mice for a moment. The mice in the lab of Mark Davis, director of the Psychoimmunology Lab at the University of South Carolina, received the human equivalent of 850-1700 mg of quercetin for their skeletal muscle and brain boost. The quercetin increased the number of mitochondria in their cells by 30% much like exercise does. The mitochondria are known as the "powerhouse" or energy producing components of the cells.

Mega-cycler Lance Armstrong swears by quercetin as a supplement for energy-boosting purposes. Perhaps quercetin was the key to his many triumphs on the Tour de France.

More human studies using quercetin as an energy booster are obviously needed, but if Lance Armstrong is any indication of the benefits of quercetin, we're on the right track. Other energy boosting compounds include carnitine and lipoic acid.

Quercetin...does an apple a day *really* keep the doctor away? Well, maybe 100 apples a day might do the trick. It's been a well-known fact for many years that if you exercise too much you get sick. The immune system just can't take it, and infections occur at a much higher rate.

Researchers at Appalachian State University in Boone, NC, decided to see if quercetin could protect people who are considered heavy exercisers.

They gave 40 male cyclists either 1 gram of quercetin per day (the equivalent to 100 apples) or a placebo, for 3 weeks. During this time, the cyclists spent a three-day period training at maximum intensity for 3 hours each day. By the time they were done, they were too pooped to pedal. Two weeks later, nine of the cyclists in the placebo group had succumbed to illness vs. none in the quercetin group. Implications abound. The U.S. military is especially interested as the troops become ill with infections more than injuries when in war zones. So, back to 100 apples a day…or at least a quercetin pill. (David Nieman, Appalachian State University, Boone NC) (*New Scientist* 18 August 2007)

Quercetin and cancer. More recent studies have indicated that an intake of quercetin may reduce the risk of colon and lung cancer by modulating signal transduction pathways that are associated with the processes of inflammation and carcinogenesis. (Murakami A, Ashida H, Terao J. Multitargeted cancer prevention by quercetin. *Cancer Letters* 2008; 269 (2):315–325)

Quercetin and chronic pelvic pain. In a study reported in the journal *Urology* (54:960, 1999), 500 mg of quercetin twice a day reduced the symptoms of chronic pelvic pain syndrome in 10 of the 15 men taking the supplements. Only 3 of the 13 placebo-taking patients received any relief.

Quercetin and viral infections. Quercetin may also boost the immune response against viruses. Studies in military recruits found that the recruits who were given 1,000 mg per day were much less likely to catch colds or other viral infections. (*Med. Sci. Sports Exercise* 2007; 39:1561)

Quiche. In Marseille, quiche is a slice of bread spread with anchovies, olive oil, and other selected toppings, and toasted in front of the fire. It is also known as "poor man's cake."

Quince. Quince is the yellow fruit of a tree native to Asia. In Europe, it is used to make confectionery (candies), liqueurs, and jam.

Quinoa. Pronounced "keen-wah,", this ancient whole grain was a staple of the Inca Indians for many centuries. Quinoa means "mother grain" in the Inca language. Its ability to grow in the high altitudes of the Andes knocked wheat and corn right off the dinner table for the Incas. It's cultivated in Colorado in the U.S. today.

Often referred to as a *superfood,* quinoa has an excellent nutritional profile. Each 220-calorie cup contains 5 grams of fiber, 8 grams of protein, and 15% of the daily iron recommendation. It's packed with the essential amino acid lysine and also contains magnesium phosphorus and zinc. It's a great option for patients with celiac disease because it's gluten-free. Cooked quinoa has a fluffy, slightly crunchy texture with a subtle nutty flavor. Quinoa seeds can enhance many dishes: you can add some seeds to salads such as tabouli, or substitute quinoa in recipes requiring rice or couscous. Quinoa flour works well as a wheat flour substitute in muffins or cookies.

Even NASA scientists were "keen" on the advantages of quinoa (before the space program took a nose dive). A NASA paper, written in 1993, stated quinoa would be a perfect crop for "meeting the needs of humans on long-term space missions."

By the way, even though it's considered a whole grain, quinoa is not a true grain in the botanical sense; close relatives include beets and spinach.

I like rice. Rice is great if you're hungry and want 2,000 of something.
—Mitch Hedberg

Raspberries. The botanical name for raspberry is Rubus Idaeus—the rubus for red and the Idaeus for "belonging to Ida"...well, who, pray tell, is Ida? Folklore has it that the original raspberry was white until the mother of Zeus, that would be Ida, pricked her finger while picking raspberries for little Zeus. As the story goes, the blood from her finger prick dripped onto the white raspberries, turning them red forevermore. As an FYI: the red raspberry is the most common; however, raspberries come in many colors including black, purple, orange, yellow, and the original white. Betcha' also didn't know that loganberries and boysenberries are raspberry hybrids.

So, are raspberries a good source of nutrients? One cup of raw raspberries contains 8 full grams of dietary fiber (one-third of the recommended Daily Value), 32.2 mg of vitamin C (54% of the recommended Daily Value), 9.6 mcg of vitamin K (12% of the recommended Daily Value), 25.8 mcg of folate (6% of the recommended Daily Value), 27 mg of magnesium (7% of the recommended Daily Value), 8 mg of manganese (41% of the recommended Daily Value), and 187 g of potassium (5% of the Daily Value).

ASPARAGUS TIP

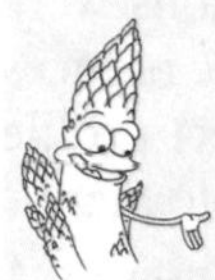

Raspberries are highly perishable. Purchase and eat the within a day or two. Refrigerate them unwashed in a single layer covered with plastic wrap.

Red Bull and energy drinks (see Energy drinks, Chapter E).

Red dye number 3. Is it safe to eat foods colored with red dye number 3? Foods such as red M&Ms, red cough drops, red pistachios, and maraschino cherries? "Yes" is the simple, concise answer. There was a big brouhaha a few years ago about a group of lab rats developing thyroid cancer after consuming amounts of red dye number 3 that would be roughly equivalent to a human eating all the cherries in 2,000 cans of fruit cocktail every day for 70 years. Reason has finally prevailed and our government has declared red dye number 3 to be safe for human consumption.

Red Herring. So, how did the term red herring become associated with a false lead? The term dates back to when the upper class would go on hunts in their private forests, and poachers figured out a way to snatch the goods from right under their noses. The trick: Getting between the hunting dogs and the prey they were chasing, and leading the dogs off the scent. So, the poachers would drag a pungent red herring across the trail. Why the red herring? Trainers often used the red herring to teach the hounds how to follow a scent. The dogs would follow the trail that smelled more familiar, leading the hunters away and giving the poachers a clear shot at the game.

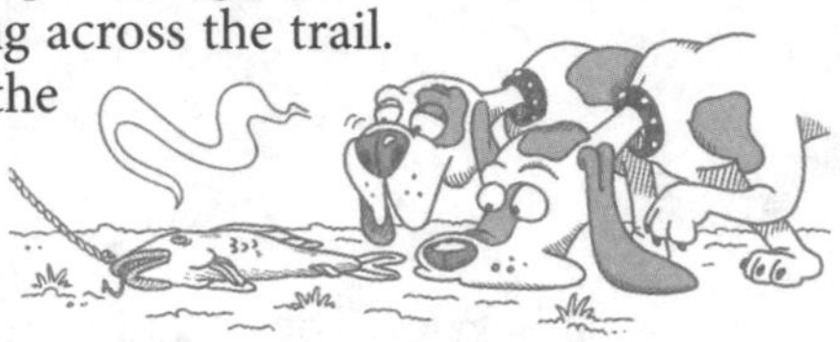

Red Yeast Rice. This over-the-counter dietary supplement is white rice fermented with red yeast. And yes, the rice turns red when the red yeast is added. It has been used in China for over 2,000 years and it continues to be a dietary staple in many Chinese diets. Its primary claim to fame is its ability to lower moderately elevated cholesterol levels. The active ingredients in red yeast rice are monacolins, compounds that inhibit an enzyme in the liver known as HMB-CoA reductase. This enzyme converts cholesterol into LDL-cholesterol, the bad cholesterol that is eventually deposited into main arteries that supply the heart, brain, legs, and kidneys. One of the monacolins, monacolin K is lovastatin, the active ingredient in the prescription cholesterol-lowering drug known as Mevacor.

In a small study red yeast rice (1800 mg) was compared to placebo. The mean LDL level was reduced from baseline by 27.3% at week 12 and 21.3% at week 24 in the red yeast rice group. The placebo group reductions were 5.7% and 8.7% respectively. It's unknown as to whether red yeast rice reduces cardiovascular events, but the authors state that since the side effect profile is negligible it might be worth trying if purchased from a reputable manufacturer. (Becker DJ et al. Red yeast rice for dyslipidemia in statin-intolerant patients: A randomized trial. *Ann Intern Med* 2009 Jun 16; 150:830)

A five-year study in China found that red yeast rice reduced not only the risk of heart attacks, but also the risk of death, the rate of angioplasty and the rate of heart surgery compared to placebo. And, the dose of the red yeast rice extract used was less than half of the lovastatin/Mevacor dose used today in clinical practice. Red yeast rice lowered the risk of heart attack-related deaths by 30% and the need for heart surgery by 33%. In addition, there was a 20 percent decrease in LDL-cholesterol and a 4% increase in HDL-cholesterol. (*American Journal of Cardiology,* April 2008)

Actually lovastatin is rarely used today as more potent "statin" drugs are on the market—including atorvastatin/Lipitor, simvastatin/Zocor, and rosuvastatin/Crestor.

Ok, should we all throw our statins out the window and head for the Red Yeast Rice in the health food stores? Not so fast. Once again, supplements are not regulated by the FDA and they don't contain a standard amount of monacolin. Studies have shown wide disparities in monacolin content in various brands of Red Yeast Rice. A July 2008 study by Consumer Labs noted that the combined level of lovastatin and its hydroxyl-form (the most potent form) varied by as much as 100-fold in the ten capsules tested. In addition, four of the ten compounds tested contained a compound known as citrinin, known to be toxic to kidneys in animal studies. The muscle aches and pains observed in statin takers are just as likely to be found in red yeast rice takers. So if you're chucking your statins for the red yeast rice to reduce these side effects, it's doubtful that you'll experience any relief. Bummer. (Robb-Nicholson C. *Harvard Women's Health Watch,* October 2008) (*Environmental Nutrition.* February 2011)

Reference values. The Food and Drug Administration definitions say that to be a good source of a nutrient, the reference amount of a food must provide 10 to 19 percent of the Daily Value. For example: Let's look at nuts as a possible source of calcium. The Daily Value for calcium is 1,000 milligrams (mg), and the reference amount for nuts is 30 grams, or about one ounce. A one-ounce serving would have to supply 10 to 19 percent of the Daily Value or, in the case of nuts, at least 100 mg of calcium. Unfortunately, for nut's sake, an ounce of almonds, for example, only contains 75 mg of calcium so it wouldn't quality as a "good source" of calcium for the average American.

Refrigeration. Keep the fridge between 39° and 40° F, and the freezer between 0° and 5° F. If your settings are 10° colder, the cost of running the refrigerator will be 25% higher than it needs to be.

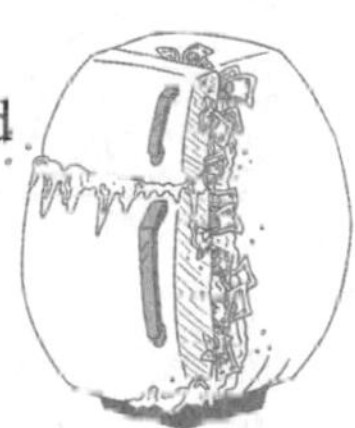

Resveratrol. Resveratrol is an antioxidant found in the skin of red and purple grapes, as well as in blueberries, cranberries, peanuts, peanut butter, pomegranates, and green tea. It is identified as the "healthful" component in red wine. It's a potent antioxidant that may aid in the prevention of cancer and heart disease, diabetes, and neurodegenerative disease. It has been shown to increase the number of mitochondria in muscles (which translates into increased energy) and to reduce fat deposits throughout the body. Should it be used for weight control? Some naturopaths recommend 125 mg daily in supplement form for energy and weight control. (Dr. Mark Stengler, *Natural Healing,* January 2009)

A study in the July 2010 issue of the American Journal of Clinical Nutrition found that resveratrol helps block immature fat cells from developing and functioning. In addition, it also appears to stimulate glucose uptake into fat cells and blocks molecules from converting into fat. These findings suggest that resveratrol may help prevent obesity and other metabolic effects that increase the risk for cardiovascular disease.

New research shows that it might behoove you to SIP your red wine instead of guzzling it. Resveratrol is largely inactivated by digestive enzymes and liver enzymes before it reaches the systemic circulation. If the red wine is consumed slowly, more resveratrol can be absorbed via the mucous membranes in the mouth. However, more research needs to be done to see if this is actually beneficial. It's unknown just how much red wine is absorbed through the mucous membranes so this might not be that effective. (Alcoholism: Clinical & Experimental Research. September, 2009)

Is resveratrol found in white wine? Yes, but not nearly as much as the amount found in red wine. If you are a white wine drinker, you may want to do a switcheroo on occasion and drink a bit of red for the benefits of resveratrol.

Can grape juice provide as much resveratrol as a glass of red wine? Sadly, yes.

Four to 16 ounces of red grape juice daily (watch out for added sugars) is just as effective as 6 ounces of red wine for women and 12 ounces of red wine for men. Doesn't work for me.

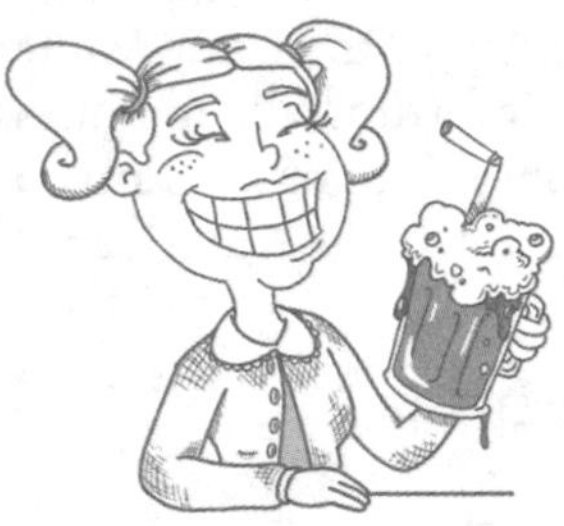

Root Beer. Root beer is less corrosive to the teeth than other sodas. In fact, it's the least acidic, according to a study of 20 regular and diet soft drinks. Pepsi, Minute Maid Orange Soda, and Coke are the most acidic. Enamel loss increased with prolonged exposure to soda. Either give up soda or drink it through a straw. (*American Academy of General Dentistry*, March 2008)

Rum. Rum received its name in 1651 when a traveler to Barbados remarked that the islands inhabitants were fond of "Rumbullion alias Kill Devel." Both rumbullion and rumbustion, two early dialect names, may have referred to the violence that the drink was said to cause. Rum became the favorite American alcoholic beverage until the Revolution.

Why does Sea World have a seafood restaurant? I'm halfway through my fish burger and I realize, oh my God...I could be eating a slow learner.
— Linda Montgomery

Saccharin. Saccharin (Sweet 'n Low) was discovered in 1879 by two chemists at Johns Hopkins University in Baltimore, Maryland. They were both working on oxidation of a coal tar derivative. The story goes that both scientists went home for dinner and both tasted a sweet residue on their fingers. (This immediately brings the question to mind, why didn't he wash his hands after working with chemicals? Well, this was 1879, after all, and hand washing wasn't in vogue.) Back to the story—when they returned to work the next day, they discussed the sweet-tasting residue and decided to characterize its chemical structure. They found a calorie-free, artificial sweetener that they named saccharin. Their findings were published in 1880. By 1907 officials tried to ban its use, but President Teddy Roosevelt put the kibosh on the ban, as he was a big fan of the artificial sweetener as a substitute for sugar. It just so happened that President Teddy Roosevelt also had diabetes.

Injurious to health? Anybody who says saccharin is injurious to health is an idiot. —President Theodore Roosevelt

---

Since that momentous occasion saccharin has been used to sweeten everything from Tab cola to ice cream and candies. Saccharin really caught on in the 1960s, but as early as 1951 scientists were discussing its carcinogenic potential. In 1977 the Canadian government published a study showing that it caused bladder cancer in male rats. One of the problems with the study was the dose of saccharin used. Those poor rats were exposed to a dose of saccharin that would have caused a bladder tumor in a hippopotamus. Nonetheless, this study set off a maelstrom of controversy that continues to rage throughout the world of artificial sweeteners.

Saccharin was delisted in 2000 from the U.S. National Toxicology Program's *Report on Carcinogens,* where it had been listed since 1981 as a substance reasonably anticipated to be a human carcinogen. In 2000, President Bill Clinton signed a bill to remove warning labels from saccharin.

The diet soft drink industry no longer uses saccharin. Aspartame (NutraSweet, Equal) has dominated the market for years and is found in more than 1,500 products and 90 countries. Aspartame does not cause cancer, and doesn't have that bitter aftertaste that saccharin leaves in the mouth. Remember Tab cola?

Saffron. Saffron is the most expensive spice on earth. It comes from the word zafaran, Arabic for yellow. The stigma of the crocus flower (Crocus sativa) are handpicked from each flower, dried and sometimes ground into a powder. It's an exhaustive process that in part explains its high cost. In fact, it takes 70,000 flowers to amass one pound of spice. In Greek mythology saffron is spoken of in the tale of Crocus and Smilax, where the nymph Smilax turns her spurned lover into a flowering saffron crocus. Persians believed that saffron induced sleep, cured melancholy and could be used as an aphrodisiac, which explains why they sprinkled saffron in the beds of newlyweds. Other historical uses of saffron included the treatment of anxiety, fevers, organ trouble (not sure which organ), arthritis, bruises and abrasions. Today saffron is used to add a beautiful yellow color to dishes—the most well known is Spanish paella. Iran grows most of the world's saffron supply, but Iranian usage is so high that Spain has become the world's top exporter of saffron.

Saliva notes. Approximately 1 to 1½ liters of saliva are secreted by our salivary glands each day. Saliva is mostly water but it contains enzymes that help to initiate the process of breaking down food, IgA to help protect against pathogens such as bacteria, viruses and fungi, and it lubricates the mouth so that we can speak and swallow.

HISTORICAL HIGHLIGHT

Salisbury Steak. Dr. James Salisbury was a late-nineteenth-century British physician who practiced and preached preventative medicine long before it became the fashionable thing to do. His major suggestion for disease prevention was to eat well, and that "well" meant to eat well-cooked ground beef three times per day. He claimed that this regimen would prevent or cure just about everything that "ailed ya" at the time, including tuberculosis, heart disease, gout, colitis, asthma, bronchitis, cognitive decline, rheumatism and pernicious anemia. His other "must do" for prevention was to drink a glass of warm water before and after every meal.

Most of this saliva is secreted during the day, with very little (about one-tenth) secreted at night. The bacteria that reside in our mouths know this important fact and, of course, being the opportunists that they are, they divide more rapidly when we are asleep and our mouths are dry. And just to let you know that they have been busy throughout the night, they leave a nice film covering your teeth as well as a healthy dose of halitosis.

If you don't produce enough saliva, you will, of course, notice mouth dryness. You're probably producing enough saliva if you can chew a dry cracker and swallow it easily.

Salivary flow can also be measured by the Lashley cup, a device that fits over the opening of the parotid duct (the primary duct of the major salivary gland, the parotid gland). Salivary flow is stimulated with a citric acid solution that is applied to the borders of the tongue with a cotton swab. Saliva is then collected. A healthy adult should produce between 0.5 ml and 1.2 ml of saliva (about one-tenth to one quarter of a teaspoon) per minute per gland when stimulated.

If you have a dry mouth, you can chew sugarless gum and suck on sugarless hard candies. Hard lemon drops are a good choice because the sourness stimulates more saliva. Drink more water or suck on ice cubes to moisten your mouth and increase fluid intake. Use a dry-mouth toothpaste such as Biotene. It doesn't stimulate saliva flow, but it may relieve burning sensations in the mouth and is less likely to irritate dry tissues in the mouth than other toothpastes. It also has mild antiseptic properties, which can help prevent tooth decay or gum infections. Avoid mouthwashes with alcohol. Alcohol dries tissues in the mouth. If you use a mouthwash, buy an alcohol-free version—and use it only once a day.

Saliva is also one of the body's innate barrier defense mechanisms. It contains antimicrobial proteins as well as protective secretory IgA antibodies. These natural protective effects help to explain why HIV is not easily transmitted by kissing or by dental procedures. A new finding provides an additional protective property of saliva—the lack of significant amounts of salt. In fact, saliva has one-seventh the amount of salt of other body fluids. When pathogens are placed in a salt-free environment, the intracellular concentration of salt in the pathogen provides a strong osmotic "pull" from the water-based saliva. Water enters the pathogen causing the cell to literally blowup from water overload.

My doctor told me to stop having intimate dinners for four. Unless there are three other people. —Oscar Wilde

---

Salmon, farm-raised and PCBs (polychlorinated biphenyls). Just when you thought it was safe and healthy to consume salmon for heart and brain protection, you must think again. The Pew Charitable Foundation tested over 2 tons of salmon from around the world and found that both farmed and wild salmon were contaminated with the chemicals. However, the farm-raised salmon contained nearly 10 times the amount of PCB and other contaminants than the wild salmon. The most significant differences among the farmed raised salmon and the wild salmon depended on the source. Contaminants in fish were highest in fish farmed in Northern Europe (Germany, Norway, Scotland, England and France), followed by farmed salmon from the U.S., Canada and Chile.

The culprit is salmon feed: The pellets of ground fatty fish that helped farmed salmon fatten fast also concentrate pesticide residues and industrial byproducts. High concentrations of chlorinated organic contaminants and other organic chemicals in farm-raised salmon from the U.S. and Europe warrant limiting consumption of this "heart-healthy" fish to no more than one time per month. (P.S. The contaminants in fish actually come from industrial chemicals that were banned in 1976, such as DDT. In other words, those contaminants are everywhere and they are not disappearing fast from the oceans and other bodies of water.)

Remember that wild salmon can also contain PCBs since they eat large numbers of smaller fish that contain PCBs. That being said, wild-caught Pacific salmon is less contaminated and can be eaten at least 2 to 4 times monthly without significantly increasing cancer risk. Do the risks for cancer outweigh the heart-healthy benefits? The answer is no, the risk of cancer is low compared to the benefits of the omega-three fatty acids that help to protect the vascular system.

However, if you or your patients are concerned—here's some friendly advice from nutrition experts around the world.

1) Don't give up on salmon altogether, however read the labels and choose North American or South American farmed salmon over European farmed salmon.
2) Eat various types of seafood—all seafood contains at least some omega-3 fatty acids. How about a can of sardines? Sardines are a rich source of omega-3s and are safe to eat.
3) Choose wild salmon over farmed—but expect to pay out the wazoo for it.
4) Look for "WildCatch" brand canned and fillet salmon, which comes from Wild Alaskan salmon. If it is stamped with the Marine Sterwardship Council label, it's from a healthy, non-endangered population of fish. Head to Whole Foods or Wild Oats for this "WildCatch" salmon.

Calcimar (calcitonin), literally means "calcitonin from the sea." This drug is used to treat osteoporosis and is obtained from salmon, whose calcitonin is compatible with that of humans.

Bring your checkbook and the credit card with the least amount of debt on it.

5) Buy canned salmon—it contains lots of omega-3 fatty acids and it's good for ya'.

Farm-raised salmon. Globally more than 1 billion kilograms (2.2 billion pounds) of salmon are farmed each year. That's a lot of salmon and that's a lot of PCBs. In the U.S. more than 90 percent of the fresh salmon consumed is farmed.

Salmonella. This species of bacteria is named after Daniel Salmon, an American veterinarian who isolated the bacteria from pigs in the late 1800s. *Salmonella* inhabits the gastrointestinal tract of humans and animals and is generally kept "in check" by all of the other bacteria competing for the same nutrients. Only when the number of *Salmonella* bacteria increase dramatically do they cause infection. This infection is referred to as *Salmonellosis,* and the GI tract is the major source of the symptoms. *Salmonella* infections have reached epidemic proportions in the U.S., responsible for two to four million cases of human illness per year.

If you become infected with *Salmonella enteritidis,* the usual food-borne type of *Salmonella*, you'll typically develop fever, abdominal cramping, and diarrhea within 12 to 72 hours. The usual course of the disease is 4 to 7 days of pure misery. Most people don't require treatment, just bed rest, a bathroom, and plenty of fluids. However, if the diarrhea is severe and you can't keep up with the fluids necessary to replace the lost fluids, hospitalization is necessary with IV fluids.

HISTORICAL HIGHLIGHT

Oregon's Rajneeshee cult has the clear distinction of causing one of the first bioterrorism attacks on U.S. soil, even though it took years to realize exactly what happened. In 1984 the Rajneeshees wanted to disrupt a local election that was voting on a referendum that could give their commune the boot out of an area known as The Dalles, Oregon. The chief of the commune's germ warfare division was a nurse from the Philippines, Ma Anand Puja (Diane Ivonne Onang). Her nickname was rather ominous—"Nurse Mengele" because of her obsession with poisons, germs, and disease.

The "germ warfare committee" bantered about various ways to disrupt the election and finally decided on using a strain of *Salmonella* typhimurium that would be debilitating but not fatal. Members of the commune sprayed the *Salmonella* on salad bars at numerous restaurants throughout The Dalles. At least 751 people contracted the *Salmonella* infection and the diarrhea was rampant. The good news is that the diarrhea didn't keep anyone from voting, and the commune was given the boot.

How do we get *salmonellosis*? Uncooked food contaminated with animal or human feces is the usual source. Cooking destroys the *Salmonella* but food can still become contaminated if it comes into contact with raw food that harbors *Salmonella* (cutting boards used for both raw meat and vegetables) or if a food handler doesn't wash their hands adequately after using the restroom.

Eggs are a well-known source of *Salmonella*. Just one in every 20,000 eggs is contaminated but that really isn't the point. If that egg happens to land on your kitchen table, you won't be a happy camper. Chickens raised in cage-free facilities have less contamination with *Salmonella*.

Reptiles can also be a source of *Salmonella*. Turtles, lizards such as iguanas, and snakes have all been known to harbor the little fella called *Salmonella*. Keep all reptiles away from children under the age of six. Even baby chicks and ducklings can pass the bacteria to children, so not only are petting zoos out of the question for the little tykes, but so are baby chicks for Easter.

Sandwich. It is estimated that over 300 million sandwiches are eaten every day in the United States.

The origins of the sandwich may actually go back even further than the story of the Earl of Sandwich. According to Jewish tradition, Hillel the Elder made the first sandwich in the first century B.C. A few hundred years before that the Hittite Empire served their soldiers meat between two slices of bread as their rations.

If you want to save a few calories when eating a sandwich, replace mayonnaise with mustard and save 100 calories. Drop the cheese and save another 100 calories. Which sandwich do you order most often? As far as healthy eat-

HISTORICAL HIGHLIGHT

The invention of the sandwich is popularly credited to John Montagu, the Fourth Earl of Sandwich in 1762. Montagu was a gambler known for his gambling marathons. On one particular occasion he had been gambling for twenty-four hours and was presumably on a winning streak. He didn't want to take the time to eat, so he asked his servant to bring the food to the gambling table. He asked that the meat be served between two slices of bread so that he could have one had free to continue betting. The other version says that he liked the sandwich because he could eat it without getting grease on his fingers from meat, making it a suitable snack while playing cards. Montagu was born on November 3, 1718, so November 3 has been officially declared as annual Sandwich Day.

ing (with a meat alternative) is concerned, the best bet is a turkey sandwich, no cheese, hold the mayonnaise, add a dab of mustard, and "sandwich" it between two pieces of whole grain bread.

Salt. Salt is considered to be the single most important of all spices. Salt has been harvested since at least 2700 B.C. and most likely for millennia prior to that. Salt allowed humans to preserve food, giving them the opportunity to migrate beyond their available food sources. Salt was exchanged in Greece for slaves (those who were underperforming were deemed "not worth his salt") and used as salary and tax payments in Rome. Salary is actually derived from the Latin "payment in salt." Salt is mined from dry underground mineral beds or taken directly from sea sources. One of the most famous is the Sel de Mer from France.

For centuries salt was served in a bowl, not a shaker. It couldn't be shaken, since it absorbs water and the salt crystals stick together. The Morton Salt Company changed that in 1911 by covering every grain with magnesium carbonate (now calcium silicate) to keep it free-flowing even in humid weather—thus Morton Salt Company's famous slogan, When It Rains, It Pours, and the picture of a little girl with an umbrella. This slogan and picture have been on Morton's blue salt packaging since 1914.

How much salt should the average American consume in a 24-hour period? The FDA recommends that one should consume no more than 96 mg per hour, or 2,300 mg in a 24-hour day. Exceptions to this rule include African-Americans ages 29 to 39, all Americans over 40 without hypertension and all people with existing hypertension or taking hypertensive medications. These groups should aim for lower—1,500 mg of sodium in a 24-hour period. (*American Heart Association*, 2012; *Centers for Disease Control, MMWR*, March 27, 2009)

Since the average American tends to not listen to the FDA, what is the average daily intake of salt? It is approximately 3,436 mg per day, a 'tad' above the recommended amount. (*American Heart Association*, 2012) Obviously Americans take this advice with a "grain of salt" (with skepticism).

Salt and fast food restaurants. Researchers from the New York City Health Department studied the amount of sodium contained in a single meal at fast-food chains in and around the Big Apple. The mean sodium content consumed in a single-meal by the average New Yorker was 1,751 mg. Given that the recommended daily allowance for sodium is 2,300 mg for most of us, a single meal contributed to 75% of the daily allowance. This single meal contributed to over the recommended daily allowance for patients with hypertension—1500 mg per day.

SHAKIN' OUT THE SALT FACTS...

* We can never run out of salt. There's enough salt in the oceans to cover the world 14 inches deep in a salt layer.
* Every human takes in about 1.6 pounds of salt per year.
* We each have about 8 ounces of salt inside us. It's absolutely vital for regulating muscle contraction, heartbeats, heart rhythms, nerve impulse transmission, protein digestion, and the exchange of water between cells.
* If you eat more than 4 ounces of salt at one meal, it will be your last meal. You'll die from an overdose of salt.
* Cutting out all processed food as well as added salt from your diet reduces salt intake to around one-tenth of an ounce a day. Do this for 5 days and your body can release up to two-and-a-half pints of excess water stored in tissues, which can lead to a weight loss of nearly three pounds.
* Just for the record, only 6% of the sodium the average American consumes per year comes from shakin' the salt shaker at the table. Another 5% is added during cooking and 12% occurs naturally in foods. How then, does the other 77% worm its way into the American diet? Processed foods are the culprits. (Centers for Disease Control and Prevention; Mattes RD, et al. American College of Nutrition)
* Salt is sacred in many cultures. It was once placed on a baby's lips during baptism in reference to Jesus calling his disciples the "salt of the earth" in Matthew's gospel.
* Throwing a pinch of salt over one's shoulder after spilling some salt is a long held superstition stemming both from salt's historical costliness and its properties as purifier and preservative, making the mineral a symbol of a good and long life.

Johnson and colleagues found that fried chicken outlets including KFC and Popeye's are the worst offenders when it comes to sodium content. Fifty-five percent of the meals bought at those fast food restaurants surpassed the recommended daily intake of 2,300 mg of sodium. Another 28% were between 1,500 and 2,300.

Pizza and hamburger chains put less sodium in their foods, with about half of the meals from these fast food restaurants containing less than 1,500 mg of sodium. McDonald's had the lowest count of high-sodium meals: 36.1% with 1,500 mg to 2,300 mg, and just 9.3% with 2,300 mg or more. It also had the lowest mean among all meals, at 1477 mg.

Did any chain have meals containing less than 1,000 mg of sodium? Yes, as a matter of fact, Au Bon Pain, had more than 7% of the meals containing less than 600 mg of sodium. But to balance that positive entree, 46% of their meals had more than 1,500 mg of sodium.

"Take-out message"? Bypass KFC and Popeye's if you're watching your salt. Stick with a quick hit from Mickey D's but don't do it often. (Johnson C, et al. "Sodium content of lunchtime fast food purchases at major U.S. chains." *Arch Intern Med* 2010; 170:732-34.)

Salt in the pills that you take. The following pills contain salt and may increase blood pressure in salt-sensitive individuals or may worsen symptoms in patients with chronic heart failure:

- Antacids
- Aspirin—One 325 mg tablet of aspirin contains 70–90 mEq of sodium.
- Zegerid (omeprazole) has 304 mg of sodium per capsule
- Alka-Seltzer Original has over 500 mg per tablet
- Most oral meds come as a sodium salt, such as levothyroxine sodium or pravastatin sodium. These will not increase blood pressure.

Salt content and various foods. The following foods are packed with salt. If you indulge, remember portion control.

- Cheese, butter, margarine
- Pickles, sour kraut, olives
- Condiments, sauces (ketchup, mustard, soy sauce, spaghetti sauces and salad dressings)—one tablespoon of ketchup contains 167 mg of sodium
- Salad dressings (regular fat, 2 tbsp contain 110 mg to 505 mg of sodium)
- Canned foods—one cup of canned lima beans contains 810 mg of sodium
- Packaged meals/frozen meals/entrees—one cup of packaged macaroni and cheese contains 837 mg of sodium
- Cheerios—one ounce provides 333 mg of sodium
- Wheaties—one ounce provides 370 mg of sodium
- Soups—one can of Campbell's Chicken Noodle Soup contains a whopping 980 mg of sodium
- Meats—ham, bacon, sausage, luncheon meats. A sandwich with cold cuts on a 6 inch roll contains 1,651 mg of sodium)
- Chips, pretzels (chips 1 oz = 120 mg to 180 mg vs. pretzels with 290 mg to 560 mg)
- Tomato juice (canned, V8) (340 mg to 1040 mg per 8 oz)
- Fast foods (see above section on Salt and Fast Food Restaurants)
- Use Lite salt (Morton or Cardia salt)—50% less sodium

Salt hints for reducing sodium intake…

- Taste food before salting—use the pepper shaker for salt (smaller holes in the pepper shaker)
- Use reduced sodium products (25% less sodium than original product); low sodium (140 mg or less/serving); very low sodium (35 mg/ or less/serving); sodium free (5 mg—YUCK); no salt added (still contains sodium that is the natural part of the food—REALLY YUCK)
- So, if you have a can of regular vegetables, simply rinse the vegetables before using.

ASPARAGUS TIP

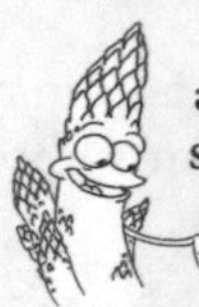

The U.S. would save about $18 billion in annual health-care costs and quality of life would improve for millions if we would cut our daily sodium intake to no more than 2,300 mg sodium. Meeting national sodium guidelines could eliminate 11 million cases of hypertension per year and extend the lives of thousands per year. (*Am J Health Promotion*, September 2009)

- When you purchase "enhanced" beef, chicken or pork products you may be purchasing beef injected with salt water and other additives to "enhance" the flavor. You're getting an unnecessary load of salt for a premium price. For example, a four-ounce serving of "enhanced" pork tenderloin contains 272 mg of sodium, compared to only 58 mg of sodium in a four-ounce regular pork tenderloin. The flavored pork tenderloins are even worse—a teriyaki flavored pork tenderloin has 463 mg of sodium in four ounces. Buy the regular pork tenderloin and season it with your favorite non-salt spices and save yourself hundreds of milligrams of sodium.

Salt and allergic dermatitis. If you've tried everything for your child's eczema and/or allergic dermatitis, try switching her drinking water to bottled water instead of tap water. Tap water contains lots of salt, whereas bottled water does not, and in a few cases it has been shown to be the difference, even after trying antihistamines, soothing lotions, and cortisone treatments.

Salt and hypertension. Should everyone reduce salt intake, even if their blood pressure is normal? A recent meta-analysis conducted by researchers receiving financial support from none other than the MmmMmm-Good Campbell's Soup Company reviewed the data collected from 56 clinical trials. Half of the clinical trials involved participants *with* hypertension, and interestingly enough the other half of the clinical trials involved participants *without* high blood pressure. Most of the studies alternated low-sodium diets with regular high-sodium diets.

The gist of the research is as follows: Individuals with hypertension received the greatest benefit from low-sodium diets, especially those over the age of 45. Younger individuals with hypertension as well as individuals with normal blood pressure, received little (if any), benefit from sodium restriction. (*Journal of the American Medical Association*, May 22/29, 1996).

Salt and osteoporosis. Urinary calcium increases by approximately 23 mg for every teaspoon of salt consumed. An uncompensated calcium loss of 23 mg/day is large enough to dissolve one percent of the skeleton per year. Reducing sodium intake to 1,600 mg/day would lower calcium excretion by one-third. Keep this in mind if osteoporosis is a concern.

Especially those easy to pop-in-the-microwave frozen dinners or pizzas, as well as hot dogs, bacon, processed American cheese, canned or dried soups (with Campbell's MmmMmm Good soups being the absolute worst offenders—although they have backed off the salt in recent years), salad dressings, canned meats, and restaurant and fast foods, just to name a few of the culprits. Let's take a look:

- Campbell's Vegetarian Vegetable soup–8 oz. contains 790 mg of sodium, vs. Campbell's Healthy Request Vegetable soup with 500 mg of sodium per 8 oz.; a can of Campbell's Chicken Noodle Soup contains a whopping 980 mg of sodium.
- Celeste Pizza for One, cheese (6.5 ounces) with 1,070 mg of sodium, vs. Weight Watcher's Three Cheese Pizza (6 oz.) with 350 mg sodium.
- Hardee's Chicken Fillet Sandwich at 1,100 mg of sodium, vs. McDonald's McGrilled Chicken Sandwich with 680 mg of sodium.
- Del Monte Whole Kernel Corn, canned (½ cup) with 360 mg sodium, vs. fresh or frozen corn (½ cup) with 14 mg of sodium.

Salt—getting it out of your diet in painless ways.

1) Compare sodium content in food products at the grocery store. A jar of prepared pasta can have 40 mg per serving or 800 mg per serving, depending on the brand. READ THE LABEL.
2) Prepare your own meals—wow, a novel idea. Easier said than done, but if done, the sodium content is drastically reduced.
3) Pile on the fruits and veggies.
4) Stay away from deli meats—any meat that is processed, smoked, and cured.
5) Dining out? Check out the menu before you get there so you'll know what to order.
6) Snack on whole foods such as fresh fruit or a handful of unsalted nuts.
7) Portion control. Portion control. Portion control.
8) Note that condiments are high in salt—ketchups, soy sauce, salad dressings can all be packed with sodium. Cut back.

Salt and sugary drinks. According to a study in the journal *Hypertension,* if you want to reduce the amount of sugary drinks consumed by your kids, work on what they eat. Those with the highest salt intake consume the most sugary drinks. By halving the salt in their diet, they could end up drinking two cans fewer per week. (*New Scientist* 23 February 2008;5)

One way to start reducing the salt in the diet is to nix the canned veggies and serve fresh. Canned veggies have 40% more salt vs. fresh vegetables. Did you also know that a bowl of Wheaties contains twice as much sodium as a bowl of potato chips? I'm not actually recommending the chips over the cereal…it's just surprising that some of the foods we think are so "healthy" have large amounts of sodium lurking within.

Salt substitutes. Will a salt substitute help lower blood pressure? Yes. A study in reported in *Hypertension Research* (2009), found that using a salt substitute for a year resulted in a significant reduction in systolic blood pressure—an average of 7.4 mmHg. In addition, arterial stiffness was reduced. Both benefits lower the risk of cardiovascular disease.

Salty and sweet. Why do we love salt and sweets when they are packaged together? Chocolate-covered pretzels are an excellent example of this combination. Another tasty combination is an order of French fries followed by a soft ice cream cone from Dairy Queen. It appears that salt blocks the bitter flavor of foods, allowing the more desirable flavors such as sweetness to tickle the taste buds. Have you ever noticed that some people salt their grapefruit? This practice enhances the sweetness of the fruit.

SAM-e and depression. SAM-e (S-adenosylmethionine) is a compound found naturally in the body that is involved in a wide range of essential chemical reactions. Is it an anti-depressant? Can it lift your "occasional moodiness"? Maybe. Several small studies have shown that a dose of 800–1600 mg may lessen the symptoms of depression. More studies are needed, and it's rather costly. The effective dose range can set you back $35 to $70 USD per week. Another study showed that it was as effective as Celebrex in alleviating osteoarthritis pain of the knee; however, it took a month longer to work. (*Nutrition Action Healthletter*, May 2009)

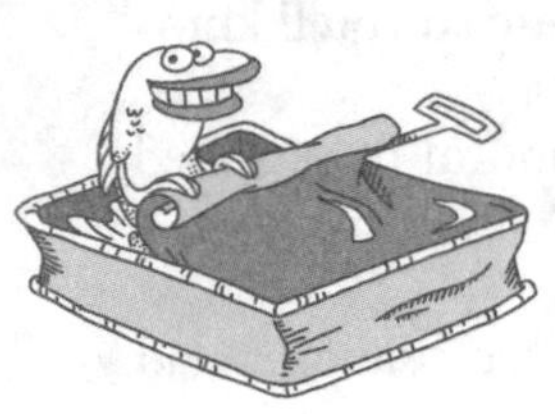

Sardines. It may come as a shock to many food aficionados, but there is no such fish as a sardine. The term "sardine" is a generic name for a number of small fish including herring and smelt. A small fish does not become a sardine until it has been canned. During the canning process certain oils, brines, and sauces are added, which give the small fish its characteristic sardine flavor. Without these additives, sardines would not be palatable to the average American. As it is, sardines are not that palatable to the majority of average Americans anyway. But they are good for you and they do contain a passel of omega-3 fatty acids.

Sauerkraut. Sauerkraut is a fermented cabbage commonly found in German cuisine. Fermented foods provide healthy bacteria for the gastrointestinal tract. It's a natural probiotic. Fermented cabbage in Korea is called kimchi. Miso is fermented soybeans used in Japanese cooking and soups.

Krauts. An American nickname for Germans, taken from their love of sauerkraut.

Sausage. The English word *sausage* comes from the Latin *salsus,* meaning "salted." Salt is necessary for a good patty or link because it dissolves the muscle fiber in meat so the fat can float in a chewy protein matrix. Add spices and a bit of blood protein and you have a yummy piece of sausage.

The Roman word for sausage, *botulus,* is the origin of the word *botulism.* The production of sausage provides a warm, moist, anaerobic environment ideal for the growth of *Clostridium botulinum,* the bacteria that produces the botulinum toxin.

Nitrates used to cure sausage are capable of killing the *Clostridium botulinum.* And that's the good news. The bad news is that the nitrates combine with amines, the natural breakdown product of proteins in the meat, to form cancer-causing nitrosamines.

Scombroid fish poisoning. SCENARIO: A husband and wife eat grilled mahi-mahi and pasta salad for dinner, washed down with a little white wine and a glass of water. Their canine companion eats the leftover mahi-mahi. Within 45 minutes, the husband and wife vomit. The dog vomits. The husband and wife develop diarrhea, headache, fever, rapid pulse and continue to vomit. The dog does the same. All three members of the family improve after taking Benadryl.

What's the scoop? Is this a food allergy?

This phenomenon is known as scombroid fish poisoning. Of all varieties of fish, the scombroid species (tuna, bonito, and mackerel) as well as dark-meat fish, such as mahi-mahi, are most likely to develop high levels of histamine. When fresh scombroid fish is not continuously iced or refrigerated, bacteria may convert the amino acid histidine, which occurs naturally in the muscle of the fish, to histamine.

Since histamine is heat-resistant, cooking the fish generally will not prevent illness.

In the case study described above, the fish was imported from Taiwan through California, and shipped frozen to Albuquerque where it was subsequently thawed and sold from a refrigerated case. Presumably somewhere along the line there was a lack of continuous freezing, allowing the histidine-to-histamine conversion.

Seafood. The average American ate16.3 pounds of fish and shellfish in 2007, a 1% decline from the 2006 consumption figures of 16.5pounds.
(www.noanews.noaa.gov/stories2008/20080717__seafood.html)

Seeds. We're talking about a powerful punch in the world of nutrition. Seeds are filled to the brim with nutrients, including vitamin E, folate, magnesium, copper, manganese and fiber. Seeds are one of the best vegetarian sources of protein, iron and zinc. Does any particular seed stand out? You bet. Sesame seeds are particularly high in calcium, but they also contain copper, manganese, magnesium, iron, thiamine (B1), zinc and B6. Other good choices include ground flaxseed, pumpkin and squash seeds, and sunflower seeds. Remember that seeds are also packed with calories, so you don't want to eat them by the bushel basket. Up to an ounce a day appears to be a practical suggestion. The runner-up in the seed world is the sunflower seed. It has vitamin E, selenium, manganese, copper, pantothenic acid, folate, B6, niacin, and zinc as the bonus ingredients, besides the obvious fiber, protein, and fat content. One ounce of sunflower seeds, shelled and dry roasted, has 165 calories in it, the same as sesame seeds.

SELENIUM

Selenium in the new millennium. The RDA for selenium for adults over 19 years of age is 55 μg with the Tolerable Upper Intake Level of 800 μg daily. Most multivitamins contain less than 70 μg. Selenium has antioxidant properties and it appears to lower cancer risk, especially of the lung, prostate, and colon with doses of 200 μg daily. In addition, selenium boosts apoptosis of cancer cells. Apoptosis is the process by which all cells are preprogrammed to self-destruct, a type of cell suicide. Selenium may also activate antitumor substances in cells and/or it may just give the immune system a needed boost to fight cancer. On the other hand, taking 200 μg per day may increase the risk of diabetes. (Meyer F, et al. Antioxidant vitamin and mineral supplementation in the SU.VI.MAX trial. *Int J Cancer* 2005;116:182–186)

Selenium is found in high concentrations in foods grown in soils rich in this mineral. Animals grazing on grass grown in selenium-rich soils also have higher concentrations in their meat. Animals may even become toxic on selenium.

In areas of the U.S. where the selenium content is low, such as the coastal areas, the rate of prostate cancer is unusually high. Recent research has shown that the incidence of prostate cancer in men who take 200 mcg supplement of selenium is only one-third as high as that of men taking a placebo. In a second study, researchers determined the amount of selenium found in toenail clippings and found that men's clippings containing the highest amounts of selenium had the lowest risk of prostate cancer. (Meyer F, et al. Antioxidant vitamin and mineral supplementation in the SU.VI.MAX trial. *Int J Cancer* 2005; 116:182–186)

Finland recently mandated that selenium be added to all farm fertilizers to reduce the overall risk of cancer. Studies have shown that selenium can also reduce the risk of cancer of the lung, stomach, colon, and rectum by as much as 50%. When populations with a low intake of selenium start getting sufficient amounts, a reduction in the amount of cancer begins to become evident after three years.

Patients with chronic hepatitis may also want to listen up. Researchers at the National Taiwan University in Taipei studied more than 7,000 chronic hepatitis patients over a 5-year period and found that selenium levels were significantly lower in those who progressed to liver cancer, as compared to controls. (*American Journal of Epidemiology,* August 1999)

Selenium and HIV infection. Consider selenium 50–200 mcg per day to decrease the transmission of the AIDS virus, HIV (Human Immunodeficiency Virus). A team of Kenyan and U.S. researchers found that women with a selenium deficiency were three times more likely to have HIV shedding in their genital mucosa, which may increase their infectivity potential.

The decline in selenium occurs even in early stages of the disease when malnutrition or malabsorption cannot be a problem. (Lancet. July 2000).

What is known about selenium and HIV:

- Less and less selenium is seen as T-cell counts drop.
- People with HIV who also have a selenium deficiency are 20 times more likely to die of HIV-related causes.
- Low levels of selenium are a greater threat to survival than low T-cell counts.
- Selenium deficiency poses more of a risk to survival than low levels of any other nutrient.

Selenium levels. Levels above 10 times the normal amount causes hair thinning and loosening of the toenails and fingernails. Most of us get plenty of selenium from our diet, so if you are considering a selenium supplement, make sure that your total intake, including diet and other supplements such as a multivitamin, does not exceed 800 mcg per day. (*Lancet* 1998; 352:715.)

Selenium and foods. The foods containing the highest amounts of selenium are Brazil nuts (4 nuts = 436 mcg), light tuna (3 ½ ounces = 80 mcg), and flounder (3½ ounces = 58 mcg) followed by pork, clams, dark turkey meat, white turkey meat, cooked pasta, whole wheat pita bread, Special K cereal, eggs, sunflower seeds, granola, Cheerios, English muffins, tofu, whole

HISTORICAL HIGHLIGHT

Marco Polo reportedly was one of the first to report the effects of selenium poisoning during his historical trip to China. After feeding on selenium-rich plants, his horses became so ill the hooves of those most severely affected literally fell off.

wheat bread, pinto beans, and navy beans. As you can surmise from the list, it's not difficult to get adequate amounts of selenium in our diet in this country.

Selenium and thyroid medication. Dr. Theodore Friedman, chairman of internal medicine and chief of endocrinology, UCLA School of Medicine, advises to eat foods rich in selenium to improve the function of medications used for hypothyroidism. Selenium helps convert thyroid hormone into a more usable form. (www.GoodHormoneHealth.com)

Serving size. Lest you forget from the P Chapter section on portion distortion—a serving is a specific, standardized quantity of food based on nutritional need. A portion is whatever is presented to you at any given meal. Standard daily servings generally are much smaller than portions served in restaurants or even at home. Here are some easy ways to estimate the recommended serving size:

One half cup of cereal, pasta, potatoes or vegetables is about the size of a small closed fist, a tennis ball, or a billiard ball.

Three ounces of meat, fish, or poultry is about the size of your palm, a deck of cards, cassette tape (does anybody even know what these look like anymore?), or mayonnaise quart jar lid.

One ounce of cheese is a chunk about the size of your thumb, five dice, or a ping pong ball.

One teaspoon of peanut butter, butter, mayonnaise, or sugar is about the size of your thumb's first joint.

One ounce of snack food is one handful of small foods like nuts, or two handfuls of larger ones like pretzels.

One medium piece of fruit is the size of a baseball or a tight fist.

One medium potato is the size of a computer mouse.

(National Heart, Lung, and Blood Institute. 2007)

Serving size of spaghetti.

Everything you see I owe to spaghetti. —Sophia Loren

Ooh la la, sis boom bah. This statement says it all. Ladies, forget the Botox, chemical peels and liposuction—let's lick the spaghetti bowl. Remember though, a serving size of spaghetti is only the size of a tennis ball.

Sesame seed. Contrary to popular belief, sesame seeds have been around a lot longer than McDonald's all beef patty, lettuce, cheese, pickles and onions topped with a sesame seed bun.

HISTORICAL HIGHLIGHT

Don't forget about Ali Baba gaining entry to the treasure cave of the 40 thieves by repeating their access code "open simsim (sesame)" in 1001 Arabian nights.

In fact, sesame seeds have been around for over 5000 years. The seed of the flowering plant Sesamum indicum has been treasured throughout the Middle East, Asia, the Mediterranean and Africa, both as a nutty flavoring and for its oil. Sesame reached the New World in the 1600s with West African slaves. The seeds are vitamin rich and its phytochemicals are potent antioxidants.

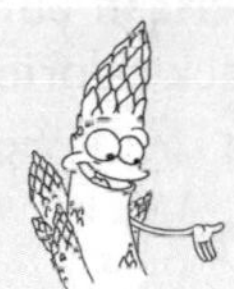

ASPARAGUS TIP

Who knew that 178 sesame seeds are on top of a McDonald's Big Mac bun?

Seven-UP, the history. In October 1929, just before the stock market crash, St. Louis businessman Charles L. Grigg began marketing a beverage called Bib-Label Lithiated Lemon-Lime Soda. His slogan: "Takes the 'Ouch' out of grouch." The drink was a huge success during the Depression, perhaps because it contained lithium—in other words, lithium was the UP part of the 7-UP. The 7-stood for its 7-ounce bottle. The 'UP' actually stood for 'bottoms up,' or for the bubbles rising from its heavy carbonation, which was later reduced. The lithium was listed on the label until the mid-1940s.

Shrimp. Shrimp is a great source of protein (18 grams per serving), vitamin B12, selenium, niacin, iron, phosphorus and zinc. However, shrimp is not a great source of omega-3 fatty acids. A serving of shrimp contains only 295 mg of total omega-3s, about one-sixth the amount in a comparable serving of salmon. See the blurb on cholesterol and shrimp in Chapter C.

Smell. Ninety percent of the ability to detect food flavors can be attributed to smell. To check your sense of smell, splurge on 10 different flavors of gourmet jelly beans. With your eyes closed, have another person feed you one flavor at a time and record what flavor you think it is. If you can detect six or seven of the flavors, your sense of smell is probably fine. If you can identify only two or three, see your friendly health practitioner.

Your sense of smell is sharpest in your 30s, 40s and 50s, with a drop-off beginning around age 60. About 50% of people over age 65 suffer some loss of the ability to smell. One of the earliest signs of Parkinson's disease is the complete loss of smell, known as anosmia.

SNACKING

Snacking. Eat a snack 90 minutes before mealtime to take the edge off your appetite. This results in fewer calories consumed at the subsequent meal and throughout the day. However, if snacking occurs just 30 minutes before the meal, the opposite effect occurs and you will consume more than the normal intake for that meal.

What size should that snack be? Shoot for 100 to 200 calories and a snack that is a good source of carbohydrates and protein. How about a little Greek yogurt with fresh fruit, hummus and veggies, almond butter on apple slices, or cottage cheese with raisins and cinnamon? The average American currently consumes about 500 snack calories per day vs. only 200 snack calories per day in the 1970s. (Jill Weisenberger, M.S, R.D, C.D.E, Diabetes Weight Loss—Week by Week, 2012)

Snacking and kids. One of the explanations for childhood obesity may be sitting right in front of you—easy access to the 'fridge. A study reported in the April 2002 issue of the *Journal of Pediatrics* examined snacking habits from three surveys conducted in 1977 to 1978, 1989 to 1991, and 1994 to 1996. The number of snacks per day increased during the study period from 24% to 32%, with the mean daily calorie intake from snacking increasing by 30%. Overall, 77% of children snacked in 1977, and 91% did so in 1996. Hispanic and white children snacked more than black children; a greater proportion of children from higher-income and more highly educated families snacked. Snacks were more energy-dense than meals. Calcium intake declined, and iron intake increased significantly in both snacks and meals. Because snacking is so entrenched as a dietary pattern, parents should make a concerted effort to ensure that their children snack on more healthful, less energy-dense foods.

Snacking late-at-night and weight gain. The time that you pick to eat may play a major role in weight gain. In a study in mice, one group was fed a high-fat diet for a 12-hour period during their usual sleeping hours, and the other was fed the exact same diet for the same period of time during their normal waking hours. The mice that were fed during their normal sleeping hours increased their weight by 48%. Those fed during their natural wakeful hours increased their weight by only 20%.

This study is one of the first to document the relationship between the time of day and weight gain. This research may be especially applicable to shift workers, whose schedules present many challenges, especially eating and sleeping patterns. Shift workers may have an easier time controlling their weight if they did not eat at times that conflicted with their body's natural rhythms.

Caveat: This study was done in mice. Studies in humans have not corroborated these findings. (Turek FW. Circadian timing of food intake contributes to weight gain. *Obesity* 2009)

Sniff your patients. Using the old "schnoz" can be a boon to clinical diagnosis if you know the smells you're sniffing around for. The usefulness of the clinician's nose as a part of the physical exam has been known for over 2,000 years. Hippocrates was one of the first proponents of the use of smell for diagnostic purposes.

Some examples of historical uses of odors in diagnosis include the following:

DESCRIPTION OF THE ODOR	DISEASE
Butcher shop	Yellow fever
Freshly baked brown bread	Typhoid
Freshly plucked feathers	Rubella
Putrid	Scurvy
Rotten straw	"Miliary fever" (TB)
Sour or musty bread	Pellagra
Sweetish	Diphtheria

- **Acetone.** The odor of acetone is the hallmark of diabetic ketoacidosis, a complication of type 1 diabetes mellitus. It is described as "fruity," whereas pure acetone is not fruity, but smells like nail polish remover. Theoretically, acetone could be smelled in starvation ketoacidosis (such as those folks on the Dr. Atkins diet); however, these patients are not starving long enough to exhale detectable amounts of acetone.
- **Alcohol.** Because pure ethanol is odorless, it is not possible to smell it on the breath. "Alcohol on the breath" is a term that is misused in all emergency rooms by nurses and physicians alike. What one actually smells is the juniper berry in gin, fusel oil in whiskey, the bouquet of the fermented grape in wine, the hops (a type of flower) in beer, or the acetaldehyde metabolite of alcohol.
- **Ammonia.** Chronic renal failure and liver failure have a characteristic "ammonia" breath; however, the two may be distinguished. In renal failure the kidneys are not capable of excreting dimethylamine and trimethylamine, both of which have a fishy component. In hepatic failure, the breath has a musty, ammonia smell due to mercaptans, dimethyl sulfide, and dimethyl disulfide.

- **Sewer breath.** Anaerobic bacteria lurking anywhere along the GI tract, from periodontal disease or peritonsillar abscesses to an intestinal obstruction, can cause the odor of sewage. Pulmonary infections such as bronchiectasis and pulmonary abscess can also result in this noxious odor.

Soda consumption. The average American drinks 50 gallons of soft drinks per person per year—about twice as much as the amount consumed in 1977. If you drink a 12-ounce soft drink containing 150 calories every day on top of your normal diet, you'll gain approximately 15 pounds per year. In 2004 soft drinks were the single largest contributor of calories in the U.S. according to a study published in the *Journal of Food Consumption and Analysis*. (*Environmental Nutrition*, June 2010). Today it appears to be French fries. See Chapter F.

Sorbitol and diarrhea. Halloween diarrhea is a common malady due to the large amounts of sorbitol used as an artificial sweetener in a wide variety of candies. Sorbitol acts as an osmotic diuretic, pulling fluids and electrolytes into the bowels and sending them to the toilet. Diabetics may also consume large amounts of artificial sweetener, and may also have diarrhea due to sorbitol. Diabetic diarrhea is usually attributed to autonomic neuropathy; sorbitol is often overlooked as a cause. One clue to autonomic neuropathy as the cause is nocturnal, or nighttime diarrhea. Having to bolt out of bed from a sound sleep for a diarrhea attack is usually due to neuropathy—not to excess sorbitol.

Sodium bicarb and a full stomach. Sodium bicarbonate (i.e., Arm & Hammer Baking Soda) should not be taken on a full stomach. Case in point: a young gentleman consumed two margaritas, one order of nachos, and a large Mexican combination plate for dinner. Upon arriving home, feeling like a stuffed taco, he gulped ½ teaspoon of baking soda in a glass of water. Within one minute he experienced severe abdominal pain. Emergency surgery revealed a ruptured stomach. It was assumed that once the sodium bicarb hit the hydrochloric acid in the over-bloated stomach, the combination of the two produced a carbon dioxide gas that was unable to exit the stomach and, BAM!

"Soteltes." Soteltes, or subtleties, are dishes of fantasy food served at French and English banquets. These dishes were not served to satisfy hunger, but were served to entertain and amuse the guests.

The tradition is said to have evolved in order to spice up the boring, meatless days of Lent. Chefs sculpted pie-dough castles, dyed green fish eggs to imitate peas, decorated cakes to look like fish, served checkerboards of tinted jellies—all for the amusement of diners.

The most well-known "soteltie" is taken from the nursery rhyme, "four and twenty blackbirds baked in a pie." Across Europe at the end of the fifteenth century, live birds were slipped into a baked pie shell through a hole cut in the bottom of the pie. Once an unsuspecting diner cuts into the pie, the birds are released, much to the delight of the guests at the table.

SOY

Soy protein. Soy products contain phytoestrogens, also known as plant estrogens. Two major classes of phytoestrogens have been defined—isoflavones and lignins. Isoflavones are found primarily in soy products and lignins are found primarily in flax seeds, whole grains, and some fruits and vegetables. Tofu is essentially a cheese made from the "milk" of soybeans. Tofu is a staple food in many Asians countries, but it has not cracked the top 10 favorite foods list in the U.S. as of this printing.

The isoflavone content of various soy products is as follows:

roasted soybeans (47 mg per ½ cup)
tempeh (37 mg per 3 ounces)
veggie burgers and soy hot dogs (5 –10 mg per burger/hot dog)
tofu (20 mg per 3 ounces)
soybean oil (0 mg per 1 Tbsp–good source of heart healthy omega-3s)
soy flour (44 mg per ¼ cup)
soy milk (30 mg per 1 cup)
soy noodles (8.5 mg per 3.5 ounces)
soy nuts (35 mg per ¼ cup)
soy yogurt (21 mg per ½ cup)
(USDA—Iowa State University Isoflavones Database, 2008)

Isoflavones are potent proteins that have proven benefits in lowering total cholesterol and LDL-cholesterol, while raising HDL-cholesterol. The FDA has approved a health claim for soy protein that indicates 25 grams per day, along with a diet low in saturated fat and cholesterol, may reduce the risk of heart disease. One serving of soy foods, such as 1 cup of soy milk or ½ cup of tofu, soybeans or edamame, provides at least 6.25 g of soy protein. (*Environmental Nutrition*, February 2011)

Soy and estrogen-dependent cancers. In recent years the relationship between soy foods and breast cancer has become controversial because of concerns based mostly on lab and rodent data that soy may stimulate the

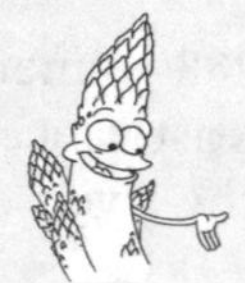

ASPARAGUS TIP

The soybean is the most widely grown and utilized legume in the world.

growth of existing estrogen-sensitive breast tumors. The studies are numerous and the data is conflicting.

New information about estrogen receptors suggests that soy isoflavone activity may be tissue-specific, allowing soy isoflavones to have minimal effect in breast tissue. Prior to 1996 it was assumed that there was only one type of estrogen receptor, estrogen receptor alpha (ERα). However, researchers discovered that there was a second estrogen receptor, and they cleverly named it estrogen receptor beta (ERβ). The original ERα occurs at higher levels in tissues in the breast and uterus. The ERβs are located in the cardiovascular system, central nervous system, osteoblasts of the bone, urinary tract, ovaries, testes, kidneys, and colon.

Phytoestrogens, such as soy, have a greater affinity for ERβ, allowing them to benefit certain tissues more than others. The discovery of ERβ may explain why phytoestrogens such as soy isoflavones appear to provide some of the beneficial effects in the bones, brain, and heart, while not causing some of the side effects associated with estrogen excess, such as breast and uterine cancer.

As mentioned earlier, soy products are a mainstay of the Asian diet and their intake is postulated to be a major reason breast and uterine cancer rates are so low in women from Japan, China, and other Eastern countries. The typical Japanese woman living in Japan (vs. living in the United States as a Japanese-American), consumes soy products daily, primarily in the form of tofu produced from soy milk. Numerous studies support the anti-estrogen effects of soy products on the development of estrogen-dependent malignancies in Asian women. Interestingly, when an Asian woman migrates to the U.S., their breast cancer risk increases over several generations and approaches that of U.S. Caucasian women.

A BRIEF DIGRESSION: This may sound a bit confusing. If soy is a plant-based estrogen, how does it have "anti-estrogen" effects? It is postulated that when bacteria in our intestines metabolize the phytoestrogens, the breakdown products exert a weak but significant estrogenic effect on various tissues in the body. However, these estrogenic effects are different from our own natural estrogens. One theory is that plant-based soy products block the effects of our own natural estrogens on our tissues. When acting as a partial blocker, the soy isoflavones compete with our own potent estradiol for estrogen receptors on breast and endometrial tissue. In addition, the plant estrogens appear to lower the overall circulating levels of natural estrogen by tricking the hypothalamus and pituitary gland into believing that the body has enough estrogen. This message is relayed to the ovaries and the ovaries slow down the production of natural estrogen.

A study reported in the October 4, 1997 *Lancet* compared 288 women, half of whom had been recently diagnosed with early-stage breast cancer. The others acted as the control group. Researchers compared the levels of various isoflavones in the urine of both groups and found much higher levels in the control group.

A more recent study in the *Journal of Clinical Oncology,* April 1, 2008, links higher blood levels of a soy isoflavone, genistein, with a 33% *reduction* in the development of breast cancer. Women with the highest genistein levels consumed about 3.5 ounces of tofu per day. The study was done in Japan, where tofu is a main staple of women's diets. ***Warning:*** Isoflavone supplements *do not* have the same effects on breast tissue. In fact, isoflavone supplements may *promote* the risk.

A meta-analysis by Wu et al. found a dose-dependent statistically significant association between soy food intake and breast cancer reduction in Asian women. There was an approximately 16% reduction per 10 mg of isoflavone intake per day. Age at exposure was found to be a co-determinant of risk: adolescent intake demonstrated a stronger effect on risk than intake during adulthood. Soy intake was unrelated to breast cancer risk in Western populations in which the average intake of soy isoflavones was low (less than 1 mg per day) and exposure is mainly in the form of soy components added as fillers/extenders to typical Western foods. (Wu AH, et al. Epidemiology of soy exposures and breast cancer risk. *Br J of Cancer.* 2008; 98:9–14; Korde LA et al. Childhood soy intake and breast cancer risk in Asian American women. *Cancer Epidemiology, Biomarkers, & Prevention.* 2009 (April);18: 1050)

A study by Messina and Wood found that there was little clinical evidence to suggest that isoflavones increase breast cancer risk in healthy women or worsen the prognosis of breast cancer patients. The epidemiologic data are generally consistent with the clinical data, showing no indication of increased risk. (Messina MJ and Wood CE. Soy isoflavones, estrogen therapy, and breast cancer: analysis and commentary. *Nutrition Journal.* 2008 (7):17)

Isoflavones appear to be more potent than lignins in terms of protecting the ductal tissue of the breast and the uterine linings. The lignin-containing foods, particularly whole wheat, rye, and flax seeds, are also high in fiber and *may* contribute to lowering overall estrogen levels by increasing their elimination from the bowel and reducing intestinal absorption of estrogen.

Should we all rush out and purchase barrels of tofu for immediate consumption? Well, perhaps not barrels, but it may be prudent to gradually add a bit of soy for an overall healthy diet. The goal should be to work up to 25–45 mg of isoflavones per day taken in food (not supplements). Note that tofu is 50% fat, so you may want to adjust your fat intake accordingly. The amount of tofu (3.5 ounces) that provides 33.7 mg of isoflavones also provides 9 grams of fat, as compared to 3.5 ounces of chicken breast, which provides 3.6 grams of fat. On a happier note, tofu has less fat than 3.5 ounces of cheddar cheese (33 grams of fat) and/or extra lean ground beef (16 grams of fat/3.5 ounces). So, how about a tofu burger, hold the cheddar?

Soy and the heart. The isoflavones in soy (genistein, daidzein, and glycitein) are the active ingredients. Consuming soy protein vs. animal protein significantly reduces total cholesterol (9.3%), LDL-cholesterol (12.9%) and triglycerides (10.5%) while increasing HDL-cholesterol only 2.4%. Genistein acts as an antioxidant, potentially limiting oxidative damage to LDL-cholesterol. Genistein has also been shown to reduce clot formation and to inhibit rapid proliferation of cells following balloon angioplasty.

People with cholesterol levels higher than 240 mg/dl may want to consume 25–50 grams of soy protein daily in place of other protein to reduce their cholesterol levels. The November 14, 2000, issue of Circulation published the first study on the beneficial effects of soy protein consumption to be judged conclusive by the American Heart Association. The study reviewed the latest 38 clinical trials on soy intake and found that 25–50 grams of soy protein per day can safely reduce LDL-cholesterol by up to 8%, reduce triglycerides, and increase HDL-cholesterol by 2.4%. The researchers found that soy protein has no effect on cholesterol levels under 200 mg/dl.

Continued research by the American Heart Association confirms soy protein's cholesterol lowering effects. Compared to control subjects, consumption of soy protein is associated with significant mean reductions in total cholesterol levels and LDL-cholesterol levels of 9.45 mg/dl and 7.12 mg/dl respectively. (Samuel P et al. Abstract 3273: Meta-analysis confirms soy protein's cholesterol lowering efficacy. *Circulation.* 2008; 118:S-1122)

> ***John Harvey Kellogg, health guru and cereal king, introduced soybean products in the 1920s as healthful substitutes for milk and meat.***

Soy and osteoporosis. Could the neck of your femur use a little tofu burger? If you live in China, yes. A recent study found that a moderate daily intake of soy—the amount found in about 1.75 ounces of tofu—was associated with a 21% to 26% reduced risk of hip fractures among women in the Singapore Chinese Health Study. Well, that's great for Chinese women, but we don't live in China nor do we eat anywhere near that amount of tofu on a daily basis. Interestingly the findings in this study did not apply to the Chinese men. (Koh W et al. *Am J Epid* 2009)

Ten more studies support soy and the prevention of vertebral osteoporosis using isoflavone supplements. A meta-analysis found that spine bone mineral density increased significantly with isoflavone intake of more than 90 mg/day and with treatment lasting six months. (Ma DF, et al. Soy isoflavone intake increases bone mineral density in the spine of menopausal women: Meta-analysis of randomized controlled trials. *ClinNutr* 2008; 27(1):57–64)

Soy and sperm counts. A diet rich in soy is associated with lower sperm concentrations, according to a cross-sectional study published online in *Human Reproduction* (2008). Researchers analyzed sperm concentrations and self-reported intake of 15 soy foods in some 100 men attending a fertility clinic with their partners. After multivariable adjustment, they found that a high intake of soy in the previous 3 months was associated with a reduced sperm concentration. Men who reported eating the most soy had an average of 41 million sperm/mL less than those who did not eat soy. The effect was even more pronounced in men who were overweight or obese.

ASPARAGUS TIP

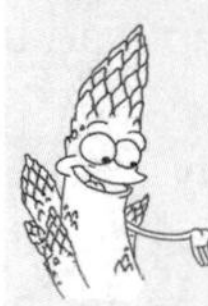

Eating as little as a single serving of soy per day (1 cup of miso soup or a single serving of tofu) can cut sperm counts in half from 80 million to 40 million (still within normal range). (Jorge Chavarro, Harvard School of Public Health, *New Scientist*, October 17, 2007)

Soy and the thyroid. The FDA has released words of wisdom and words of warning concerning the interaction of soy and thyroid hormones. It appears that soy can interfere with the production of thyroid hormone. Women with Hashimoto's thyroiditis should minimize their intake of soy products or avoid them altogether, and avoid isoflavone supplements as well. (Wold RS, Lopez ST, Yau LY, et al. Increasing trends in elderly persons' use of nonvitamin, nonmineral dietary supplements and concurrent use of medications. *J Am Dietetic Assoc* 2005; 105(1). Bonakdar, R. Herb-drug interactions. *Patient Care* 2003; January: 58–69)

Inhabitants of underdeveloped nations and victims of natural disasters are the only people who have been happy to see soybeans. —Fran Leibowitz

---

Soybean oil in generic drugs and allergies. The use of generic drugs has increased throughout the U.S. and Europe in recent years. The main regulatory requirement for generic drugs is that they have the same amount of drug as the brand name drug—in other words, that the generic drug is the bioequivalent of the branded drug. However, the problem seems to be the "filler" that is used in some of the generic forms of drugs. One of the filler's used recently in a generic omeprazole was soybean oil.

In a study from Spain, researchers reported on two women who presented with anaphylaxis a few minutes after ingesting generic omeprazole capsules. In both women the systolic blood pressure fell to less than 90, and both had a sudden onset of difficulty breathing. Both women had previously taken a brand name omeprazole and neither had problems with hypotension or difficulty breathing.

And, here's the problem. Many of the generic drug labels don't include what is added as a "filler" or additive. The active ingredients of the drug are clearly labeled, but the additives or "fillers" are not. The additives are displayed as "excip. c.s. which basically tells you nuttin', zero, zilch, nada. So bottom line?

The researchers suggest that all patients who have hypersensitivitiy reactions to drugs should be tested for soy allergies. (Duenas-Laita A, Pineda F, Armentia A. Hypersensitivity to generic drugs with soybean oil. Letters to the editor. *N Engl J Med* 2009;36 (13): 1318)

Space medicine—preparing for the 3-year round-trip to Mars. Space flight "speeds up aging." Astronauts experience accelerated bone loss, accelerated muscle loss, and a greater chance of DNA mutations that can lead to cancer.

The loss of bone density in space flight equals to approximately 1% per month. The bone loss begins within hours of weightlessness, and is especially pronounced in the weight-bearing bones of the ankles, hips and spine. Using foods with a long shelf life exacerbates the bone loss problem. Shelf-stable foods that would be necessary for such a long flight require large amounts of sodium to remain stable, unlike refrigerated and frozen foods. Unfortunately, more sodium equates to a greater calcium loss from bone. The kidney filters the sodium and it competes with calcium for excretion. Calcium wins the competition and is excreted into the urine; sodium remains in the body. But, until the refrigeration problem is solved, high-sodium shelf-stable foods continue to be the major dietary staple of the astronaut of today.

The lack of the protective ozone layer results in tremendous oxidative damage to an astronaut's DNA, ultimately increasing the risk of loss of growth control and thus cancer. Providing an antioxidant cocktail containing vitamins C and E, as well as isoflavones from plants, may be beneficial.

The risk of colon cancer may be particularly high in the astronaut cohort. Combining the massive oxidative stress with the "fear of flying fiber" provides a fertile soil for DNA mutations and the development of colon cancer. Fiber has been the forbidden food of space shuttles past and present. The prevailing theory was obvious. It would create an overabundance of fecal material with a paucity of disposal space. So the astronauts were given only 0–1 gram of fiber per day, hardly enough to stimulate one centimeter of peristalsis hence, the major complaint of all astronauts was a serious case of constipation.

Adding fish oil to the antioxidant cocktail may help prevent the oxidative damage to cells. Fish oil can potentially prime the cell membrane to signal the rest of the cell that it should prepare to undergo apoptosis, or programmed cell death. This process of apoptosis prevents the precancerous cell from uncontrolled growth and the formation of a malignant tumor.

A second step is necessary to prevent cancer from developing. The fish oil only *prepares* the cell for apoptosis; it doesn't actually cause the death of the cell. Enter our friend fiber to the tune of approximately 20–25 grams per day. The microflora of the colon feed off the fiber, and actually form short-chain fatty acids such as butyrate. Butyrate is the "trigger" for the initiation of cell death.

Iron overload is another potential problem on a long space trip. During space travel, astronauts lose approximately 20% of their blood volume. The body compensates by reducing the number of red blood cells, which in turn reduces the amount of intracellular iron. More iron circulates in the blood as "free" iron. Unfortunately, this free iron may infiltrate organs, resulting in iron overload and tissue damage similar to the inherited condition known as hemochromatosis.

Muscle atrophy resulting from the lack of exercise and lack of gravity may be prevented by taking an amino acid supplement. This supplement may also be useful for the elderly who also experience muscle mass atrophy due to disuse and travel. Space travel sounds exciting, but after realizing all of the potential medical problems, perhaps it's not all it's cracked up to be.

SPAM. Every four seconds, somebody in the world opens a can of SPAM, the number one canned luncheon meat sold around the world. The word SPAM comes from the combination of two words, SPicedhAM. It consists of a loaf of molded ground pork shoulder with some added ground ham, salt, water, sugar, and sodium nitrite. The amount of sodium in one 2-oz serving of SPAM is enough to make any blood pressure skyrocket. This 2-oz serving contains 750 mg of sodium and 170 calories, with 140 of those calories from saturated fat. SPAM is, by all intents and purposes, death in a can.

Ahhhh, not so fast, you exclaim. The makers of SPAM have developed a variation on the theme, known as SPAM LITE. It's 25% less sodium, and 140 calories, 90% of which are saturated fats. Remarkably, SPAM does not make the top-10 food list at Weight Watcher's or any other weight loss program. In fact, it doesn't make anyone's top 10 list as a nutritional powerhouse.

The George A. Hormel Company of Austin, Minnesota, manufactures SPAM. Who eats SPAM? No one admits they eat SPAM, but there must be a few million closet SPAM eaters in this world because eighty-five million pounds of canned SPAM are sold per year! SPAM corners 75% of the canned luncheon meat market in the U.S. and overseas. I repeat my question, Who eats SPAM?

The island of Guam wins the prize for the most SPAM consumed in the world per year and per capita. Guam has 135,000 citizens, but consumes 1.5 million cans of SPAM per year. You do the math.

The pork packers of the world also think highly of SPAM. In their journal, Squeal, an article touted the introduction of SPAM to the world as "as historic as the first rifle shot at the Battle of Lexington." In the "What's on the Menu" section of the journal, the following recipes were found: Polynesian baked SPAM, sweet and sour SPAM, SPAM enchilada breakfast casserole, spaghetti carbonara with SPAM, and cool SPAM, cucumber, and avocado sandwiches. If you don't have the current issue of Squeal on your coffee table, you can go to your local bookstore and purchase the comprehensive cookbook on every SPAM recipe known to man. Dorothy Horn has published a SPAM cookbook with over 500 recipes.

SPAM is making a comeback... Yes, sales of this "death in a can" luncheon meat have increased by 9% since January 1, 2008. Why? It appears as if SPAM must be the only food item that hasn't increased its prices, thus people with limited food budgets are buying it by the caseload. So, in the short haul, food bills will either decrease or remain the same; however, in the long haul health insurance claims will skyrocket as the consumption of SPAM in any amount can be hazardous to your cardiovascular health.

The week of November 19, 2010 was an especially memorable week for the passengers on the cruise ship, Splendor. An engine room fire left the 3,299 vacationers stranded off the coast of Mexico with no hot water, hot food, or working toilets for days. The first food that was airlifted in to the stranded cruise liner was SPAM.

SPINACH

Spinach. Each one-cup serving of cooked spinach provides 140% of the day's worth of vitamin A, 30% of a day's worth of folic acid, 15% of a day's iron and vitamin C, and 10% of a day's potassium—and the best part: all of this and more for only 20 calories. The combination of vitamin C in the spinach is especially nutritive. Vitamin C reduces the loss of folate during the cooking process, and it enhances the body's absorption of the iron in spinach. Popeye was obviously on to something over 70 years ago.

"Spinach poisoning." Spinach contains nitrates that are converted via innate mechanisms in the stomach to nitrites. Nitrites, in turn, react with proteins to form nitrosamines, some of which are known or suspected carcino-

HISTORICAL HIGHLIGHT

Popeye made his first appearance in the comic strip Thimble Theatre in 1927. Popeye was not considered to be a major character when he was first introduced. In fact, the original comic strip revolved around his future "goil," Olive Oyl and her family.

Popeye's spinach obsession began in the Thimble Theater comic strip; however, it became an indispensable plot device during his later role as Popeye the Sailor. Spinach growers in the U.S. credited Popeye with a 33% increase in spinach consumption, literally saving the spinach industry from ruin.

In 1937, Crystal City, Texas, the spinach capital of the world, erected a statue to commemorate Popeye and his creator, E.C. Segar, and their influence on the spinach-eating habits of the American population.

gens. Before you panic and eschew spinach for the rest of your born days, realize that this natural chemical reaction presents no known problems for the healthy average American adult. But, when nitrate-rich vegetables (beets, celery, eggplant, radishes, collard and turnip greens, and of course, spinach) are cooked and left to stand at room temperature, bacterial enzyme action (and perhaps some enzymes in the plants) convert the nitrates to nitrites at a much faster rate than normal. These higher-nitrite foods may be hazardous to infants; several cases of "spinach poisoning" have been reported among children who ate cooked spinach that had been left at room temperature for a long period of time.

Stevia (Stevia rebaudiana), the "sugar herb." If you are uncomfortable with the artificial sweeteners aspartame and saccharin, Stevia just may be your sweet savior. The FDA allowed Stevia into the country in 1995 with the provision that it must be sold as a dietary supplement, not as an artificial sweetener. The FDA considers it as an untested food additive, although the raw leaves have been used in South America for a few centuries, and processed Stevia has been on the shelves of Japanese grocery stores for more than 30 years without adverse effects.

This little green plant, native to Paraguay, is the sweetest known natural substance. The human body does not metabolize the sweet glycosides from the stevia leaf or any of its processed forms so there is no caloric intake. Stevia doesn't adversely affect blood glucose levels and may be used freely by diabetics. Stevia is an ingredient in the products PureVia and Truvia.

Stevia is 10–15 times as sweet as table sugar, although varying extracts can range from 100–300 times sweeter. If you are going to substitute Stevia in recipes, the conversion rate is one *teaspoon* of Stevia for one *cup* of sugar. Obviously a mistake here with a one-to-one *cup* ratio would be disastrous for any dessert-loving aficionado.

You can purchase processed Stevia at health-food stores in a concentrated powder or liquid form. You can also grow your own with seeds or plants purchased from your friendly local nursery for about $2 to $6 each. Mature leaves can be dried and ground into a green powder to be used in cooking or to sweeten your favorite beverage.

HISTORICAL HIGHLIGHT

Count Paul Stroganoff was one of the last members of the wealthy Stroganoff family in early nineteenth century Russia. He was famous for his ability to throw lavish dinner parties, many of which featured his now famous signature dish consisting of sautéed beef, onions, mushrooms, sour cream, and a few other family secrets. That famous dish is eponymously known as Beef Stroganoff.

> *Anybody who believes that the way to a man's heart is through his stomach flunked geography.* —Robert Byrne

Sugar. The amount of sugar in one 12-ounce can of soda is 10 teaspoons. Ouch.Ten teaspoons multiplied by 4 grams of sugar per teaspoon gives you 40 grams of sugar from that one 12-ounce beverage. How about calories from sugar in that beverage? To convert a level teaspoon of sugar to calories multiply by 15. You don't need a calculator—10 x 15 = 150 calories. Non-diet soda is an obvious sugar source, as are cookies, ice cream, cakes, pies, and candy, any candy—candy bars, candy canes, candy pieces. The not-so-obvious places will surprise you. Barbecue and steak sauce may have as much as 12–14 grams of sugar per teaspoon. Ketchup has 4 grams; however, all brands have varying amounts. A spoonful of jam can give you as much as 14 grams of sugar. Read the labels on cereals. Even some of the so-called all-bran cereals are packed with sugar. Raisin Bran has up to 20 grams of sugar compared to Wheat Chex with has five grams of sugar. Commercial salad dressings have 5–7 or more grams, and tomato sauces between 11 and 14 grams. Lots of so-called fat-free products are packed with sugar. JELL-O's fat-free pudding snacks contain 17 grams of sugar. Manufacturers of some fat-free products increase the sugar content to make up for the flavor lost when fats are eliminated, making many of these "diet, fat-free" snacks higher in calories than the original snack food that contains fat. So, if you are attempting to cut down on your sugar intake, you must, once again, read the label.

Sugar and lipid levels. Consuming higher amounts of added sugars is associated with lower levels of HDLs and higher levels of triglycerides, which are important risk factors for cardiovascular disease. (Welsh et al. Caloric sweetener consumption and dyslipidemia among US adults. *JAMA* 2010; 303 (15)

Sugar recommendations—hot off the press from the AHA. The American Heart Association has made the definitive statement on the absolute amount of sugar one should consume on a daily basis. Women should have no more than 6 ½ teaspoons daily (100 calories) and men, no more than 9 ½ teaspoons daily (150 calories) of added sugars. Most average Americans average 22 to 28 teaspoons of sugar per day. That's 350 to 440 empty calories per day. This new recommendation includes soft drinks, Hershey kisses, M&Ms,and other delicious candies, but it does not include sugars that occur naturally in fruits and other foods.

In other words, the average apple contains the equivalent of 6 teaspoons of sugar; however, this doesn't count toward your daily teaspoon recommendation since it is a "natural" sugar. (*American Heart Association,* 2009)

HISTORICAL HIGHLIGHT

Dentists invented cotton candy and chewing gum, both of which tickle the sweet tooth. Dr. William Morrison, a Nashville dentist in the late 1800s, invented the Fairy Floss candy machine that made sugar-laden cotton candy. About the same time, an Ohio dentist, Dr. William Semple patented the first chewing gum. He anticipated that chewing gum would help clean the teeth…humm. For more fascinating facts on dentistry, visit the National Museum of Dentistry, 31 South Green Street (at Lombard), Baltimore, Maryland, 410-706-8313.

Many new sweets were developed around the turn of the twentieth century. Until that time sugar was very expensive. When the sugar tariffs were lifted in the 1880s, the price of sugar dropped and more people could afford to buy it and experiment with it.

Sugar—the following are some uncommon uses for sugar: (*Cook's Illustrated*, January/February 2012)

…..Burn your tongue on a hot drink? Press your tongue directly against a spoonful of sugar. The sugar crystals will immediately begin to dissolve and pull heat from the tongue, reducing the pain.

…..Want to preserve the chewiness of cookies for a couple of days? Add two sugar cubes to a closed container of the fresh, soft, and chewy cookies. Sugar absorbs the moisture from the air and keeps the cookies from drying out. Cookies retain a just-baked freshness for two days.

…..Want to get rid of the garlic or onion smell on your hands? Wash you hands with warm water, sprinkle your hands with a tablespoon of granulated sugar, rub for 60 seconds, and rinse off your hands. The sugar crystals act like a big ol' porous sponge to absorb the odor of the onion and garlic.

Sulfites and food allergies. Sulfites (sulfur dioxide, sulfur bisulfite, etc.) are chemicals added to various foods to 1) enhance the flavor (canned tuna, for example), 2) to keep foods from turning brown as they dry (sliced apples, apricots, dried bananas, dried dates, dried figs, dried peaches, dried pineapple, commercially prepared potato salads, dried prunes, and raisins), and 3) to prevent the growth of microorganisms that might turn white wine into vinegar. People sensitive to sulfites can have severe allergic reactions, including anaphylactic shock, if they consume these products. In a perfect world, all products containing sulfites should be banned; however, reading the label will provide additional reassurance.

Sulfur and ulcerative colitis. Sulfur in food plays a role in contributing to the abdominal pain and in the frequent hurried trips to the bathroom in patients with ulcerative colitis. One way to help patients with symptomatic ulcerative colitis is to advise them to reduce the amount of dietary sulfur by decreasing the following: whole milk, cheese, ice cream, soy milk, eggs, mayonnaise, red meat, Brussels sprouts, cabbage, broccoli, cauliflower, nuts, and wine.

Sunflower seeds. Sunflower seeds are a great snack food, plus you can add them to soups, salads, omelets, and cookie batters. These little seeds pack a powerful punch of fiber, protein, B vitamins, magnesium, copper, and folate. Yes, they are high in fats—but low in saturated fat and high in polyunsaturated fat. So, grab a handful of UN-salted sunflower seeds the next time you need a little "crunch" in your diet.

Super Bowl Sunday. Super Bowl Sunday is the second-biggest day for food consumption in the U.S., trailing only Thanksgiving Day. In total, Americans will eat 30 million pounds of snacks. On average, each viewer will consume 1,200 calories during the game. Here's a snapshot of consumption on the big day…

…..13.2 million pounds of guacamole (26 million avocados)
…..28 million pounds of potato chips
…..8 million pounds of popcorn
…..450 million chicken wings (90 million pounds)
…..49.2 million cases of beer
…..10 million slices of pizza

Sushi. Is sushi healthy? Absolutely, if you choose your sushi wisely. Examples of sushi rich in healthy omega-3 fatty acids include freshwater eel, Spanish mackerel, salmon, salmon roe, red snapper, oysters, scallops, crabs, squid, sea urchin, and lobster. Is eating sushi dangerous? Well, since many of your seafood choices for sushi are raw, yes, eating raw fish can be dangerous. Of course, one way to avoid that is to choose sushi products that contain cooked seafood, such as the California roll made with cooked crab, avocado, and cucumber. If you're going to eat raw sushi, make sure you eat it at a reputable Japanese restaurant that freezes the fish to very low temperatures for an extended period of time to kill the parasites. This is a common practice at reputable Japanese restaurants.

Don't forget that adding a heavy dose of soy sauce can be hazardous to your health as well. Americans tend to dunk their foods in soy sauce. Japanese tend to brush the soy sauce on the sushi. Too much salt in the soy sauce can negate the healthy benefits of the omega-3 fatty acids. Step away from the soy sauce, or just brush it lightly on your nigiri, maki, or chirashi ushi.

Swallow. The average volume of a single swallow of any fluid is as follows:

- Child (age 1 ¼ to 3 ½ years): 4.5 mL
- Adult male: 21 mL
- Adult female: 14 mL
- Average: 0.27 mL/kg

(Jones DV, Work CE: Volume of a swallow. *Am J Dis Child* 102:427, 1961)

Sweet on sweets. A survey of 400 Americans aged 18 or older shows that nearly 77% think about dessert between one and eight times per day, and 9% have visions of sugarplums dancing in their heads more than eight times per day. In fact, nearly 60% of Americans admit to eating a meal just so they can have dessert, and 41% would rather skip the meal and go right for the grand finale. In 1984, the amount of sugar (cane and beet sugar, corn syrup, and glucose) sold in the U.S. was about 125 pounds per person. By 1998, despite the increased use of the artificial sweetener aspartame, the amount of sugar sold per person in the U.S. was 156 pounds. In just 14 years Americans had increased their sweets intake by a remarkable 25%! This averages out to 20 teaspoons per day for the male or female adult and 34 teaspoons per day for the average teenage boy. (Nutrition Action Newsletter, September 1999).

According to another survey, 35% of U.S. men and women are not about to abandon all sweets for the sake of the waistline compared to 25% who refuse to give up meat (especially steak) and 14% who draw the line at giving up pizza. A whopping 93% said that they would never consider giving up that good old American staple—the greasy burger.

A woman is like a tea bag—you never know how strong she is until she gets in hot water.
—Eleanor Roosevelt

Take Control. Take Control is a cholesterol-lowering margarine substitute containing a stanol ester derived from soybeans. The fatty base is canola and soybean oil. Like Benecol, Take Control blocks the channels in the intestine through which dietary cholesterol passes back into the bloodstream. If cholesterol can't go back into the bloodstream it has only one way to go—into the toilet. Take Control tastes and feels just like regular margarine; however, it cannot be used in cooking since it loses its cholesterol-lowering activity when heated. This is also not considered to be a "weight-loss" product, since it contains as much fat as the usual "dose" of margarine. It works best for borderline high cholesterol (in the range of 200–240 mg), and it is not intended to replace cholesterol-lowering drugs. Both Take Control and Benecol work best if the diet contains lots of cholesterol, and neither product is effective if you are already on a low-animal-fat diet.

Tapeworms. Tapeworms derive their name from the fact that the adult worm is long and ribbonlike. The baby worm you accidentally ingest attaches to the wall of the small intestine and has the capacity to grow to be 60 feet long. Tapeworms can be found in raw meat, under cooked pork, and fish.

Gefilte fish, a Jewish delicacy, is prepared by boiling ground pike, carp, whiting, or other fish that has been seasoned and molded into balls. Gefilte fish is also a well-known source of tapeworms. When gefilte fish is cooked insufficiently, tapeworm larvae survive and enter the GI tract of the unsuspecting diner. So many Jewish maids have developed the tapeworm infection while preparing the gefilte fish and taste-testing the partially cooked fish, that the name "Jewish Maid Syndrome" has been coined for this particular tapeworm infestation.

Taste. Four tastes have been traditionally described in the world of taste physiology: sweet, sour, bitter, and salty. However, the taste physiologists have just added a fifth taste to the traditional foursome: umami. U-whoey? Yes, umami (pronounced oo-mommy.) Actually, the American taste physiologists have arrived just a tad late for the discovery of umami. No less than 1,200 years ago, Japanese cooks described a flavor that they called umami. This flavor is so difficult to describe that it doesn't have a true definition. Some say that it has a "savory characteristic" or that it has a "quality of deliciousness." Other terms used are "rich," "well-rounded," "savory," "full-bodied," and "more chickenlike." The compounds that are responsible for umami have been identified, but each compound has little taste or flavor on its own. However, when added to foods, the natural flavors are enhanced, as is the "quality of deliciousness."

One of the compounds responsible for umami is glutamate or glutamic acid, an amino acid ubiquitous in nature. Amino acids can be combined to form proteins, or they function as a single amino acid. When glutamic acid is not bound to other proteins, it gives food the umami taste. The tomato taste is enhanced by glutamic acid, as are certain cheeses and soy sauce.

MSG, monosodium glutamate, the sodium salt of glutamic acid, has been added to Asian cooking for centuries to enhance the flavors. When MSG is added to meat broth, the overall taste is enhanced and the broth is more flavorful and has a meatier taste. In the 1960s, MSG was reported to be responsible for a collection of symptoms known as the "Chinese Restaurant Syndrome." The symptoms included numbness at the back of the neck and a feeling of pressure in the chest and face. Over the years, MSG has been one of the most intensely studied food additives, but subsequent scientific studies have failed to link these symptoms with MSG. As a result of these studies, the American Medical Association's Council on Scientific Affairs, the National Academy of Sciences, and the U.S. Food and Drug Administration have designated MSG safe for human consumption.

Taste buds. The life-span of a taste bud is about 10.5 days. According to the April 2000 issue of *Psychology Today,* the winter depression brought on by lowered amounts of sunlight can also temporarily blunt the taste buds, making sweet and sour flavors less distinguishable—another reason to be depressed by the lack of winter sunlight.

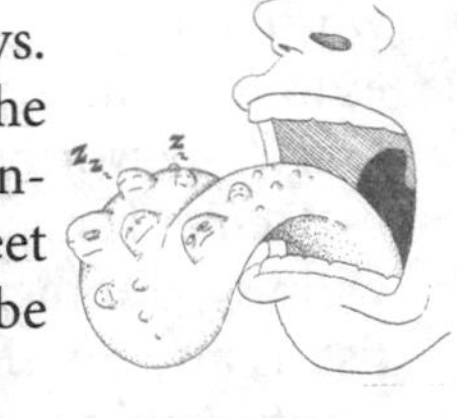

Taste-altering drugs are the most common cause of taste problems. Some examples include: Captopril (Capoten), Ampicillin, Tetracycline, Cisplatin, Methotrexate, amitriptyline (Elavil), fluoxetine (Prozac), imipramine (Tofranil), pseudoephedrine, clonidine (Catapres), hydrocortisone, levodopa, propranolol (Inderal), albuterol, cromolyn, nifedipine, statins, cholestyramine, clofibrate, gemfibrozil (Lopid), hydrochlorothiazide, baclofen, dantrolene, and nitroglycerin patches.

Taste test. To determine your taste perception, place the following in your mouth, one at a time: sugar for sweet, lemon juice for sour, instant-coffee granules for bitter, and salt for salty. If you have trouble detecting any of the four, see your health practitioner.

TEA

Tea. The Chinese emperor Shen Nung in 2737 B.C. first discovered tea. He was boiling water outside when some leaves from a nearby bush, the *Camellia sinensis* plant, fell into the kettle. As he was frantically attempting to retrieve the leaves from the boiling water, he started smelling a sweet aroma wafting up from the kettle. He tasted it, found it to be delicious, and green tea was invented.

Tea is the second most consumed beverage in the world, water is the first. It has been estimated that approximately 2,020,000 metric tons of tea are consumed worldwide each year. This equates to 855 billion cups consumed by everyone around the globe per year. The number one country in the world for producing tea is Kenya, Africa.

There are many types of tea to choose from today. Green tea, black tea, and oolong all come from the same *Camellia sinensis* plant, but are processed differently. Green tea is made from leaves that are dried soon after harvesting while the leaves are still green. This process gives a delicate flavor to the tea. Black tea is made from leaves that are allowed to ferment after harvesting. The process causes the leaves to oxidize, resulting in brownish-black tea leaves and a more intense flavor. Oolong tea is made from leaves that are allowed to ferment for only a short period of time. The taste of oolong tea is somewhere in between green tea and black tea. Black tea is further divided into teas with varying grades of black tea leaves. Souchong, pekoe, and orange pekoe are types of black tea with round leaves, short, round wiry leaves, and wiry leaves, respectively. White tea is made from the youngest tea leaves and contains slightly more antioxidants than green tea. Unfortunately white tea is not widely available and it's also more expensive.

The tea plant is a good source of the B vitamin folate. Teas are also high in fluoride, with some tea plants averaging a fluoride concentration of 100 ppm (parts per million). By comparison, fluoridated water has a concentration of 1 ppm. A 5-ounce cup of tea contains an average of 12 μg of folate, and 0.3–0.5 mg fluoride. Tea also contains a couple of other chemicals called hexanes that inhibit bacterial production of glucans in the mouth. Glucans are a sticky material containing sugar that allows the bacteria to bind to the teeth and cause decay and also contribute to gingivitis and plaque formation. Also, hold a swig of tea (preferably green to reduce staining) in your mouth for 30–60 seconds to reduce plaque formation. The levels of plaque are significantly decreased even in the absence of brushing and flossing.

Tea also contains methylxanthine stimulants similar to coffee and chocolate. Methylxanthine stimulants include caffeine, theophylline, and theobromine. Coffee has more caffeine, and tea has more theophylline. A 5-ounce cup of tea contains 40–60 mg of caffeine, compared to a 5-ounce cup of drip-brewed coffee, which contains 139 mg of caffeine. Theophylline, by the way, is a drug used to open the airways of patients with asthma and chronic obstructive pulmonary disease. Unfortunately, the relatively low concentrations found in a cup of tea are not therapeutic during an asthma attack.

Green tea has also been shown to increase thermogenesis. In other words green tea helps burn more calories contributing to weight loss. People who drink green tea or take green tea supplements can have a 3% to 4% increase in metabolism. A study of moderately obese individuals found that those who took green tea supplements for three months had reductions in body weight of 4.6%, on average, and nearly a 5% decrease in waist circumference.

What happens if you drink too much tea? Too much tea can trigger a thiamine deficiency and a B12 deficiency and can bind calcium and iron into insoluble compounds that your body cannot absorb. The tannins in tea are primarily responsible for these side effects and should be a concern, especially for children drinking too much tea. Tea also contains oxalates that can bind calcium and potentially contribute to calcium-oxalate kidney stones in those individuals unlucky enough to be predisposed to kidney-stone formation. If you can drink your tea with a bit of milk, the casein in the milk inactivates the tannins. Also, adding lemon to the tea will inactivate the iron-binding properties of tea.

Teas have been used for medicinal purposes for hundreds of years. Hippocrates recommended a tea made from the bark and leaves of a willow tree for analgesic (pain-killing) purposes. The bark of the willow tree contains salicylic acid, the precursor to acetylsalicylic acid, or aspirin. Tea is a stimulant and mood elevator because of the caffeine it contains. Tea may protect the heart as a result of the B vitamin content.

Since green tea is less processed than black tea, it may explain why it is an even richer source of antioxidants than black tea. Green tea contains a substance known as epigallocatechin (EGCG) that inhibits an enzyme required for cancer cell growth. In January 1999, Purdue University scientists documented green tea's cancer-protective effects. The researchers went so far as to recommend drinking four cups of green tea per day to reduce the overall risk of developing a malignancy.

Research since that time has produced conflicting results concerning cancer-protective properties of green tea. The FDA in a June 30, 2005 statement found that green tea is unlikely to reduce the risk of cancers. Other studies are currently underway testing the effectiveness of green tea extracts in the treatment of chronic lymphocytic leukemia. (Lee YK, et al. VEGF receptor phosphorylation status and apoptosis is modulated by a green tea component, EGCG in B cell CLL. *Blood.* 2004; 104(3):788–94)

Paradoxically, the antioxidant properties may actually have the potential to interfere with cancer chemotherapy. Some types of chemotherapy use the process of oxidation to kill cancer cells. Green tea should be used with caution by patients on chemotherapy. (Block KI, et al. Impact of antioxidant supplementation on chemotherapeutic efficacy: A systematic review of the evidence from randomized controlled trials. *Cancer Treatment Reviews.* 2007)

Other benefits of green tea include decreasing LDL-cholesterol, decreasing blood pressure, boosting mood, weight loss, and decreasing periodontal disease. Three cups of green tea daily has been shown to decrease heart attacks by 11% and strokes by 21%. (Maron DJ, et al. Cholesterol-lowering effect of a theaflavin-enriched green tea extract: a randomized controlled trial. *Arch Intern Med.* 2003; 163(12):1448-53; Yang YC, et al. The protective effect of habitual tea consumption on hypertension. *Arch Intern Med.* 2004; 164(14):1534–40)

Green tea notes:

To make sure that more than 80% of the catechins from green tea are released, steep the leaves for five minutes. A squeeze of lemon also seems to preserve catechin levels. Don't reuse tea bags—most of the catechins are released in the first cup. Instant tea provides insignificant levels of catechins. (Lester A. Mitscher, PhD, University of Kansas, professor of medicinal chemistry, 2009)

Three eight-ounce cups of green tea daily is the minimum amount found to be helpful in most clinical studies. Green tea supplements (300 mg to 400 mg daily) will give the same benefits as drinking the green tea.

Green tea can interact with anti-coagulants, some antibiotics, antipsychotics, and one of the lipid-lowering drugs, simvastatin (Zocor). The green tea increases the bioavailability of drugs, potentially resulting in toxic side effects. Consult with a health care professional before consuming copious amounts of green tea

Green tea contains approximately 30 mg of caffeine per cup. Green tea supplements contain caffeine in varying amounts, depending on how they are prepared. Decaffeinated green tea contains 2 mg per cup and also lower levels of antioxidants.

ASPARAGUS TIP

It takes 16–24 hours for the bacteria in the mouth to produce the plaque that contributes to gingivitis and periodontal disease. Therefore, brushing after every meal to prevent plaque is an unnecessary expenditure of time and energy. If you brush properly in the a.m. and p.m. and throw in one flossing episode with either, and swish around a mouthful of green tea once a day, plaque problems will be history.

Tea, hold the milk for vascular benefits. In a study of 16 postmenopausal women, those who drank about two cups of black tea without milk had a greater than four-fold increase in nitric oxide induced vasodilation from baseline in the forearm brachial artery. Nitric oxide is the MOST potent vasodilator known to man. However, those who drank a mix of 90% black tea with 10% skim milk had no more of an increase in vasodilation than if they

HISTORICAL HIGHLIGHT

July, 1860. Notes on Nursing—Author, Florence Nightingale. "When you see the natural and almost universal craving in English sick for their 'tea,' you cannot but feel that nature knows what she is about. But a little tea or coffee restores the quite as much as a great deal; and a great deal of tea, and especially coffee, impairs the little power of digestion they have. Yet the nurse, because she sees how one or two cups of tea or coffee restores her patients, thinks that three or four will do twice as much. This is not that case at all. The only English patients I have ever known to refuse tea, have been typhus cases; and the first sign of their getting better was their craving again for tea."

had consumed two cups of hot water. Milk in the tea is the problem. It appears as if three milk proteins—alpha casein, beta-casein, and kappa-casein blunt nitric oxide production. Other milk proteins did not interfere with nitric oxide. (Stangl V. *European Heart Journal.* January 2007)

Tea bags. The tea bag was an accidental invention as the result of a marketing gimmick. In 1903, New York tea merchant, Thomas Sullivan, devised a new method of distributing tea samples to his customers. He originally sent tea samples in small tin cans to his customers, but this became quite expensive. He decided to save money by putting a sample of tea into a small silk muslin bag that he personally stitched. Customers receiving the bags simply poured the hot water over the bags instead of removing the tea from the bag. Customer feedback for the "tea bags" was so overwhelming that Sullivan decided to sell the bags commercially. He changed the silk bag to a cotton gauze bag—not for cost-saving purposes but because the silk mesh was too fine. He received a patent in 1903 and by 1920 tea bags were all the rage in the U.S. At some point paper replaced cotton gauze and a string was added to "steep" the tea bag. Tea bags didn't "cross the pond" to England until 1953 when Joseph Tetley and Company introduced them to the English tea drinkers.

Tea, herbal. The popular herbal teas are made from the dried leaves or flowers of non-tea plants such as mint or chamomile. The vast majority of research into the health effects of tea has been done on the traditional teas derived from the C. sinensis plant. Herbal teas are not a major source of health benefits.

Teeth, George Washington's. Contrary to historical myth, George Washington did ***not*** wear wooden dentures. In the 1700s, the most common ma-

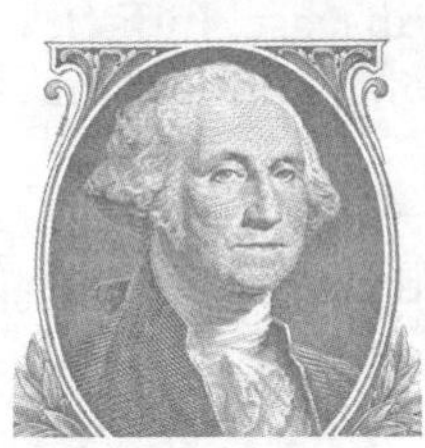

terial used to form the plates in which the teeth (human or animal) were anchored was ivory, often taken from hippopotamus tusks. Over time, ivory develops hairline cracks along its surface, between the mineralized prisms of which it is made. Years of eating, drinking, and smoking can stain these cracks dark. Apparently someone mistook the pattern of staining for wood grain, and a legend was born.

Thyroid health and diet. Raw cruciferous vegetables, such as Brussels sprouts, cabbage, and broccoli, can worsen thyroid health in people with thyroid disorders. However, cooking these vegetables deactivates their anti-thyroid properties. Wheat can also interfere with thyroid health. Many people with thyroid disease state they feel better when they avoid wheat. (Starbuck J, ND. University of Montana, guest lecturer, Past President of the American Association of Naturopathic Physicians, July 2009)

TOFU

Tofu. Just exactly what is tofu? You hear about it, you talk about it, you may or may not devour it with a passion, but where does it come from? Tofu was first produced more than two thousand years ago. It is essentially a cheese made from the "milk" of soybeans, and it has traditionally been a staple of the Asian diet for centuries. The consistency of tofu is determined by the amount of water left in the curd after pressing. Firm and extra-firm tofu are similar to the tofu produced in China; silken and soft tofu are similar to those produced in Japan. Tofu is an excellent source of protein. It contains no saturated fat or cholesterol, and has a higher amount of fiber and phytochemicals than animal proteins. It is also low in calories and sodium. Anything else? Yes, iron, manganese, magnesium, phosphorus, copper and selenium.

Tofu—new use. Toilet manufacturer's once used small plastic balls to test their commode's flushing capacity. But the new substance of choice is properly shaped tubes of miso, which is made primarily from cooked soybeans. It's a very good indicator of commode flushing capacity," says an official at Kohler. And most average Americans would agree that this is the best use for tofu. (*Wall Street Journal,* 2006)

TOMATO

Tomato. "You say tomato, I say tomah-to." No matter how you say it, you should add tomatoes and tomato-based products to your diet, pronto. Tomatoes are rich in lycopene, the pigment that gives tomatoes their beautiful red color. Lycopene is a carotenoid, a plant-based antioxidant compound that may provide some protection against cancer and heart disease. In fact, lycopene is more powerful than beta-carotene, the best-known antioxidant of the yellow-orange-red pigmented bunch.

Should you eat fresh tomatoes for this protective effect, or should you pop open a can of tomato paste? This is one case in which canned and processed tomatoes are better than fresh tomatoes. Processed tomatoes are cooked, which makes it easier for the body to absorb the lycopene. In fact, canned tomato sauce has five times more lycopene than one large fresh tomato. Lycopene develops as tomatoes ripen on the vine. Tomatoes grown for canning are harvested at a riper stage than those sold fresh off the vine. In fact, yellow, orange, or green tomatoes are not good sources of lycopene.

Eating fresh tomatoes? Lycopene is fat-soluble, so drizzle a little olive oil on fresh tomatoes to help boost lycopene absorption.

Prior to 2005, lycopene was hyped as the magic bullet against prostate cancer. It seemed like such a simple and inexpensive way to protect the prostates of the world—almost too good to be true, and unfortunately it was. A study published in Cancer Epidemiology, Biomarkers & Prevention (May 1, 2007), dashed the hopes of lycopene as the magic bullet. This study looked at 28,243 men between the ages of 55 and 74, free of cancer at the start of the study who were participating in the National Institutes of Health-funded Prostate, Lung, Colorectal and Ovarian Screening Trial. Of this group, 692 were diagnosed with prostate cancer up to eight years after entering the study; 270 were aggressive cases. The cancer patients were matched with 844 randomly selected controls without cancer. No association was found between blood levels of lycopene and either total prostate cancer risk or risk for aggressive cancer. But interestingly, high beta-carotene levels were linked to a greater risk of aggressive cancer. The researchers reached two conclusions from this study:

1) Lycopene or tomato-based regimens are not effective for prostate-cancer prevention and,

2) Continue eating carrots and other vegetables high in beta carotene, but be cautious about taking beta-carotene supplements, especially in high doses.

TOMATO tips.

- Europeans shied away from the tomato, a New World fruit, fearing that it was ripe with poison.
- The average tomato travels 1,300 miles from farm to salad bowl. (*Environmental Nutrition,* April 2001)
- La Tomatina is held every August for a week in Bunol, Spain. Having grown from a brawl near a tomato stall in 1945, it now claims to be the biggest food fight in the world. The tomato fight lasts exactly one hour. The rules? The tomato must be squashed before being thrown to minimize injuries. The target? Anything that moves.

Tootsie Roll. In 1896, Leonard Hirschfield, a candy maker in his twenties with a young daughter named Tootsie, introduced the first paper-wrapped candy, the chewy Tootsie Roll.

Tongues. Pink flamingo tongues were considered to be a delicacy in ancient Rome, and blackbird tongues were popular in the middle Ages. Today, the ox tongue (roughly 4½ pounds worth), the calf's tongue, pig's tongue, and lamb's tongue are used for cooking ragouts, stews, and sauces. The calf's tongue is considered to be superior in quality and quicker to cook.

Total parenteral nutrition. Total parenteral nutrition (TPN) is a method of feeding patients through the veins (also referred to as intravenous). In general, TPN is indicated when the gastrointestinal (GI) tract is not functioning properly or bowel rest is necessary for a prolonged period of time. The procedure will benefit patients with various GI ailments such as inflammatory bowel disease, including Crohn's disease and ulcerative colitis, fistula (abnormal connection between bowel loops), and hypermetabolic states with tissue breakdown. Some surgeons will also use TPN for seven days prior to surgery in order to "build up" the severely malnourished patient. This preoperative procedure has been shown to significantly decrease the rate of surgical complications in this patient population.

TPN provides the patient's daily fluid and caloric needs. Generally it contains free water as well as dextrose (sugar or glucose), lipids (fats), and amino acids (proteins). Dextrose provides 30–70% of the patient's total caloric needs. The total glucose concentration in the TPN solution should not exceed 35%. Higher percentages increase the risk for clotting and thrombophlebitis. Lipids contribute approximately 30% of the nonprotein calories and provide the essential fatty acids. Providing protein in the form of amino acids helps to prevent muscle breakdown. Electrolytes are also added, and include sodium, potassium, chloride, calcium, magnesium, phosphorus, and acetate. Other supplements include multivitamins, trace metals, selenium, and possibly vitamin K (if the patient has liver dysfunction with a prolonged clotting time). Either cimetidine (Tagamet) or ranitidine (Zantac) is also added to help prevent gastric ulcers from excess gastric acid secretion. Insulin is usually added to the final solution to help regulate blood glucose. Most TPN solutions cause hyperglycemia (a secondary diabetes), so insulin is needed to move the excess sugar from the blood into the cells. And finally, heparin may or may not be added, depending on the physician ordering the solution. Heparin has the potential benefit of preventing clots from forming from the hypertonic solution. (Gupta K and Copra SC. Total parenteral nutrition. *Journal of Anaesth Clin Pharm* 2008; 24(2):137–146)

Trans fats. Trans fatty acids found in fast foods such as French fries and packaged snacks are artificially created by the partial hydrogenation of unsaturated fats. This process transforms liquid fatty acids into an artery-clogging semisolid. Trans fats also turn HDLs into LDLs—good cholesterol to bad cholesterol. Trans fats are also inflammatory…is it any wonder why these have received the thumbs down? The FDA has mandated that all nutrition labels indicate the amount of trans fats. New York City and Denmark have passed legislation to eliminate trans fats from restaurants and food supplies.

Triclosan. Triclosan is an ingredient added to many consumer products to reduce or prevent bacterial contamination. It may be found in products such as clothing, kitchenware, furniture, and toys. It has also been added to antibacterial soaps and body washes, toothpastes and some cosmetics. Triclosan is not hazardous to humans but it's also really not necessary—it doesn't provide any extra health benefits over soap and water.

An antibacterial product called *Microban* is a trademarked product that incorporates the chemical triclosan as one of its ingredients. *Microban* can be permanently imbedded into cutting boards and even dish towels to inhibit the growth of bacteria like *E. coli O157:H7* and *Salmonella.*

Don't let this lull you into a false sense of antibacterial security. While antibacterial products can help keep bacteria at bay, there is no substitute for proper hand washing and other safe food-handling practices. A major concern is the possibility of bacteria developing resistance to yet another antibacterial product. (FDA, Triclosan: What consumers should know. www.fda.gov)

Triglycerides. Did you realize that even a modest weight loss can drop triglycerides by 20 percent? Reducing added sugars, eliminating trans fats, increasing fiber and monounsaturated fats, and limiting alcohol can drop triglycerides by another 20 percent. Well, that seems obvious. Eliminating everything you love from your diet will cause any level of anything to drop. ☺ Fish oil with omega-3 fatty acids can also lower triglycerides. Ye' ol' rule of thumb for fish oil is as follows:

One gram/ day of marine-based omega-3 fatty acids lowers triglycerides by approximately 5 to 10 percent. Patients can use up to 4 grams per day if tolerated. See your primary care practitioner before gulping 3 to 4 grams of fish oil per day. That amount can possibly interfere with drugs. (P*rescriber's Letter,* June 2011) Don't go overboard on the fish oil unless you talk to your cardiologist. Greater than 3 grams/day can cause bleeding due to platelet inhibition (*Diabetes Forecast* June 2007)

The most recent 2011 American Heart Association guidelines set less than 100 mg/dl as an optimal fasting triglyceride level. (Miller M et al. Triglycerides and cardiovascular disease: A scientific statement from the American Heart Association. *Circulation* 2011 May 24; 123:2292)

Truffles. Truffles, like mushrooms, are considered to be one of the most valuable of the edible fungi. What differentiates a truffle from a mushroom is that their spores form underground rather than above the ground. Genetic studies show that most truffles have actually evolved from mushrooms—a short while ago—somewhere between 85 million and 50 million years ago. However, over the years, for some unknown reason, the truffle spores began to grow underground on plant roots and produce aromatic molecules attractive to certain animals—dogs and pigs in particular. Each truffle species has its own array of aromatics. Of the thousands of truffles that exist today, only a few dozen appeal to humans. And that appeal costs you big time. The Italian White variety of truffle recently sold for $3000 per kilogram. The European black Perigord truffle is another favorite of humans. It contains androstenol, a sex hormone found in the saliva of male pigs. Based on this well-known fact truffle hunters have long used female pigs to locate the truffles underground. In fact, pigs have been documented as far back as the 15th century for truffle hunting. Pigs also have a natural affinity for rooting for food. One of the problems the truffle hunters have with the female pigs is that they want the truffle they have just found and they are unwilling to accept an alternative reward for their findings. In other words, they WANT that $3000 truffle and they won't take no for an answer nor will they accept any other treat in place of the truffle. It's a sexual thing. Truffle hunters are now using dogs ("truffle hounds") because the dogs are more willing than the pig to accept an alternative food reward, such as a simple Beggin' strip, for their sniffing efforts. Traditionalists argue that the pig has a more sensitive nose and their particular affinity for the "smell of the truffle" leads to a more devoted truffle hunter than a trained dog. (Hall IR, Gorton TB, Zambonelli A. Taming the Truffle: The History, Love, and Science of the Ultimate Mushroom. Timber Press, 2007; Trappe JM, Claridge AW. *Scientific American*, April 2010)

The Romans savored truffles and thought they were produced by thunder.

Tryptophan. Tryptophan, an amino acid, is the building block for serotonin. Serotonin is the "jack-of-all-trades" neurotransmitter. She ("Sara") helps regulate everything from sleep to mood to food intake to pain tolerance. If serotonin levels are low, people complain of insomnia, depression, food cravings (especially carbohydrates), increased sensitivity to pain, aggressive behavior, and poor body temperature regulation.

So when looking at the list of symptoms produced by low serotonin, it would only make sense that there would be a natural tendency to do everything possible to increase serotonin levels. Serotonin levels are directly related to the amount of tryptophan in the diet as well as the availability of vitamins B6, B12 and folic acid.

Paradoxically eating a protein-rich meal (full of amino acids) lowers brain tryptophan levels, while eating a carbohydrate-rich snack increases brain tryptophan levels. You would think it would be just the opposite, since tryptophan is an amino acid and a protein-rich meal gives you a bolus of tryptophan.

A protein-rich meal provides many other amino acids, as well as tryptophan. The other amino acids compete with tryptophan for entry into the brain. Tryptophan gets the short end of the stick, so to speak, and loses the competition for entry into the brain. If tryptophan is unable to enter the brain, serotonin levels remain low. When serotonin levels are low, a person will crave carbohydrates.

A carbohydrate-rich meal facilitates the entry of tryptophan into the brain. The carbohydrate load stimulates the release of insulin from the pancreas. Insulin causes the competing amino acids to enter body tissues, leaving tryptophan free to enter the brain without competition. Tryptophan is available as the substrate for serotonin production and serotonin levels increase in the brain. The person feels calm, less irritable, happy, and sleepy.

Sugar also triggers the release of insulin from the pancreas. Insulin lowers the serum levels of most large amino acids and increases blood levels of tryptophan. The tryptophan is able to cross the blood brain barrier and induce a short-term increase in brain serotonin levels. That's why a bag of M&Ms gives you a quick burst of "feelin' good."

Tube feedings and *Clostridium difficile* infection. Tube feedings increase the risk for *Clostridium difficile* threefold. *C. difficile* is now the leading cause of nosocomial diarrhea in the U.S., accounting for 30% of patients with antibiotic-associated diarrhea, 70% of those with antibiotic-associated colitis, and most cases of pseudomembranous colitis.

The incidence of diarrhea is highest in patients with the feeding tubes that have the tips placed beyond the pylorus (the sphincter between the stomach and the duodenum.) Critically ill patients commonly have impaired upper gastrointestinal function with poor motility and ileus. Feeding tubes placed in the stomach appear to benefit from the acidity of the stomach environment.

Although tube feedings have long been associated with diarrhea, it is no longer safe to automatically assume that all diarrhea is "just due to the tube." Prompt efforts should be made, especially in cases of post-pyloric placement, to reveal any *C. difficile* infection. (Bliss D, et al. Acquisition of *C. difficile* and *C. difficile*-associated diarrhea in hospitalized patients receiving tube feedings. *Annals of Internal Medicine* 1998 (Dec 15);129:1072–1079; Stephen JD. Tube feeding, the microbiota, and *Clostridium difficile* infection. *World Journal of Gastroenterol* 2010;16(2):139–142)

Tuna, bluefin. In January 2010 a 511-pound bluefin tuna sold at Tokyo's Tsukiji fish market for a record $175,000. Sadly the total Northern bluefin population has plummeted to almost extinct levels—grouping it with the white rhino and the Asian elephant in terms of risk of extinction. Japan imports 80% of the total Northern bluefin catch in the Atlantic and Mediterranean.

Turkey. Besides the obvious role of turkey in the Thanksgiving Day ritual, turkey also has a place in the clinical laboratory. Raw turkey breasts have been used in clinical studies to test the efficacy of surgical gloves. Since turkey breasts have a texture very similar to human skin, researchers operate on turkey breasts to determine how well the gloves block bacteria during operating techniques such as cutting, suturing, and stapling.

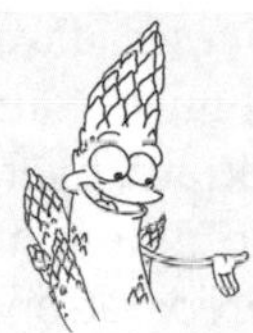

ASPARAGUS TIP

Americans eat 269 million turkeys per year,
45 million of them on Thanksgiving Day.

Turmeric to prevent Alzheimer's disease? Turmeric's active ingredient curcumin, acts as both a powerful antioxidant and anti-inflammatory agent. Recent research has supported the effect of curcumin's use to combat amyloid plaques that trigger inflammation and oxidation in the brain with subsequent destruction of neurons and surrounding supporting structures. One animal study, led by researchers at M.D. Anderson Cancer Center in Houston, showed that mice diets containing curcumin had 80 percent less amyloid plaque in their brains compared to mice fed with normal diets. What is the mechanism? Curcumin not only inhibits amyloid proteins from clumping and triggering inflammation and oxidation, but it also blocks plaque formation and weakens existing plaques and triggers their disintegration. Curcumin also increases the "good" HDL-cholesterol. In one study, participants who took 500 mg of curcumin daily for 7 days had a 29% increase in HDLs and an 11% decrease in total cholesterol. Another possible effect of curcumin is on the cells of the immune system in the brain, also known as microglial cells. The usual function of microglial cells (also referred to as macrophages) is to monitor for excess amyloid and to engulf the excess and destroy it before it is capable of forming plaques. People who develop Alzheimer's disease may have faulty microglial cells that are unable to scavenge the excess plaque formed in the brain. When studying this effect in the laboratory, researchers from the Greater Los Angeles Veterans' Affairs Medical Center placed macrophages from the brains of Alzheimer's patients into lab dishes with amyloid plaques. He found that these macrophages lacked the ability to scavenge the plaques, largely because of a reduced activity of a gene called MGAT3. Adding curcumin to the lab dish restored the plaque-clearing abilities of 50% of the macrophages and returned MGAT3 to its normal activity level. (Fiala M, *Proceedings of the National Academy of Sciences,* July 31, 2007; *Science News,* September 15,2007;(172):168.)

Tyramine-containing foods. Another well-known food-drug interaction concerns foods rich in the amino acid tyramine interacting with monoamine oxidase (MAO) inhibitors isocarboxazid (Marplan), phenelzine sulfate (Nardil) and tranylcypromine sulfate (Parnate) and the anti-tuberculin drug, isoniazid (INH), and the antibiotic, linezolid (Zyvox). Foods with high tyramine levels can trigger severe hypertensive episodes and cardiovascular events when taken with certain drugs.

Tyramine-containing foods and beverages include aged cheeses, fava beans, pickled herring, yeast extracts, overripe avocado, figs, yogurt, sour cream, raisins, fermented sausages (salami and pepperoni), sauerkraut, liver, poultry, fish and red wines, specifically Chianti. It's important to note that foods vary in their tyramine levels at various stages of food preparation. Fresh liver has a moderate amount of tyramine; however, stored liver pâté has a very high level of tyramine. Meat, poultry and fish levels of tyramine are moderate; however, after these foods are cooked and stored for a few days the tyramine levels increase considerably. A firm avocado may have a moderate level, but a ripe one (soft and ready for the guacamole dip), a high level. (Northwestern Memorial Hospital, Patient Education Diet and Nutrition, 2012)

I love Thanksgiving turkey...it's the only time in Los Angeles that you can see natural breasts. —Arnold Schwarzenegger

---

I cook using the four food groups:
canned, boxed, bagged, and frozen.
—Aunty Acid

Ullage. Ullage is the term used to describe the amount of space in a wine bottle not filled with wine.

Umami. Umami is the fifth taste classified by taste scientists. The other four are the traditional tastes of sweet (fructose, sucrose, saccharin), bitter (quercetin found in red wine, caffeine), sour (acetic acid/vinegar, citric acid/citric fruit), and salty (sodium chloride/salt). The umami taste is responsible for taste that characterizes certain vegetables, such as tomatoes and mushrooms, certain dairy products such as milk and cheese, and meat products including ham and veal. Two chemicals are believed to be responsible for umami—the sodium salt of the amino acid glutamic acid (fancy way for saying MSG), and the disodium salts of the 5'-inosine monophosphate and 5'-guanosine monophosphate molecules. (By the way, 5' is pronounced as five prime—just in case you are dining with chemists). (see Chapter T for Taste for more fascinating facts on the ability to discern various flavors.) (Nicolaou KC, Montagnon T. Molecules That Changed the World 2008.

URINARY TRACT INFECTIONS

Urinary tract infections (UTI) and cranberry juice. Like blueberries, cranberries can also be used as a urinary antiseptic. Cranberries also contain an as-yet-to-be elucidated compound that inhibits the ability of E. coli to attach to the walls of the bladder. If E. coli cannot attach to the bladder wall, it cannot trigger a urinary tract infection.

NOTE: An interesting side effect from the Viagra revolution is a 20% increase in urinary tract infections in women whose partners use Viagra. Similar to the "honeymoon cystitis" seen with increased sexual activity after marriage, these women in their 50s and 60s have also experienced an increase in sexual activity since their partner now has a functional apparatus.

HISTORICAL HIGHLIGHT

One of the first names for the cranberry was "bounce" berry. This name was derived from the fact that ripe cranberries are known to bounce when tossed onto a hard surface. The name "cranberry" was most likely derived from the blossoms (resembling the heads of cranes) on the plants inhabiting the New England bogs and was shortened from "craneberry" to cranberry somewhere along the way.

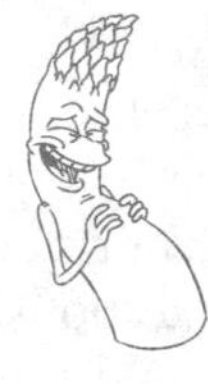

Add an ounce of Vodka to that cranberry juice and give those HDLs a boost while you're at it.

U

390

USP (United States Pharmacopoeia). Look for a USP designation on a product label, which indicates that a supplement meets five quality standards set by the USP for vitamin, mineral, botanical, and herbal supplements: 1) disintegration, 2) dissolution, 3) potency, 4) purity, and 5) expiration date. Products that say "Laboratory Tested" or "Quality Assured" don't meet the standards. Buyer beware.

Vegetables are interesting but lack a sense of purpose when unaccompanied by a good cut of meat.

—Fran Leibowitz

Valentine's day candy. Contrary to popular belief, greeting-card companies did not invent Valentine's day just to sell a zillion cutsey cards. Candy suppliers can be blamed for this annual pound-packing February 14th. In 1892, the *Confectioner's Journal,* advocated persuading customers that candy was better than any other form "cheap, grotesque" valentine's gifts. Consumers were convinced and as of 2004, more than 35 million heart-shaped boxes of candy are sold each year.

Valerian (Valeriana officinalis). This perennial herb has been used for over 2,000 years as a sleep aid, alias hypnotic/sedative. Its therapeutic uses were described by Hippocrates, and in the 2nd century Galen prescribed valerian for insomnia. According to legend, the Pied Piper enticed the rats from the village of Hamelin with valerian, whose volatile oils give it a distinctive, and to most folks, disagreeable smell. In fact, valerian is used to make "stink bombs." Animals love it, hence, the purported use by the Pied Piper.

Valerian continues to be used as an over-the-counter herbal remedy for insomnia. It is also used for mild anxiety and restlessness. It appears to work by boosting gamma amino butyric acid (GABA) levels in the brain. GABA is an inhibitory neurotransmitter that helps to calm down brain activity. Many drugs also have similar effects on GABA, including the class of drugs known as the benzodiazepines. Diazepam (Valium) is a benzodiazepine.

It takes a fairly large dose of valerian to be effective. This dose can be 50–100 drops of the tincture form, or a tea prepared from 1 teaspoon of the dried root. The dose may need to be repeated 2–3 times before the desired sedative effect occurs. It's best to start taking valerian at least one hour prior to bedtime.

Just a few caveats should be mentioned. Valerian should not be mistaken for Valium. Valerian should not be taken with Valium or any other sedative, hypnotic, or anxiety-reducing drug, including alcohol. It is not recommended for use with antidepressants either. (NIH 2011, *National Center for Complementary and Alternative Medicine:* Herbs at a glance: Valerian.)

Variety is the spice of life. The average American consumes approximately 20 different foods per day.

VEGAN

Vegan. The definition of a vegan is an individual who avoids consumption of any animal foods or dairy products.

Vegans beware. If you are a vegan and avoid any and all animal foods and dairy products, beware of even the most innocuous of food items. Marshmallows and gummy bears have beef and beef by-products in them. Lipsticks and other cosmetics, cookies, salty snacks, shampoos, and ice cream are also rife with meat by-products. Beef albumin is used in moisturizing creams, and the gelatin refined from cattle hide and bones is used in ice cream, gummy bears, and marshmallows. Desiccated liver is used as a nutritional supplement, collagen from the inner layer of the hide is used in cosmetic injections and wound balms, and tallow is used in soaps, creams, and cosmetics.

VEGETABLES

Vegetables. In 2005, approximately 32.6% of the U.S. adult population surveyed consumed fruit two or more times per day, and 27.2% ate vegetables three or more times per day. The prevalence of consuming fruit two or more times per day was 28.7% among women and 36.4% among men. Persons who were not overweight or obese (defined as a body mass index of less than 25), had the highest prevalence of consuming fruit two or more times per day (36%), and obese individuals have the lowest prevalence (28.1%). (CDC, MMWR. Fruit and vegetable consumption among adults–United States 2005. March 16, 2006; 56(10):213—217)

Vegetable cleaning (and fruits). Everyone keeps asking—how do I clean something to prevent foodborne illnesses? Like a cantaloupe for example. We all know that a recent outbreak of Salmonella from Honduran cantaloupes wreaked havoc with bowels across the U.S. So, take a clean produce brush and scrub the outside of the cantaloupe and rinse with tap water just before cutting into the fresh cantaloupe. Even tho' we don't eat the peel, bacteria on the outside can be transferred to the inside with just one slice of the knife. You can also use the commercial veggie washes. The acidity of the wash kills the pathogens. Or you can mix vinegar and water and have the same pathogen-killing capacity (see vinegar wash). You just never know where those fruits and vegetables have come from, what's dripped on top of them, what they have been washed in, or what has been on the hands of the food handlers…so be safe, not sorry, and clean all fruits and vegetables prior to consuming.

Vegetable combinations with foods. Eating your vegetables with certain foods can also help absorb the nutrients found in vegetables. Researchers from Ohio State measured blood levels of subjects who ate servings of salsa and salads. They found that when a salsa or salad was served with fat-rich avocados or a full-fat salad dressing, diners absorbed as much as 4 times more lycopene, 7 times more lutein, and 18 times more beta carotene than those who had their vegetables plain or with low-fat dressing. Of course, the diners got fat, but hey…at least they absorbed the good stuff. ☺

Vegetables and kids. Kids will eat more vegetables if you give them a zippy name? Like Laser-vision carrots, Bobble-head Broccoli, Barracuda Brussel sprouts. Keep trying to get those vegetables in. A landmark 1982 study, "I Don't Like It, I've Never Tried It," (sound familiar?) published in the journal *Appetite,* found that preschoolers took up to 10 tries over several weeks before they liked an unfamiliar food. A study in the July 2011 *American Journal of Clinical Nutrition* found that preschoolers who consumed food whose caloric density was reduced by increasing the proportion of "hidden" pureed vegetables, significantly increased their daily vegetable intake between 50 and 73 percent.

Another way to get kids (and finicky adults) to eat more vegetables is to "hide" them in foods. Whaaat? Nondisclosure? Use a little kitchen deception by puréeing, grating or dicing certain vegetables into dishes. Match the veggie color with the food you're hiding it in for the best results. Zip to your nearest bookstore and buy Jessica Seinfeld's book (yes, that's Jerry Seinfeld's wife), <u>Deceptively Delicious</u> (2008) for ideas and/or Missy Chase Lapine's <u>The Sneaky Chef</u> cookbooks.

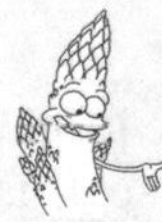

ASPARAGUS TIP

Foods that are easily pureed and/or hidden include carrots, sweet potatoes, cauliflower, zucchini, squash, green beans, broccoli, and spinach.

Vegetables and nutrients. A March 2007 study in the Journal of Food Science examined the effects of boiling, steaming, microwaving and pressure cooking on the nutrients in broccoli. Steaming and boiling caused a 22 percent to 34 percent loss of vitamin C. Microwaved and pressure-cooked vegetable retained 90 percent of their vitamin C. Be sure to microwave your vegetables in a glass or ceramic container. Microwaving in plastic containers may cause certain chemicals, referred to as hormone/endocrine disruptors, to leech from the plastic into the vegetables, and over the long haul this may be hazardous to your health.

Vegetables or shoes? The average American spends over $100 more a year on footwear than on vegetables. And that's your answer. (*The Week*, July 18, 2008)

VEGETARIAN

Vegetarian numbers. About 20% of the world's 7 billion population is vegetarian. Of that 20%, 75 million are vegetarian by choice, 500 million eat a mostly plant-based diet, and 1.45 billion can't afford to eat meat. (*New Scientist* 17 July 2010)

Vegetarians and wound healing. The diets of some vegetarians may alter their ability to heal normally. Discuss this important fact with any vegetarian planning elective surgery in the future. The vegetarian should consider supplementing his/her diet for at least one week prior to surgery with the following wound-healing nutrients:

- Albumin contained in proteins
- Glucose contained in carbohydrates
- Essential fatty acids found in walnuts and soybean and canola oil
- Vitamins A, B complex, C, and K
- Minerals including zinc, copper, iron, and manganese

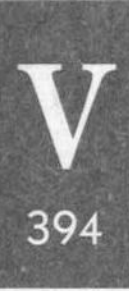

Can vegetarians eat animal crackers? —Anonymous

Vegetarians and multivitamins. Strict vegetarians may want to consider either a multivitamin or single supplements of calcium, B12, iron, and zinc. Unless a vegetarian eats fortified foods, vegetarians who exclude eggs and dairy products can have inadequate amounts of the above nutrients.

Viactiv, a calcium chewable. This is a tasty and convenient way to get 1,000 to 1,500 mg of bone-building calcium you need daily. Of course, this might be too much as a supplement, but honestly, if you are not inclined to get any calcium in your diet, this is a great way to have a tasty treat that is also a healthy treat. Each soft bite-sized candy, at 20 calories and 0.5 grams of fat, supplies 500 mg of calcium, 100 IU of vitamin D, and 50 μg of vitamin K.

Viagra (sildenafil, Pfizer) and food interactions. Viagra, also jokingly referred to as either the "Pfizer Riser" or vitamin V, should not be taken with grapefruit juice. Grapefruit juice *increases* the bioavailability of Viagra

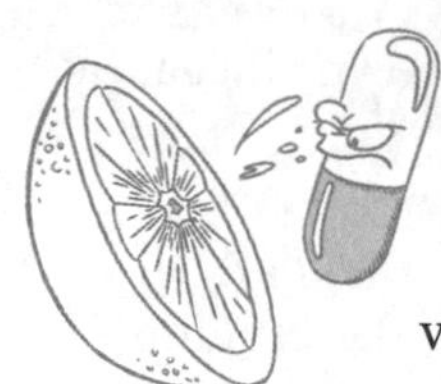

and can result in toxic side effects. Now, it may not seem as if a toxic dose of Viagra would be a bad thing to most gentlemen using this pecker-upper. However, blood pressure can fall to dangerously low levels, especially if other vasodilating blood pressure drugs are being taken at the same time.

On the other hand, a high-fat meal taken with Viagra decreases the maximum concentration of the drug by 29% and slows the timing to peak action of the drug. In other words, it may take up to one hour for the drug to work if the drug is taken with a high-fat meal. You and your partner may be waiting, waiting, waiting for something to come up, and the mood might plummet. This may result in "treatment failure" in some patients if they are not advised appropriately when the drug is prescribed. The proper advice for any gentlemen taking Viagra is to time the Viagra one to two hours after eating a high-fat meal or take Viagra with a reduced fat meal.

In other words, no Big Mac and fries at the same time as the Pfizer Riser or you *and* your partner will be greatly disappointed. What about the other two drugs for erectile dysfunction (ED)—vardenafil (Levitra) or tadalafil (Cialis) and meals? Levitra is ok with a moderate or low fat meal, but it would be wise to delay taking it by one hour after a high fat meal. Cialis has a longer half-life and is unaffected by a high fat meal and can be taken with any meal, any time, all day, any day. (Carson CC. Phosphodiesterase type 5 inhibitors: State of the therapeutic class. *Urologic Clinics of North America* 2007 November)

VINEGAR

Vinegar. The word vinegar is derived from the French words vin for wine and aigre for sour. Vinegar was discovered over 10,000 years ago somewhere in France, strictly by accident. Some unsuspecting winemaker left the wine standing for too long, and made sour wine, or vinegar. The process is slightly more refined today, but essentially requires two steps: 1) yeast changes the natural sugars of the grape to alcohol via the process of fermentation and, 2) bacteria change the alcohol to an acid via the process of acid fermentation. The wine is then exposed to air for a certain amount of time and voilà, you have vinegar.

Vinegar has been used historically as a medicine and continues to be used today for medicinal purposes. It was prescribed for everything from skin disorders to internal hemorrhaging. Vinegar has been added to water to purify it for drinking. Prior to the days of refrigeration, vinegar was used as the preservative in the pickling process.

Vinegar comes in many varieties including red wine vinegar, white vinegar, balsamic vinegar, and apple cider vinegar. There is no known difference in the health properties of vinegars. You can even make your own vinegar by adding garlic, mustard, and spices such as oregano.

Vinegar and weight loss? A study in the July 8, 2009 *Journal of Agricultural and Food Chemistry* found that vinegar may prevent the buildup of body fat and weight gain. Of course, the study only looked at mice, but the good news is that the mice fed acetic acid (the main ingredient of vinegar) gained up to 10 percent less body fat than the mice that were not given the acetic acid. How might vinegar work? The mechanism by which acetic acid works may involve activating genes that produce proteins that are involved in the breakdown of fat. So do all of those vinegar diets sold between midnight and 6 a.m. on late-night TV work? Stay tuned…but just remember—anything sold on late-night TV is most likely a ruse.

Vinegar as a vegetable wash. Tennessee State University scientists compared a produce wash, dilute vinegar and plain water and found that plain water, with a little scrubbing, can remove 98% of bacteria from the surface of fruits and vegetables. A similar test by *Cooks Illustrated* magazine gave the thumbs up for a light mist of a 25% vinegar solution, followed by washing in plain water. (*Tuft's University Health and Nutrition Letter.* November 2010)

VITAMINS

Vitamins. The term vitamin applies only to a specific group of organic compounds that medical science has shown to be necessary to survival. A vitamin has to be something your body requires for good health and normal functioning—in other words, you have to take it in your diet regularly in some amount, however miniscule, or you will become ill. Its absence from your diet must result in an identifiable and reproducible disease or disorder. In contrast, a nutrient is a component of food that nourishes our body. A nutrient can be essential to life or nonessential. A vitamin, on the other hand, can only be essential.

Vitamin deficiencies and disease. The concept of dietary deficiencies causing disease did not become widely accepted until the very late nineteenth century—1890 to be exact. In 1890, Dutch physician Christian Eijkman was investigating a disease called beriberi on the island of Java in the Dutch East Indies. He observed the causative connection between beriberi and diets high in polished or milled rice. Polished or milled rice is rice with the husks/bran removed. Ten years after his observation, he and his colleague Gerrit Grijns, proved that beriberi could actually be cured if the husks or bran were added back to the rice. This obviously proved that milling the rice removed a vital substance.

In 1912 a Polish chemist, Casimir Funk, extracted a substance from the rice bran that he believed was the "anti-beriberi" substance. He characterized it as a vital substance and he thought that it was chemical known as an amine. He coined the term "vital amine" and subsequently joined the two words into "vitamine." As research continued and other organic compounds were found that were vital but not amines, the "e" was eventually dropped and "vitamin" became the operative word. The "anti-beriberi" vitamin was named thiamine.

Casimir Funk also proposed that the other well-known historical maladies of pellagra, scurvy, and rickets were also caused by an absence of "vitamines." Each of those diseases has been relegated to the historical footnotes because of the discovery of more vitamins.

The first disease to be "cured" was scurvy—the scourge of the sailing crews around the world in the 17th and 18th centuries. In 1746 the Scottish surgeon Joseph Lind conducted the first human nutrition experiment when he gave fresh lemons and limes to sailors in the Royal British Navy. His discovery that lemons and limes prevented scurvy not only gave the Royal British Navy sailors the nickname of "limey," but also stimulated interest in the food-disease connection. Scurvy was eventually identified as a deficiency in vitamin C once vitamin C was discovered in 1907 by the Hungarian scientist, Albert Szent-Gyorgyi.

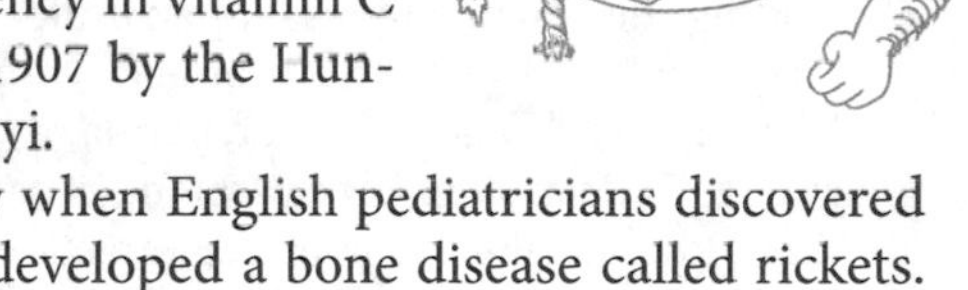

Fast forward to the 19th century when English pediatricians discovered that children deprived of sunlight developed a bone disease called rickets. Vitamin D, the "sunshine" vitamin, was not discovered until 1919.

Japanese physicians used cod-liver oil to treat night-blindness. Cod-liver oil was subsequently discovered to be a rich source of vitamin A. Vitamin A, the first fat-soluble vitamin, was discovered in 1915.

The last vitamin to be discovered was cobalamin (B12) in 1948. Ten Nobel prizes have been awarded for vitamin discovery.

Vitamin A. The RDA for vitamin A is 700 μg RAE per day for females, and 900 μg RAE for males. RDA stands for recommended daily allowance, but what on earth is the RAE? RAE stands for retinol activity equivalents. One RAE is the equivalent to 1 μg of retinol, 12 μg of beta-carotene, 24 μg of alpha-carotene, or 24 μg of beta cryptoxanthin. Beta-carotene, alpha-carotene, and cryptoxanthin are pre-vitamin A carotenoids. Good grief…do you really have time to work all that out? How about 2310 IU for women and 3000 IU for men? Neither gender should regularly exceed 3,000 μg per day. More is OK only if it's from beta-carotene. The absolute Tolerable Upper Intake Level, the most that can be consumed daily with the risk of adverse effects, is 10,000 IU of retinol. Toxic doses of vitamin A can cause liver failure.

This group of compounds is essential for proper vision, reproduction, growth and cellular differentiation of the developing embryo, immune system integrity and bone metabolism. Of the three, beta-carotene is the most important. Carrots and green leafy vegetables provide mega amounts of beta-carotene.

Kids under five are most likely to develop vitamin A deficiency, as are patients with chronic malabsorption—Crohn's disease, celiac disease, and bariatric surgery patients.

The best natural sources for vitamin A include fish-liver oil, liver, carrots, green and yellow vegetables, eggs, milk and dairy products, margarine, and yellow fruits.

The earliest symptom of a vitamin A deficiency is night blindness. Once consumed, vitamin A from carrots becomes 11-cis retinol, the essential element in rhodopsin, a protein found in the rods of the retina. The rods are the cells in the retina that help you see in the evening or night. One carrot a day provides more than enough vitamin A to maintain vision in the average American.

HISTORICAL HIGHLIGHT

Beta-carotene, one of the active carotenoids, is stored in fatty tissue, including the subcutaneous fat just under the skin. During World War II, pilots were fed huge amounts of beta-carotene to improve their night vision. Many pilots developed carotenemia, a yellowish discoloration of the skin, and an indication of beta-carotene excess. Some individuals might mistake this discoloration for jaundice (a yellowing of the skin due to excess bilirubin, the breakdown product of hemoglobin in red blood cells); however, with carotenemia, the sclera of the eye (the white membrane covering the eyeballs) does not turn yellow. Patients with jaundice have yellow sclera, yellow soft palates (the soft tissue of the roof of the mouth), and the area under the tongue (sublingual) is also yellow.

Vitamin A and lung cancer. Vitamin A has harmful effects when used as a supplement combined with beta-carotene. It *increases* lung cancer risk inadult smokers and individuals exposed to asbestos. (Greenwald P. Clinical trials of vitamin and mineral supplements for cancer prevention. *Am J ClinNutr.* 2007;85 (suppl 1):314S–317S)

Vitamin B1—Thiamine (1.1 mg/day for adult females, 1.2 mg/day for adult males). As mentioned earlier, thiamine (FYI: Thiamine can be spelled with or without the "e" at the end.) was extracted from brown rice in 1901 and has the distinction of being the very first vitamin discovered. Thiamine is a coenzyme in the metabolism of carbohydrates and amino acids.

Do not regularly exceed 50 mg on a daily basis (50 mg is almost 50 times the recommended dose). More than 100 mg of thiamine can cause reversible neurological damage. Foods rich in thiamine include unrefined cereal grains, brewer's yeast, whole wheat, oatmeal, lean pork, legumes, seeds, nuts

ASPARAGUS TIP

Excess vitamin A can cause liver failure and possibly birth defects. The normal human liver contains approximately two years' supply of vitamin A. Because large doses may be teratogenic (causing birth defects), supplementation with vitamin A should be avoided during the first trimester of pregnancy. Liver toxicity occurs in 50% of the patients taking excess vitamin A. The dosage associated with liver damage varies from 15,000 IU per day to 1.4 million IU per day, and the duration of exposure from 1 day to 30 years.

It's been a long known fact to the Inuit living in the North Pole that polar bear liver shouldn't be eaten. And, if it is eaten, *it will kill you.* Just 3 ounces (100 grams) of polar bear liver contains 2.4 million–3.5 million IU of vitamin A. Compare that to our usual consumption of 3 ounces (100 grams) of chicken liver with only 12,000 IU of vitamin A and 3 oz (100 gm) of calf liver with 14,378 IU of vitamin A.

(especially peanuts) and organ meats (liver, kidney and heart), as well as foods enriched with B1. Thiamine is a co-factor in carbohydrate metabolism, and the need for thiamine is related to carbohydrate intake. Thiamine cannot be stored in the body for any length of time so it must be taken on a regular basis.

This brings us to the individual with chronic alcoholism. Alcohol is a well-known source of carbohydrates; however, thiamine has not yet been added to alcoholic beverages. In other words, chronic alcoholics consume large amounts of carbohydrates in booze, but don't consume thiamine in nuts, organ meats, and legumes as an accompaniment. If and when thiamine deficiency occurs, the early symptoms include constipation, decreased appetite, nausea, mental depression, neuropathy, and fatigue. As the thiamine deficiency continues, confusion, ataxia (staggering gait), loss of eye coordination (the triad of symptoms known as Wernicke's encephalopathy), cardiomyopathy (disease of the heart muscle), and peripheral neuropathy occur.

Vitamin B1 deficiency, Wernicke's encephalopathy, and bariatric surgery. Jeez, I remember this obscure neurologic syndrome when learning about the trials and tribulations of alcoholics with chronic thiamine (vitamin B1) deficiency. So, what's up with the bariatric-surgery patient? Even though this is a rare complication post-surgery, 32 cases have been identified through database searches and reviews of references. Patients ranged from 23-55 years of age and most were women. The majority of cases occurred within four to twelve weeks after the surgery although the range for presentation was from two weeks to 78 weeks following the procedure. Four of the

ASPARAGUS TIP

If adding thiamine to alcoholic beverages would prevent the acute and chronic problems due to alcohol, one might wonder why this has not been on the agenda of our venerable politicians on Capitol Hill. Oh, because they are too busy trying to figure out whether or not baseball players have used illegal steroids. Well, it has been on the agenda in years past. In fact, one group that suggested the simple remedy of adding thiamine to alcoholic beverages was none other than the government's very own Veteran's Administration Medical Centers. They theorized that adding thiamine to booze would save our Federal Government hundreds of millions of dollars per year in treating veterans with alcohol-related thiamine-deficiency complications. Was this a simple solution for a complex and very expensive problem? Actually, yes it could have been.

But, it wasn't. The Jim Beams of Kentucky and Jack Daniel of Tennessee, the Bud Weisers of St. Louis, and even the Jose Cuervos of Mexico chimed in with their lobbyists. Adding thiamine to booze was going to cost big bucks to the liquor companies—never mind that they could pass those costs on to the unsuspecting consumer. So, instead of spending big bucks to add thiamine to help our veterans they started pouring those big bucksinto the pockets (known as political action committees) of certain powerful congressmen on Capitol Hill. The bill didn't even make it out of committee before it was axed.

Moral of the story: This narrative continues to prove that two neurons will never synapse at the same time on Capitol Hill.

patients also had peripheral neuropathy from thiamine deficiency. Prompt initiation of therapy with thiaminr achieved a favorable outcome in most cases; however, a few cases experienced persistent problems such as neuropathy, ataxia, psychosis, and/or cognitive deficits. (Singh S, Kumar A. Wernicke encephalopathy after obesity surgery: a systematic review. *Neurology* 2007;807–81)

Vitamin B2—Riboflavin (adult 1.1 mg for females, 1.3 mg for males per day). Do not regularly exceed 200 mg/day. The best dietary sources are fish and meat, peanuts, brown rice, eggs, and leafy green veggies such as broccoli and spinach, and turnip greens, and asparagus. Riboflavin is the vitamin that makes your urine turn bright yellow when you are taking a multivitamin.

Vitamin B3—Niacin, also known as nicotinic acid (14 mg/day for females, 16 mg/day for males). The best dietary sources for B3 are liver, lean meat, eggs, fish, whole grains, wheat germ, white meat of poultry, roasted peanuts, avocados, dates, figs, prunes, and legumes.

Vitamin B3 as a pill. Niacin, as an over-the-counter supplement, has been shown to be effective at improving cholesterol levels in high supplemental doses, ranging from 1,000 to 4,000 mg per day. Unfortunately, doses that high in over-the-counter supplement form can also cause liver problems and possibly liver failure. The recommended safe limit is 500 mg/day with this form of niacin (250 mg if it's slow-release niacin). HDL levels increase approximately 20% in patients taking extended-release niacin, also known as Niaspan. Gradually increase the dose of Niaspan by starting with 500 mg/day of extended-release niacin each night and increase the dose by 500 mg each month. The usual maintenance dose is 1,500–2,000 mg. This gradual increase and maintenance dose doesn't appear to cause liver problems.

ASPARAGUS TIP

Flushing is an annoying side effect of niacin. As little as 50 mg/day can cause flushing. Instruct the patient take an 81-mg dose of aspirin 30 minutes prior to taking any formulation of niacin to prevent flushing.

Vitamin B3 and street drugs. Emergency room physicians from around the country are reporting that patients are taking large amounts of niacin with the false belief that niacin helps to cause the urine screening test for drugs to test negative. Large doses of niacin cause the clinical signs of nausea, tachycardia (increased heart rate), vertigo (dizziness), dehydration, hypoglycemia (low blood sugar), bleeding tendencies (bruising, nose bleeds), liver toxicity (high liver enzymes) and acidosis (low pH).

In 2006, the Rocky Mountain Poison and Drug Center in Denver received 16 calls from people who admitted using niacin while attempting to dodge drug screens and 12 calls from other related niacin-questions that appeared to be drug-related as well. Niacin overdoses can be confused with allergic reactions, so a high index of suspicion is necessary on the part of ER personnel.

Vitamin B6—Pyridoxine (Recommendations vary with age; under 50: 1.3 mg for females and males; over 51? 1.5mg/day for adult females, 1.7 mg/day for adult males). The recommended safe limit is 200 mg per day. Pyridoxine is found in fortified cereals (whole grain TOTAL and Wheaties), brewer's yeast, leafy greens, chick peas, legumes, oranges, chicken breast, beef, bananas, cantaloupe, cabbage, blackstrap molasses, milk, eggs, and red pepper. Pyridoxine helps to maintain the health of the myelin covering the peripheral nerves. It also assists in lowering elevated homocysteine levels along with folic acid and B12.

Elevated homocysteine levels have been linked to cardiovascular and cerebrovascular diseases. Three vitamins have been shown to reduce homocysteine levels. The general consensus was that if you reduce homocysteine levels you would subsequently reduce cardiovascular and cerebrovascular disease. Unfortunately, the research doesn't support that theory. Even though

B6 lowers homocysteine levels, along with folic acid and B12, it doesn't reduce the risk of stroke or any other cardiovascular disease. (Albert CM et al. Effect of folic acid and B vitamins on risk of cardiovascular events and total mortality among women at high risk for cardiovascular disease: a randomized trial. *JAMA* 2008;299:2027; Ebbing M et al. Combined analyses and extended follow-up of two randomized controlled homocysteine-lowering B vitamin trials. *J Intern Med* 2010;268:367)

Vitamin B6—Pyridoxine and drugs. The anti-tuberculosis drug, INH, forms complexes with pyridoxine and decreases its availability, causing a peripheral neuropathy in some patients. Giving pyridoxine to patients treated with Isoniazid (INH) prevents this side effect. The vinca alkaloids (vincristine and vinblastine), used in the treatment of certain cancers, have also been known to induce a B6 deficiency and subsequent peripheral neuropathy. Treatment with pyridoxine has been shown to be effective. (Akbayram S, et al. Use of pyridoxine and pyridostigmine in children with vincristine-induced neuropathy. *Indian J of Pediatr* 2010 Jun; 77(6):681–683)

Pyridoxine is a safe and effective vitamin for pregnancy-induced nausea and vomiting (morning sickness). How is it used? Give pyridoxine (vitamin B6) 25 mg three times a day combined with 12.5 mg doxylamine at bedtime. Doxylamine is a sedating antihistamine and is the main ingredient in Unisom Nighttime Sleep-Aid. Pyridoxine-doxylamine is available in Canada under the trade name Dicletin (10 mg and doxylamine 10 mg) in a delayed release tablet. Diclectin typically is prescribed in a dosage of 2 tablets at night for mild morning sickness and up to 4 tablets per day for more severe symptoms. (Quinlan J, Hill DA. Nausea and vomiting of pregnancy. *Am Fam Phys.* 2003(Jul 1); 68(1): 121–128)

Pyridoxine, 2 mg, per day helps to reduce elevated homocysteine levels.

ASPARAGUS TIP

Paradoxically, pyridoxine (B6) can cause peripheral nerve damage (reversible) at doses of 200 mg or more. Interestingly, it is protective when given with drugs that predispose patients to peripheral neuropathy, but even more interestingly it can cause neuropathy if taken in excess.

Vitamin B9—Folic acid (400µg daily for women and men). Folate and folic acid derive their names from the Latin word "folium" (which means "leaf"). Leafy vegetables are a principle source. Folate is the form found naturally in foods. Lentils (dried beans and nuts), oatmeal, cantaloupe, apricots, pumpkins, avocados, carrots, asparagus, egg yolks, and dark green leafy vegetables such as spinach have the highest amount of folate. Folic acid is the form of the vitamin found most often in your body and the form added to foods and supplements. Folacin is a collective term for these and other forms of the vitamin. (Bailey RL et al. Total folate and folic acid intake from foods and dietary supplements in the United States: 2003-2006. *Am J Clin Nutr.* 2010;91(1):231–237)

Vitamin B9—Folic acid and the prevention of neural tube defects. All women with functioning ovaries should be consuming 400 μg of folic acid daily. This is especially important if she is in the mood or the mode to get pregnant. And, even if she isn't in the mood or mode to get pregnant, mistakes have been made and the shocked response is: "I can't believe I'm pregnant!" So, why is folic acid so important in women with functioning ovaries? It has everything to do with preventing a birth defect called a neural tube disorder (NTD).

The neural tube is the precursor to the development of the healthy brain and spinal cord in the embryo. Like all good "tubes," the neural tube has an opening (known as a pore) at either end—the front end and the back end. The front opening is known as the anterior neuropore and the back opening is known as the posterior neuropore. If either neuropore fails to close at the appropriate time in embryologic development, a neural tube defect occurs. The normal neural tube closure occurs between the 18th and the 26th day after conception.The critical period of neural tube development is only 8 days, and occurs during the first month of pregnancy when most women have absolutely *no* idea that they are pregnant.

The exact mechanism by which folic acid prevents neural tube defects has not been determined; however, folic acid is essential for any tissue that is rapidly dividing.

In 1992, the U.S. Public Health Service recommended that all young women who were "in the mood or the mode" to get pregnant should increase their intake of folic acid either by diet or by supplements to help prevent neural tube defects. Mandatory fortification of cereal grain products took effect in 1998. The dose to prevent neural tube defects in women in the "mood or the mode" to get pregnant, is 400 μg per day. This is one case where the supplement form is better absorbed than the natural form.

The folic acid must to be taken prior to pregnancy because, as mentioned above, the critical period of neural development occurs before most women have any idea that they are pregnant. In the U.S. 90% of all teenage girls who become pregnant are absolutely 100% totally surprised by it…in other words, many young girls are clueless as to the importance of taking folic acid prevent neural tube defects.

On the other hand, it appears as if some women are listening to the experts. The estimated number of neural tube defect-affected pregnancies in the U.S. declined from 4,000 in 1995-1996 to 3,000 in 1999-2000. This decline highlights the partial success of the U.S. folic acid fortification program as a public health strategy. (CDC. Spina bifida and anencephaly before and after folic acid mandate—United States, 1995-1996 and 1999-2000. *MMWR.* May 2004;53(17):364–365). Studies continue to support the benefit of folic-acid supplementation and the reduction of neural tube defects. (Wolff T, et al. Folic acid supplementation for the prevention of neural tube defects: An update of the evidence for the U.S. preventive service task force. *Ann Int Med* 2009;150(9):632–639).

ASPARAGUS TIP

If one-quarter of the 44 million women of childbearing age who do not currently take folic acid took 400 μg daily, neural tube defects could be prevented in as many as 600 babies annually. (The Health Impact Study IV commissioned by the Dietary Supplement Education Alliance September, 2009)

Low carb diets and serum folate levels in child-bearing women. Times have changed since the enrichment of grain products with folic acid. Low carbohydrate diets are en vogue for young women today. Since enriched grain products, typically cereals and breads, are carbohydrate dense, women have reduced their intake thinking that high carb diets are the main culprit in weight gain. (They're wrong, we know, but it's the prevailing thought in the world of Hollywood and everyone who follows the Kardashians). So, the Atkins diet, the South Beach Diet, and the other low-carbohydrate diets are taking their toll on folic acid levels in women. Serum folate concentrations declined by 16% between 1999 and 2004. (*Morbidity and Mortality Weekly Report,* January 2007)

Vitamin B9—Folic acid and the prevention of cardiovascular disease. As mentioned previously, homocysteine is an amino acid that increases the risk of heart disease. High levels of homocysteine trigger formation of atherosclerotic (fatty) plaques in the coronary, cerebral, and femoral arteries. The most important factor affecting homocysteine levels in the general population is a dietary deficiency of vitamin B6 and folic acid.

So, one would surmise that as homocysteine levels increase, the risk of cardiovascular disease would increase as well. But that's not the case, according to a 2008 report in the *Journal of the American Medical Association.* This study found that a combination pill of folic acid, B6, and B12 did not reduce a combined end point of total cardiovascular events among high-risk women, despite significant homocysteine lowering. Bummer. (Albert CM et al. Effect of folic acid and B vitamins on risk of cardiovascular events and total mortality among women at high risk for cardiovascular disease. *JAMA* 2008;299 (17):2027–36)

Other studies have supported that same findings—even though homocysteine levels are reduced with folic acid supplementation, cardiovascular events and mortality rates from cardiovascular disease remain unchanged. (Buzzano LA. No effect of folic acid supplementation on CV events, cancer or mortality after 5 years in people at increased cardiovascular risks, although homocysteine levels are reduced. *Evidence-based Medicine.* 2011 (August);16(4): 117–118)

Folic acid and masking B12 deficiency. Excessive consumption of folic acid masks neurological complications in people with vitamin B12 deficiency.

Vitamin B9—Folate and depression. Kim and associates found that lower levels of folate and vitamin B12 resulting in higher levels of homocysteine were associated with an increased risk of depression in late life. (Kim JM.

Predictive value of folate, vitamin B12 and homocysteine levels in late-life depression. *The Br J of Psych.* 2008; 192:268–274)

Vitamin B9—Folic acid and drugs. Drugs that inhibit folic acid metabolism as a mechanism of action may require folic acid supplements to overcome folic acid deficiency. Two major culprits for inhibiting folic acid metabolism are the anticonvulsant phenytoin (Dilantin) and the antimetabolite methotrexate (Rheumatrex), used for patients with rheumatoid arthritis.

Drugs containing estrogen can also lower folic acid. This estrogen-containing group of drugs includes combined oral contraceptives and estrogen replacement drugs such as Premarin, Estrace, and Estraderm. Brilliantly, a new oral contraceptive actually contains folic acid, BeYaz. It contains 0.45 mg (450 μg) of folic acid in the form of levomefolate calcium. (What does "levomefolate" mean? Levomefolate and L-methylfolate are the names for the active form of folic acid).

Even aspirin has been deemed as one of the "bad guys" when it comes to lowering folic acid. More studies are needed to determine the clinical implications of these drug-nutrient interactions; however, it wouldn't hurt to take a folic acid supplement if you're on any of these drugs for various and sundry reasons.

Vitamin B12 (Cobalamin). Vitamin B12 was discovered in 1948. The RDA for B12 is 2.4μg per day. Do not exceed 3,000 μg regularly. No, 3,000 μg is not a typing error. There is a wide margin of safety with B12 doses, unlike vitamins A and B3(Niacin). The best natural sources of vitamin B12 are liver, beef, pork, fish, eggs, milk and cheese. Then following food servings all provide at least 25% of the Daily Value of vitamin B12:

Clams.......................... 3 oz. cooked
Oysters.......................... 3 oz. cooked
King crab.......................... 3 oz cooked
Whole grain TOTAL cereal.......................... ¾ c.
Beef liver, braised.......................... 1 slice
Rainbow trout.......................... 3 oz.
Sockeye salmon.......................... 3 oz.
Lean top sirloin broiled.......................... 3 oz.
Plain skim yogurt.......................... 1 cup

The 2010 guidelines from the National Academy of Sciences recommend that B12 be taken in the synthetic form found in supplements and in food supplemented with B12.The best foods for B12 supplementation are fortified breakfast cereals and dairy products. A bowl of fortified breakfast cereal contains six micrograms of vitamin B12, more than enough for daily needs. Contrary to popular belief, B12 from meat, poultry, and fish does not appear to be as effective as supplements. Perhaps some B12 is lost in the cooking process, or the way the B12 is bound to the protein in meats may make it less available for absorption, especially in the over 55 crowd. (*American Journal of Clinical Nutrition*. 71:514, 2000)

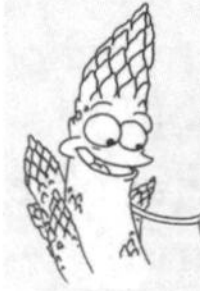

ASPARAGUS TIP

Excess consumption of B12 results in an embarrassing symptom—anal itching. So you might want to cut down on the B12 if this becomes an uncontrollable urge when you are strolling through the local shopping mall wth your significant other.

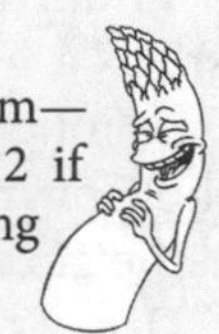

Vitamin B12 deficiency diagnosis and supplements. Vitamin B12 deficiency is diagnosed by elevated serum concentrations of methylmalonic acid (MMA test). Methylmalonic acid may be ordered by itself or along with a homocysteine test or as a follow up to a Vitamin B12 test result that is in the lower end of the normal range. If the MMA test and the homocysteine levels are elevated, then an early or mild B12 deficiency may be present.

B12 can be administered in 4 ways, and I call them the "4 Ss"— you can swallow it, suck it, snort it, or shoot it. In other words, you can swallow a pill, you can put that pill under the tongue (sublingual), you can squirt B12 up the nostrils, or you can receive a B12 injection. The choice of administration depends on the level of deficiency and the patient's symptoms. For day-to-day maintenance the pill or sublingual form is fine. Injections are used for the treatment of a B12 dementia or B12-induced peripheral neuropathy.

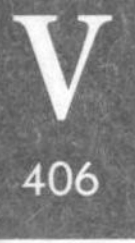

Vitamins B12 and B6 and depression. Research published online June 2, 2010 in *The American Journal of Clinical Nutrition* has found that higher total intakes of vitamins B6 and B12 may protect against depressive symptoms in adults ages 65 and older. Each 10 additional milligrams of B6 and 10 additional micrograms of B12 were associated with a two percent lower chance per year of experiencing depressive symptoms. These associations remained after adjustment for other factors such as depression, smoking, alcohol use, cognitive function, physical disability, and comorbid conditions.

Vitamin B12 absorption and intrinsic factor (pernicious anemia). Pernicious anemia develops when the stomach does not produce enough intrinsic factor to bind to dietary B12. An intrinsic factor deficiency can result from an autoimmune disease targeting and destroying it, from the partial removal of the stomach (a partial gastrectomy for severe ulcers—a surgical procedure that is no longer used), or when the stomach is too old (over 55 years—LOL) to extract the B12 from dietary sources. A deficiency of B12 due to the lack of intrinsic factor can be corrected with very large oral doses—1,000 μg per day. An estimated 1% of the oral dose (10 μg) is absorbed through the stomach mucosa by passive diffusion and may be sufficient to reverse the deficiency.

Vitamin B12 and the incredible shrinking brain. Is there no end to the benefits of vitamin B12? YES, it helps maintain a healthy production of red blood cells, and YES, it keeps your neurons happy, and YES, it helps maintain peripheral nervous system myelin, so what else is new? A study in the journal *Neurology,* (September 9, 2008), found that older people with low, but still "normal," levels of B12 were 6 times more likely to experience brain atrophy (shrinkage) than those with the highest B12 levels. The low-B12 group in the study also lost twice as much brain volume on average. WHOA!! But, before you run out and buy all of the B12 on every shelf in Walmart, Kmart, and Target, note that this study had a few flaws—1) it was an observational study and couldn't prove a causal connection between vitamin B12 intake and brain shrinkage, and 2) the sample size was relatively small (107 men and women). BUT, that being said, most of us over 55 could use a little boost of B12 and it certainly couldn't hurt, and it has all of the potential in the world to help. So…off you go to your local "Mart" for a bottle of B12.

Vitamin B12 deficiency and metformin (Glucophage). The association of metformin treatment with vitamin B12 deficiency was confirmed in a long-term trial, suggesting that diabetic patients receiving the number one oral drug for type 2 diabetes would benefit from vitamin monitoring and perhaps B12 supplementation. The B12 deficiency could be the cause of neuropathy in diabetics, so when evaluating a diabetic patient with neuropathy make sure B12 levels are included in the evaluation. Don't automatically assume that the neuropathy is due to the diabetes. (deJager J, et al. Long term treatment with metformin in patients with type 2 diabetes and risk of vitamin B-12 deficiency: Randomized placebo controlled trial *BMJ* 2010; DOI: 10.1136/bmj.c2181).

Vitamin B12 deficiency and proton pump inhibitors. The class of drugs known as the proton pump inhibitors are prescribed for gastroesophageal reflux disease, or GERD. This class of drugs has the last name "prazole"—omeprazole (Prilosec), rabeprazole (AcipHex)(Pariet in Canada), pantoprazole (Protonix, Pantoloc in Canada), lansoprazole (Prevacid), dexlansoprazole (Dexilant), and esomeprazole (Nexium, the "purple pill"). The pump that pumps acid into the stomach lumen is the same pump that pumps intrinsic factor—if the pump is inhibited to prevent acid pumping, then it only follows that the intrinsic factor pumping would be diminished as well. Long term follow up of patients on these "GERD" drugs includes checking for B12 deficiency.

Vitamin C (ascorbic acid). Vitamin C was discovered in 1907. The RDA for vitamin C is 75 mg/day for women and 90 mg/day for men. Smokers should up this amount by 35 mg/ day for both genders. The UL (upper limit) for vitamin C is 2,000 mg/day from food and supplements. If you take a dose greater than 2,000 mg per day you might be spending a considerable amount of your day on the toilet with an annoying bout of diarrhea. The rec-

HISTORICAL HIGHLIGHT

Dietary treatment for pernicious anemia (low red blood cell production caused by B12 deficiency) was first introduced in the early 1900s. Patients were required to consume at least a half a pound of liver per day as their treatment for this severe, unrelenting (hence, "pernicious") anemia. At the time this replacement treatment with liver was heralded as a lifesaving miracle, even though no one really knew the actual cause of the deficiency.

In 1928, William Castle, a research associate at Boston City Hospital, posed a very simple question: "Why don't normal people need a half of a pound of liver per day to prevent the development of pernicious anemia?" William (who, by the way, flunked his course in hematology while a medical student at Harvard) knew that the stomachs of patients with pernicious anemia were shriveled and atrophic. He proposed that this atrophic stomach may cause them to lack some very important factor that the stomach could no longer provide.

How did he approach this question? His experimental protocol consisted of two consecutive periods of approximately 10 days, during which daily reticulocyte counts were drawn. (NOTE: A reticulocyte is an immature red blood cell, the precursor to the mature red blood cell known as the erythrocyte. If the bone marrow is making adequate numbers of red blood cells, the reticulocyte count should be between 0.5 and 2%). His study had a sample size of two—himself and one other patient. During the first 10 days the patient received 200 grams of rare hamburger steak daily. His rationale for using hamburger was that it was similar in texture to liver. During this 10-day period the reticulocyte count remained the same.

During the second part of the protocol, Castle consumed 200 grams of hamburger meat. One hour later he inserted a tube through his nose in to his stomach (a nasogastric, or NG tube) to collect partially digested contents and gastric juice. He would incubate his gastric contents for several hours until liquefaction of the meat occurred. He then inserted an NG tube into the patient in the study and delivered the solution of his own gastric contents to the patient.

The result? The patient demonstrated a rise in the reticulocyte count—in other words the patient's red blood cells were being produced in the bone marrow and were being released into the bloodstream. This meant that the patient was responding to something that he received from the stomach of Dr. Castle. Castle found that neither the hamburger alone nor the gastric contents, when given alone, would help the patient; they needed to be given in combination in order for the treatment to be effective. He referred to the hamburger meat as the "extrinsic factor" and the substance in the gastric juices as the "intrinsic factor." And now you know the rest of the story. We now know that the "extrinsic factor" is B12, and intrinsic factor continues to be the name of the gastric binding protein that binds the B12 for absorption.

You might be asking yourself, "Why did the one-half pound of liver work by itself as the original treatment for pernicious anemia, but not the hamburger by itself?" Good question—here's your answer: Liver contains such abundant quantities of B12 that the mass effect of B12 given was enough to ensure sufficient passive absorption and clinical response despite the loss of the binding protein (or "intrinsic factor") in the atrophic stomach.

ommended intake for health reasons is 200 mg per day, not to exceed 2,000 mg per day for prolonged periods. Dietary levels of about 300–400 mg/day maintain body pools of vitamin C. The antioxidant dose of vitamin C is 200 mg per day or higher.

Vitamin C is widespread in plant tissues, with particularly high concentrations occurring in citrus fruits (oranges, lemons, limes, grapefruit), tomatoes, potatoes, sweet potatoes, cabbages, berries, and green peppers.

The disease caused by the lack of vitamin C is known as scurvy. Scurvy does not occur in most animals because they can synthesize their own vitamin C. However, humans and other higher primates (chimpanzees and apes), guinea pigs, most or all bats, and some species of birds and fish lack an enzyme necessary for such synthesis of vitamin C and must obtain vitamin C through the diet.

The highest risk group for scurvy today is teenagers. Dentists can pick this up pretty quickly as the classic signs of scurvy include inflammation in the interdental papillae, as well as bleeding and spongy gums.

The top foods containing vitamin C are:

½ chili pepper .... 182 mg
½ cantaloupe... 112 mg
1 cup orange juice.................................. 97 mg
½ cup sweet red pepper........................ 95 mg
1 cup grapefruit juice............................ 83 mg
1 California orange................................ 80 mg
1 Florida orange..................................... 65 mg
1 cup mixed vegetable juice .... 67 mg
1 cup grape juice.................................... 60 mg

Vitamin C is vital for the body's production of collagen, a key component of connective tissue. Without collagen, capillaries separate and leak, resulting in bleeding gums and red splotches characteristic of scurvy.

Vitamin C and the common cold. In the 1970s, vitamin C emerged as the first "megavitamin"—promoted by Linus Pauling, the American chemist who was convinced that taking 3,000 mg (3 grams) per day could prevent the common cold. Not true, but he sold a lot of copies of his book Vitamin C and the Common Cold.

More is NOT better when it comes to vitamins. If anything, some vitamins can be harmful when taken in "mega-doses," as observed with vitamin A.

Vitamin C and chemotherapy. Supplementing with vitamin C before starting chemotherapy may interfere with treatment. A group of researchers found that high levels of vitamin C supplements found in mice after supplementation negated much of the cancer-killing benefits of many chemotherapy agents. The levels of vitamin C found in mice were similar to levels found in the WBCs of people taking vitamin C supplements, suggesting that the findings may apply to humans as well—particularly with leukemia and lymphoma. The findings do not apply to the vitamin C found naturally in foods. (*Cancer Research.* October 1, 2008)

Vitamin C as an antioxidant. The antioxidant dose is 200 mg/day. Vitamin C has a direct antioxidant capacity and contributes to the protection of cells from the damaging effects of free radicals. Vitamin C prevents oxidative damage of lipids, proteins, and DNA which has been implicated as a major contributing factor in the development of chronic diseases such as cardiovascular disease, cancer, and cataracts, respectively. Vitamin C may also provide indirect antioxidant protection by regenerating other biologically important antioxidants such as glutathione and vitamin E to their active state. (Wintergerst ES, Maggini S, Hornig DH. Immune-enhancing role of vitamin C and effect of clinical conditions)

Vitamin C and the immune system. Vitamin C minimizes damage to neutrophils and lymphocytes (white blood cells) during immune activation via its antioxidant effects as mentioned above. Vitamin C may also help to mitigate the effects of glucose on cells, thus curbing complications in the patient with diabetes. (*Environmental Nutrition,* December 1997).

Vitamin C and insomnia. Even small doses of vitamin C taken late in the day can interfere with sleep, especially as we age. So, when contemplating causes of insomnia in the elderly think outside the bottle (medication and alcohol, that is), and consider the possibility of a high intake of vitamin C containing foods (glass of orange juice, tomato juice, bowl of melon or strawberries) consumed at dinner or in the evening. (*American Family Physician* 2002; 65:1184)

Vitamin C and wound healing. Vitamin C is necessary for the conversion of the amino acid proline into hydroxyproline, an essential ingredient in collagen. Collagen helps to maintain the integrity of skin, tendons, and bones. In an individual with a deficiency of vitamin C, however, taking vitamin C may or may not help to speed up the process.

Vitamin C and wrinkles? Women with high intakes of vitamin C and the essential fatty acid linoleic acid have fewer wrinkles than women with lower intakes. Why? Vitamin C is an important component of collagen synthesis and linoleic acid promotes normal skin structure. So eat your vitamin C rich fruits and veggies, such as oranges and broccoli, and chow down on foods high in linoleic acid, such as soybeans and sunflower oil. And, stop smoking, stay out of the sun, chose your parents wisely, use facial moisturizer, and sleep with a coat hanger in your mouth…

Vitamin D. It has been estimated that one billion people worldwide have a vitamin D deficiency. Roughly two-thirds of Americans are not getting enough vitamin D.

HISTORICAL HIGHLIGHT

On June 19, 1922, the New York Times reported that a team led by Dr. E.V. McCollum, a famous biochemist, had discovered an unknown vitamin, which was labeled vitamin D. Vitamins A, B, and C had already been discovered. The specific purpose of this "hormone" was to protect bone growth and to prevent the bone disease known as rickets. At the same time another group showed that direct exposure to the sun also produced vitamin D—even without its inclusion in the diet.

Since the 1930s, milk and other foods in the U.S. have been fortified with vitamin D, a measure that has almost eradicated rickets. Adding vitamin D to milk began as a way to boost milk sales.

Vitamin D production. Sunlight stimulates the production of vitamin D in the skin—in fact, 80% of our vitamin D comes from the conversion of vitamin D in the skin; however, we can't rely on the sun to meet our daily needs. Why? We have office jobs, 567 channels to choose from on cable and Dish TV, video games, long commutes, and the ever-present obsession with slathering on sunscreen with extreme SPF numbers every time we venture out into the sunlight. Sunscreens block the ability to convert vitamin D in the skin while they are protecting the skin from the harmful, cancer-causing rays of the sun. In fact, SPF-7 blocks 97.5% of vitamin D production in the skin. Also, as we age, our skin becomes 60% less efficient at converting sunlight into vitamin D.

People living north of the Mason-Dixon line also tend to be vitamin D-deficient, as do people living in cloudy climates (hello, Seattle, Portland, Vancouver, Calgary, Edmonton, Chicago, Minneapolis, Detroit, Boston) and people living in polluted air (hello, Los Angeles). In Boston, sun exposure does not trigger vitamin D conversion between mid-October and mid-March. In fact, for every ten degrees latitude north of the Mason-Dixon line, you can add another month at both ends of the season for vitamin D deficiency.

In the right location, less than half an hour outside can give you all the vitamin D you need for a week. —Dr. Susan Harris, Tufts University.

So, you say, I'll just drink more milk fortified with vitamin D. Well, you need a quart a day to get the amount you need, and unfortunately that might not be the answer, because milk is not a reliable source of vitamin D. Even though vitamin D is added to milk, each carton appears to contain varying amounts of vitamin D. Some cartons are laden with the vitamin, while others have minimal amounts.

Ok, then how about a multivitamin, plus sunlight, and consuming vitamin D containing products? This just might do the trick, but apparently not in everyone. At the end of winter, 32% of healthy students, physicians, and residents at a Boston hospital were found to be vitamin D deficient, despite drinking a glass of milk and taking a multivitamin daily and eating salmon at least once a week. They lived in Boston for Pete's sake. (Holick MF. Vitamin D Deficiency. *New Engl J Med.* 2007 (July 19);357:266–281)

Vitamin D and bones. The latest recommendations for the daily minimum requirement of vitamin D (vitamin D3 is preferred) for bone health from the Institute of Medicine (IOM) are as follows:

600 IUs from age 1 to 70 for both men and women, including during pregnancy. After age 70, the recommended daily allowance is 800 IUs for both men and women.

Controversy abounds about the above recommendations. People have squawked that these numbers are too low, but the IOM states that their guidelines are based on clinically-based medicine and are the current recommendations for maintaining bone health only. There are no recommendations about the amount of Vitamin D that could be helpful for the other presumed benefits of vitamin D—cancer protection, prevention of diabetes, cardiovascular benefits, anti-depressive benefits, dementia prevention, prevention of falls and more. (www.iom.edu)

So, what is the bottom line here? The general consensus by vitamin D experts is as follows:

Persons infrequently exposed to sun may need 800-1000 IU daily and many experts now recommend 800 IU for all postmenopausal females, regardless of your age. If you are over age 50, aim for 800 to 1,000 IU of vitamin D3 per day. (NOTE: Vitamin D3, known as cholecalciferol, can be utilized by the body better than vitamin D2, ergocalciferol). You can combine your sources with multivitamin intake, dietary sources, and a calcium supplement with vitamin D added.

Some experts have also suggested that serum levels of 25-hydroxy vitamin D ≥ 30 ng/mL may be desirable in older adults to help prevent fractures and falls. It appears as if 700 IU/day of vitamin D3, with or without calcium supplementation decreased the risk of nonvertebral fractures. (Bischoff-Ferrari HA et al. Fracture prevention with vitamin D supplementation: a meta analysis. *Lancet* 2007;370:657)

Don't take more than 2,000 IU per day. Excess vitamin D leads to hypercalcemia (too much calcium in the blood), which can cause calcium deposits in the kidneys, leading to kidney stone formation as well as calcium deposits in the arteries, contributing to atherosclerosis.

Sun-produced vitamin D has been shown to last as least twice as long in the blood as vitamin D from supplements.

Vitamin D and cancer protection. When epidemiologists Cedric and Frank Garland began looking at the geographic incidence of colon cancer in the United States back in the 1970s, they noted an interesting pattern. People who lived South of the Mason-Dixon line were half as likely to die of colon cancer than those living in the Northeast. At that time they asked the question: Could the reason have to do with sunshine and vitamin D levels? Every year vitamin D deficiency probably accounts for thousands of deaths from breast, prostate, colon, and ovarian cancer. According to researchers at the University of California, San Diego, 1000 IU of vitamin D orally reduces the incidence of these four adult cancers. If the study is validated, this may be one of the most feasible ways to reduce the risk of cancer in everyone. (*British Medical Journal* 332:70, 2006)

Dr. Michael Holick, MD, PhD, one of the nation's top experts in vitamin D research, has stated that about half of all colorectal cancers in the U.S. are believed to be preventable by raising vitamin D levels in people who are deficient. (www.DrHolick.com)

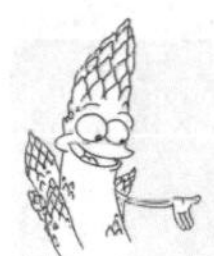

ASPARAGUS TIP

Guys, get your prostate out in the sun!!!

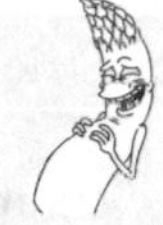

Vitamin D and cardiovascular protection. A study in the June 11, 2007, *Archives of Internal Medicine* found a "significantly higher" prevalence of hypertension, diabetes, obesity, and high triglyceride levels in individuals with lower levels of vitamin D. One of the possible reasons is the anti-inflammatory effect of vitamin D. Vitamin D lowers inflammation by increasing anti-inflammatory proteins such as interleukin-10. Research has also shown that vitamin D can lower blood pressure by inhibiting the renin-angiotensin-aldosterone system. In addition, vitamin D has been shown to reduce total cholesterol as well.

Vitamin D and the color of skin. Black and brown people, because of the natural sun-filtering effect of the dark pigment melanin, are far more likely than light-skinned individuals to have a vitamin D deficiency. What does this mean clinically? Darker-skinned individuals need to stay out in the sun longer than lighter-skinned individuals in order to obtain adequate vitamin D.

Vitamin D deficiency and diabetes. Researchers have found vitamin D receptors on just about every cell of the body and that includes the beta cells of the pancreas, the cells that produce insulin. For people with type 2 diabetes, it appears as if vitamin D allows the body to secrete more insulin. At the same time, there's evidence that vitamin D may increase insulin sensitivity.

People who get more than 800 IU of vitamin D daily may be about one-third less likely to develop type 2 diabetes. Since darker-skinned individuals tend to be vitamin D deficient (melatonin acts as a natural sunscreen), African-Americans have lower levels of vitamin D. Hmmm...can this explain why the majority of type 2 diabetes is diagnosed in darker skinned individuals such as African-Americans and Native American individuals? The number one country in the world for diabetes is India.

Children with type 1 diabetes tend to be lighter-skinned with a Scandinavian background named Sven or Inga. Kidding with the names. It is true, however, that the number one country in the world for type 1 diabetes is Finland. Since vitamin D is scant in Scandinavian countries, it makes sense that type 1 diabetes may have something to do with vitamin D deficiency.

Vitamin D deficiency, signs and symptoms. Low energy, bone pain (especially in the arms and legs) and/or lack of muscle strength can indicate a vitamin D deficiency. Osteomalacia is a softening of bone resulting from an abnormality in the bone-building and remodeling process. Patients with osteomalacia complain of throbbing and aching bone pain. Press firmly with your thumb or forefinger on your sternum or shins. If you feel pain in either area, you are most likely low in vitamin D and may have osteomalacia. Visit your friendly health care practitioner for a vitamin-D level.

Vitamin D deficiency lab values. How can you tell if you are vitamin-D deficient? The only way to know for sure is to get a blood test for 25-hydroxyvitamin D, an intermediary in the conversion of vitamin D to its active form. Who should have this blood test? Everyone, but specifically individuals over 50, or anyone who has risk factors such as living above the Mason-Dixon line, is housebound and unable to get daily or every-other-day sunlight, and/or who has chronic liver or kidney disease.Vitamin D levels are as follows:

Reference values for total vitamin D

Normal range	Above 30 ng/mL
Insufficiency	10–30 ng/mL
Deficiency	Less than 10 ng/mL
Excess	Above 150 ng/mL

(Corbett JV, Banks D. Laboratory Tests and Diagnostic Procedures. 2013. Pearson, Boston)

Dr. Michael Holick recommends exposure to sunlight three times a week—during the period of 10 a.m. to 3 p.m. (virtually no vitamin D is produced at other times)—spend one-quarter to one-half the amount of time in the sun that it takes you to get the beginning of a sunburn. For someone with dark skin, this might be 30 minutes three times weekly. If you're fair-skinned, five to 10 minutes might be enough. Expose your arms and legs—and, if possible, your abdomen and back—to sun. When you're not doing a timed exposure , cover all exposed skin with sunscreen to prevent sunburn. However, if you live above the 33° latitude (roughly any area north of Atlanta), you cannot produce any significant vitamin D from sun exposure during the winter. (www.DrHolick.com)

Vitamin D blood levels around the world:

African-Americans with Multiple Sclerosis	2 ng/ml
Men in Finland	13 ng/ml
Veiled Tunisian women (ages 20-60)	14 ng/ml
Elderly African American men in U.S.	19 ng/ml
Danish girls taking 600 IU per day	24 ng/ml
Elderly Afro-Caribbean men living in Tobago	35 ng/ml
Healthy black children in South Africa	37 ng/ml
Elderly people in Florida taking 2,000 IU per day	43 ng/ml
Lifeguards in Missouri	65 ng/ml

Vitamin D and infections. Vitamin D boosts a natural antimicrobial compound known as cathelicidin produced by white blood cells. Cathelicidin targets bacteria, viruses, and fungi. It has a lytic function—in other words, it punches holes in the external membrane of a microbe causing the microbe to rupture. The production of this chemical is ramped up by the active form of vitamin D—1,25-cholecalciferol, or 1, 25-D. This active form of vitamin D literally ramps up the genes that produce cathelicidin. Cathelicidin is also produced in the skin, making it a perfect antimicrobial to regulate the skin's response to pathogens. The active form of vitamin D is also produced in the skin, thus the two go hand-in-hand for fighting microbes. A researcher from Sweden, Mona Ståhle, administered an ointment containing a drug mimic of 1, 25-D to the skin of four healthy people. The ointment hit the jackpot, so to speak. Where the ointment had been applied, cathelicidin-gene activity skyrocketed as much as 100-fold and the local concentrations of cathelicidin increased. (Ståhle, *M. Journal of Investigative Dermatology*, May 2005)

Cold-weather coats, gloves, and hats, as well as the sun's angle in the winter sky, limit how much ultraviolet light reaches the skin. This adds up to a deficiency in vitamin D production in the winter, which might explain why respiratory infections are common and severe in the winter.

Vitamin D and tuberculosis. What is the role of vitamin D in fending off tuberculosis? The role has been known for over a century, as the treatment for "consumption" (the old name for TB) in the early 20th century was to "go up on the mountain if you have consumption." Studies from microbial immunologist Robert Modlin and colleagues of UCLA studied the macrophage, the most important cell in fending off TB and other microbes. Modlin's team showed that just before making cathelicidin, the macrophages briefly boosted their production of vitamin D receptors and an enzyme that converts the vitamin D prehormone into 1,25-D. The data also found that significant concentrations of 1, 25-D would develop only in the presence of the TB bacteria. He also found that black people, because of the sun-filtering effect of dark pigments in their skin, are far more likely than whites to be vitamin D deficient. Furthermore, blacks tend to be more susceptible to TB than whites and to develop a more severe illness when infected. The macrophages from black patients produce 63% less cathelicidin and were less likely to kill the TB when compared to macrophages from Caucasians. (*Science News.* October 16, 2004:248; *Science News.* November 11, 2006:317)

Vitamin D and osteoporosis. It is just as important to have adequate amounts of vitamin D as it is to have adequate amounts of calcium to prevent and to treat established osteoporosis. Vitamin D is essential for the absorption of calcium and for the maintenance of bone mineralization. Some new studies have concluded that as a population, Americans are woefully deficient in this "sunshine vitamin."

Vitamin D and rickets. This condition is rare in the U.S.; however, it is occurring more often in breast-fed babies who are not receiving vitamin D supplements or who don't get enough sun. African American babies have an increased risk due to decreased vitamin D metabolism secondary to the pigment melanin. Kids with rickets also experience more infections than kids without rickets.

ASPARAGUS TIP

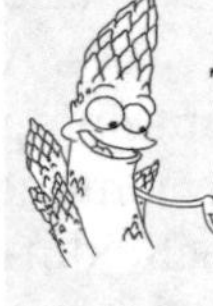

Take a vitamin D supplements with your largest meal of the day. Taking the supplement with the largest meal of the day increases absorption by 57%. This is most likely due to the fact that the largest meals of the day have the most fat content, boosting absorption of this fat-soluble vitamin. (Angelo Licata, MD, Cleveland Clinic, *Journal of Bone and Mineral Research*)

So, what are the food sources that provide vitamin D? Natural food sources include:

Cod liver oil, 1 tsp .... 400-1,000 IU
Fresh wild-caught salmon, 3.5 ounces .... 600-1,000 IU
Catfish, 3 ounces , cooked .... 571 IU
Shrimp, 3 ounces, cooked .... 171 IU

Canned tuna (in water), 3.5 oz. .... 236 IU
Sun-dried shiitake mushrooms, 3.5 oz. .... 1,600 IU
Egg yolk .... 20-41 IU

Fortified food sources of vitamin D include:

Milk, 8 oz. .... 100 IU
Orange juice, 8 oz .... 100 IU
Yogurt, 8 oz. 100 .... IU
Cereal, one serving .... 100 IU

Margarine, 3.5 oz. .... 429 IU
Quaker Oatmeal Nutrition for Women, 1 packet .... 140 IU
Slim-Fast Shake, 1 can, 11 oz. .... 140 IU
Dannon Fruision Smoothie, 10 oz. .... 140 IU

Pharmaceutical and supplement sources of vitamin D:
Multivitamin ....400–1,000 IU
Vitamin D catch-up pills ....400–50,000 IU

(Source: Holick MF, et al. *J of Clin Endo & Metabol,* July 2011.

Vitamin E. Vitamin E is actually a complex group of eight related compounds that may be especially important in the aging process. The eight related compounds include four tocopherols and four tocotrienols (in both cases called alpha, beta, gamma, and delta). The recommended daily intake is 15 mg (22.5 IU). Stick with a multivitamin that contains no more than 100 IU. Almonds are the best natural source of vitamin E, with 11 IU in three tablespoons. Other dietary sources include walnuts, vegetable and seed oils. To E or not to E, that is the question.

Vitamin E in food, which is mostly gamma-tocopherol, acts as an antioxidant. The vitamin E found in supplements is primarily alpha-tocopherol, which may actually block the antioxidant effect of gamma-tocopherol and may actually have a pro-oxidant effect in the body. This is a revolting development as far as the vitamin E proponents are concerned. The latest studies have not been kind to vitamin E supplementation. (*The Medical Letter.* 2011 (December 12/26);53(1379/1380:101–102)

Vitamin E and mortality. A Cochrane review of 26 trials with over 100,000 subjects found that vitamin E supplements with or without beta carotene and vitamin A was associated with a higher risk of death. (Bjelakovic G et al. Antioxidant supplements for prevention of mortality in healthy participants and patients with various diseases. *Cochrane Database Syst Rev* 2008;2;CD007176)

Vitamin E and bleeding. Bleeding complications from vitamin E are quite rare, and are virtually unheard of when the dose is kept at or below 800 IU per day. High doses of vitamin E may interfere with vitamin K metabolism and platelet aggregation (clumping). One note of caution: When other antiplatelet drugs and anticoagulant drugs are used in addition to vitamin E, the dose of vitamin E at which bleeding occurs may be less than 800 IU. So, keep in mind drugs such as aspirin, warfarin (Coumadin), ibuprofen (Advil and others), ginkgo, and garlic may increase the risk of bleeding when vitamin E is added to the pot, so to speak.

Vitamin E and prostate cancer. Well, this one came out of nowhere. Another meta-analysis of over 35,000 men found that vitamin E (400 IU/day) had a statistically significant increase (17%) in the risk of prostate cancer, compared to those taking placebo. (Klein EA et al. Vitamin E and the risk of prostate cancer; the Selenium and Vitamin E Cancer Prevention Trial (SELECT). *JAMA* 2011;306:154)

Vitamin E and heart disease. Three randomized trials found the supplementation with vitamin E did *not* reduce the risk of major cardiovascular events. (Sesso HD et al. Vitamins E and C in the prevention of cardiovascular disease in men: the Physician's Health Study II randomized controlled trial. *JAMA* 2008; 300:2123; Lee IM et al. Vitamin E in the primary prevention of cardiovascular disease and cancer: the Women's Health Study: a randomized controlled trial. *JAMA* 2005;294:56)

Vitamin E and stroke. One big meta-analysis of over 150,000 patients found that vitamin E was of zero benefit in preventing any type of stroke. And, a second study found that vitamin E increased the risk of hemorrhagic stroke by 22% and reduced the risk of ischemic stroke by 10%. (Bin Q et al. The role of vitamin E (tocopherol) supplementation in the prevention of stroke: a meta-analysis of 13 randomized controlled trials. ThrombHaemost 2011; 105:589; Schurks M, et al. Effects of vitamin E on stroke subtypes: meta-analysis of randomized controlled trials. *BMJ* 2010;341:c5702)

Vitamin E—synthetic or natural? The recommended daily allowance for vitamin E is 15 mg per day for adults. To get this amount, you need 22 IU of natural vitamin E (also known as d-alphatocopheroll) or 33 IU of synthetic vitamin E (also known as dl-alpha-tocopherol). Why the difference in amounts? Natural vitamin E is more potent than synthetic, so less is needed.

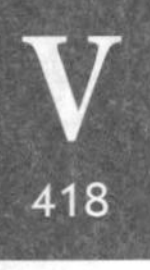

Vitamin K. The current Daily Value is 80 μg/day for men and 60 μg/day for women. Most multivitamins have less than this because vitamin K can interfere with anticoagulants such as warfarin/Coumadin.

There are two types of vitamin K–K1 and K2. Vitamin K2 is also known as menaquinone and its primary function is to help maintain bone strength. The higher the vitamin K levels, the lower the incidence of bone fractures. Vitamin K2 has also been linked to a reduced risk of atherosclerosis. Vitamin K2 is found primarily in chicken, beef, organ meats, egg yolks, and milk as well as fermented foods such as hard cheese and sauerkraut.

Vitamin K1, also known as phylloquinone, is obtained from plant foods such as green leafys, broccoli, Brussels sprouts, and asparagus. About 10% of K1 is converted to K2 in the body.

Vitamin K1 and K2 both play a role in the production of coagulation factors such as prothrombin. Women should strive for 60 μg per day, and men should shoot for 80 μg per day. Rich sources of Vitamin K1 include most dark green leafy greens (kale, lettuce, spinach, and Swiss chard), asparagus, broccoli, brussels sprouts, cabbage, cauliflower, and some oils like canola and soybean.

Since Vitamin K plays a major role in the production of prothrombin, should individuals reduce their intake of vitamin K-containing foods if they are on the anticoagulant warfarin (Coumadin)? See below. The general answer to that question is no if their intake remains consistent. However, there may be some situations where your vitamin K intake may increase enough to require an adjustment in Coumadin dosing. What are those situations?

You don't eat a lot of salads in the winter, but as soon as summer comes around, salads become a daily habit. Be consistent! Consistency is the RULE.

You have started a new diet and have increased your vegetable and salad consumption considerably.

You are taking *Viactiv.* (Each *Viactiv* chew contains 50 μg of vitamin K.)

Vitamin K and warfarin. The interaction between warfarin (Coumadin) and vitamin K-containing foods has been well documented in the literature. Vitamin K is an essential co-factor in the hepatic production of clotting factors II, VII, X, and X. As a result of vitamin K antagonism, warfarin inhibits the production of the above four clotting factors. Given orally, it is widely used for the long-term prevention of thromboembolic disease.

Since vitamin K and warfarin are antagonists, the amount of vitamin K in the diet can diminish warfarin's anticoagulant effects. The most important concept concerning the vitamin K-warfarin effect is consistency. Remind patients to adhere to a steady diet of vitamin K-containing foods, and their INR levels should not be a concern. Advise patients to report any significant changes in their dietary vitamin K intake in order to maintain a therapeutic INR.

The foods with the highest vitamin K content are as follows:

Vegetables: Broccoli, Brussels sprouts, beet greens, cabbage, collard greens, endive (raw), kale (raw leaf), kohlrabi, lettuce (bib, red leaf), mustard greens (raw), parsley, spinach, turnip greens (raw), watercress (raw), Swiss chard

Oils and fats: mayonnaise, canola oil, soybean oil

Beverages: Tea (green tea) (Brewing the green tea may alter the vitamin K content; however, this is controversial.)

The foods with moderate amounts of vitamin K include:

Vegetables: asparagus, avocado, red cabbage, green peas, dill pickles, iceberg lettuce

Fats and oils: margarine and olive oil

The foods with the lowest amount of vitamin K include:

Vegetables: Green beans, carrots, cauliflower, celery, corn, cucumber (sans peel), eggplant, mushrooms, onions, green pepper, potato, pumpkin, sauerkraut (canned), tomato

Fruits are low in vitamin K as are meat and dairy products.

Oils and fats: corn oil, peanut oil, safflower oil, sesame oil, sunflower oil.
Beverages: coffee, cola, fruit juices, milk, tea (black).

(Clotcare Online Resource; www.clotcare.com)

Vitamins—prenatal vitamins and birth defects. Does the use of prenatal vitamins *increase* the rate of birth defects? What??? In 2000, a group of researchers found that the risk of having an infant with multiple congenital anomalies was increased in women who took periconceptional multivitamins containing folic acid. (*Am J Med Genet* 2000;93:188). This finding piqued the interest of a group of CDC researchers who subsequently analyzed data using the 1992-1997 Atlanta Birth Defects Risk Factor Surveillance study. They found 96 infants with at least 2 major birth defects. They compared this group with 334 infants with no birth defects from the same population and time period. After adjusting for a zillion variables, including maternal age, educational level, family history, prepregnancy body mass index (BMI), and alcohol or cigarette use, Moms who reported using periconceptional multivitamins (with at least 200 mg of folic acid) had an increased risk for giving birth to an infant with multiple congenital anomalies. When the analysis was limited to infants with no first-degree relatives with major birth defects, the increase in risk in regular multivitamin users was statistically significant. Whoa. Why, you might ask? Who knows, I might answer. However, as always, researchers have their ideas and explanations for the findings. One hypothesis is that multivitamin use decreases the likelihood of spontaneous loss of fetuses with malformations, thus increasing the odds that a fetus with multiple congenital anomalies will survive to birth. Folic acid is still recommended to prevent neural tube defects, but the possibility that multivitamin exposure might be associated with a risk for birth defects is a REAL possibility and can no longer be ignored. More to come. (Yuskiv N, et al. *Am J Med* Genet 2005 July;136:1–7)

Vodka. Vodka, meaning "little water," was first distilled in Russia in the sixteenth century from the most abundant local grain of the time, rye. Later, in the nineteenth century, potatoes were employed for distillation. Currently maize and wheat are also used for the distillation of vodka in Russia. By 1861 taxes on vodka provided 45% of the revenue of the Russia. Throughout the nineteenth century, more than 70% of the expenditures for the Russian army were paid for by vodka taxes.

Now that food has replaced sex in my life, I can't even get into my own pants.
—Anonymous

WAIST SIZE

Waist size. Where do you officially measure waist size? Official guidelines:

Locate the top of the right iliac crest (the hip bone); where it intersects with a line dropped vertically from the middle of the right axilla (the armpit) is where you place the paper tape measure (cloth tape measures are too easy to stretch.)

What should your waist size be? As a general rule the average American man should have a waist size of 40 inches or less and the average American woman should have a waist size of 35 inches or less. This number can be deceiving though. Think about it…what if you are only 50 inches tall and your waist size is 40 inches…hum. In other words, if we can jump over you faster than we can run around you, this is not a good waist size. The best way to determine your waist size is to measure your height and divide that by two. Your waist should be one-half of your height. So, if you're 62 inches tall your waist should be 31 inches.

Waist size and diabetes. The bigger the belly, the higher the risk for abdominal or visceral fat, insulin resistance, and subsequent risk of type 2 diabetes. Compare your waist size to the list below and you may want to determine what your next course of action might be.

The risk of diabetes is 2.5 times greater with a waist size of 30–31 inches.

The risk of diabetes is 4 times greater with a waist size of 32–33 inches.

The risk of diabetes is 4.5 times greater with a waist size of 34–35 inches.

This risk of diabetes is 5.5 times greater with a waist size of 36–37 inches.

The risk of diabetes is 6 times greater with a waist size of 38 inches or greater.

Guys, what are you laughin' at? Put the TV remote down, get up off the couch, and grab that paper tape measure from your wife. Here are your numbers:

A waist size of 34-36 doubles the risk of diabetes in men.

A waist size of 36 to 38 nearly triples the risk of diabetes in men.

A waist size of 38 to 40 inches is associated with a five times greater risk.

A waist size of 40 to 62 inches is associated with a 12 times greater risk.

(Warner J. "Waist size predicts diabetes risk: Men should aim for waist size of 37 inches or less." *WebMD Health News.* March 10, 2005)

The above numbers are for the average American, not for the average European or the average sub-Saharan African. The 2009 International Diabetes Federation recently published consensus cutoff points for waist circumference for other populations, and here they are:

Europeans, Japanese, sub-Saharan Africa, Eastern Mediterranean, and Middle Eastern—male (36.7 inches); female (31.3)

South Asian—China, Malaysia, Asian-Indian population), ethnic South and Central American—males (35.2), females (31.3)

HISTORICAL HIGHLIGHT—THE WAKE

In the 1500s lead cups were used to drink whiskey and other forms of alcohol. The combination of the lead in the cup with the whiskey or ale would sometimes knock a person out for a few days. When found in that inebriated condition, they were often thought to be dead. They were laid out on the kitchen table and the family would gather around and eat and drink and wait to see if they would wake up; hence the custom of holding the "wake."

Wafers and Holy Communion. Often overlooked as a source of wheat gluten, the wafers given out during Holy Communion can be the source of an acute diarrhea attack in individuals with gluten hypersensitivity. Even the wafers classified as "gluten-free" may still contain sufficient gluten to cause diarrhea. Most of the individuals sensitive to wheat gluten are classified as having celiac disease—an allergy to gluten that results in malabsorption and diarrhea.

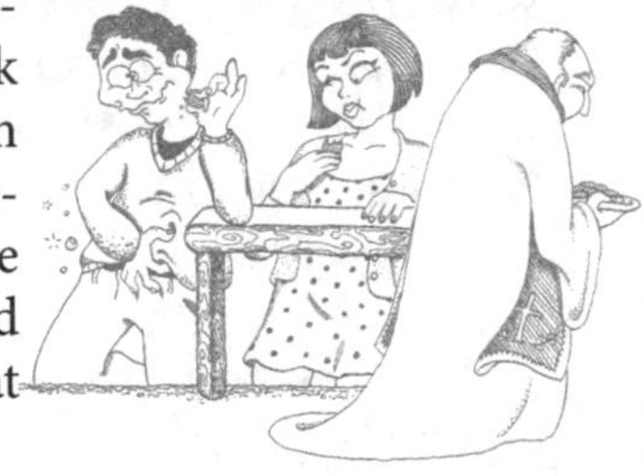

WALNUTS

Walnuts. Walnuts have been described as "food for the gods" by the ancient Romans. In the 16th and 17th century walnuts were used for headaches, boosting cognitive function, and reducing anxiety.

Of the nine varieties of nuts, walnuts pack the most powerful antioxidant punch. Walnuts are also a great source of protein, fiber, and polyunsaturated fat. Walnuts are the only nut that supply significant amounts of alpha linolenic acid, which the body converts to heart-healthy omega-3 fatty acids. They also contain some saturated fat and are relatively high in calories, but the overall consensus is that a handful of walnuts a day can keep the cardiologist and perhaps the oncologist away. Remember, antioxidants slurp up free radicals. Free radicals build up and have been implicated in heart disease, cancer and a myriad of other chronic health conditions. So, grab a handful of nuts (about 14 walnut halves, ¼ cup or 1 ounce of shelled pieces) and say cheers to your overall health! (*American Chemical Society,* March 2011)

"Walnutrients:"
1 ounce = 14 halves = ¼ cup shelled pieces
Calories: 185
Fiber: 2 grams
Magnesium: 45 mg
Copper: 45 µg
Manganese: 1 mg
Phosphorus: 98 mg
Alpha-linolenic acid: 2.6 grams (163% of adequate intake for men; 235% for women)

HISTORICAL HIGHLIGHT

President George Washington blamed all of his dental problems on years of cracking walnuts shells with his teeth.

Warfarin (Coumadin) and nutritional supplements. Many herbs have natural anticoagulant effects that can potentiate the effect of warfarin (Coumadin), and others can counteract its effect. In addition, foods containing vitamin K, a natural antagonist of warfarin, can weaken its effect. Examples include:

- Garlic, dong quai, dan shen, and ginseng can antagonize the effects of warfarin.
- Ginkgo biloba is known to contain a potent inhibitor of platelet activation, so that its use with warfarin can cause bleeding.
- Vitamin E has weak antiplatelet effects and is generally not considered to be a problem when taken with warfarin if the dose is less than 800 IU/day.

Green tea has one of the highest contents of vitamin K. If taken with warfarin, the patient should limit the intake to only two to four cups of green tea per day. Other vitamin K-rich foods include dark green leafy vegetables such as spinach, collard greens, Brussels sprouts, and broccoli. Patients can still eat these foods as long as they consume relatively constant amounts, since titration of the warfarin dosage takes this consumption into account. Some multivitamin preparations and nutritional supplements such as Ensure and Isocal also contain vitamin K.

Patients should be asked to stop taking any herbs, drugs, or nutritional supplements that potentiate or interfere with the action of warfarin. Those who insist on taking any herb concomitantly with the drug should have an international normalized ratio (INR) measurement within a week of starting to take the herbal product.

The interaction of warfarin with alcohol is an interesting one. Acute alcohol consumption can decrease warfarin metabolism and increase warfarin effect, whereas chronic alcohol consumption can induce warfarin metabolism and decrease warfarin effect. Due to the increased risk of bleeding or clotting with acute or chronic alcohol use, patients should be advised to reduce or avoid alcohol consumption while on warfarin.

Wasting food in America. The average American household wastes up to 15% of the solid food it purchases. The total food wasted in the U.S. would be enough to feed the population of Canada. And it should come as no surprise, especially to children, that the food most commonly wasted is vegetables.

WATER

Water. Water is your best choice for replenishing the fluids that are used daily in all bodily functions. Water can even help you lose a little weight. Water is absorbed faster than any other beverage, and of course doesn't have any calories. However, don't forget that you get water in foods as well as from drinking a glass of water. Fruits and vegetables contain 80–95% water, milk is 90% water, cooked cereal such as oatmeal is 85% water, an egg is 75% water, pasta is 65% water, fish/seafood is 60–85% water, meats are 45–65% water, cheese is 35% water, bread is 35–40% water, nuts are only 2–5% water, and oil is zippo, zero, zilch, nada. Foods that are liquid at room temperature can also be counted as fluids. This includes popsicles, sherbet, ice cream, and there's always room for JELL-O. What about booze? No. Booze inhibits anti-diuretic hormone and causes you to lose more fluid that you take in. How about coffee and soda? Yes, they can be counted since contrary to popular belief, caffeine is not considered to be a diuretic.

How do you know how much water to drink? First of all, don't rely on your thirst mechanisms to tell you when to take a swig. If you are thirsty, you have waited too long for that drink. By the time you feel thirsty, you are about two cups low and may already be mildly dehydrated. As we age we also lose our thirst mechanism, so we can't even rely on that to tell us when we are mildly dehydrated. So, here are a few ways to keep your water balance where it should be:

1) Hop on a scale, weigh yourself, and divide your weight in half. That number, in ounces, is your recommended daily fluid intake. Adding a slice of lemon or lime is a good way to vary the taste of bottled water. (Cory SerVaas, M.D.)
2) Drink 2/3 ounces of water per pound of body weight per day if you're active and 1/2 ounce per pound if you are a couch potato. (International Sportsmedicine Institute, West Los Angeles, California.)
3) Another general rule is to drink a quart of water for every 1,000 calories you burn. (*Environmental Nutrition,* May 1998.)
4) And yet another group has chimed in...The Institute of Medicine advises that men consume roughly 3 liters (about 13 cups) of total beverages per day and women consume 2.2 liters (about 9 cups) of total beverages. Note: TOTAL BEVERAGES, not specifically water. (http://www.mayoclinic.com/health/water/NU00283)

The average American drinks approximately 16,000 gallons of water in a lifetime. We should—most of the body consists of water. Water constitutes 55% of a woman's body and 60% of a man's body. The infant's body is 78% water. The brain consists of 70% water. (*Science Illustrated.* January/February 2012)

Some people in developing countries only get 7.9 gallons of water for all of their daily needs—the equivalent of a five-minute shower in an average American household.

How long can we go without water? Seven days at most. We can go without food for a month.

What about that old *myth* that you need to drink at least 8 glasses of water per day? Well it's just that—a myth. It was a 1945 recommendation that we consume 1 mL of water per calorie of food—but most people didn't read the next sentence. "Most of this quantity of water is contained in prepared foods." No evidence exists to support the 8-glass a day rule; drinking typical amounts of milk, juice, and other liquids should suffice. Besides, too much water can cause water intoxication, hyponatremia (low sodium), and even death from electrolyte imbalance. (Vreeman RC, Carroll AE, *British Medical Journal* 2007; 335:1288–1289)

Water, bottled. Are you addicted to bottled water? Americans spend more than 7 billion dollars on bottled water per year, paying from 120 to 7,500 times as much per gallon for bottled water as for tap. Ouch. If that's not enough to make you think twice the next time you pick up a 6-pack of Evian or other bottled water beverage, you might want to check the label. The Natural Resources Defense Council (NRDC) tested over 1,000 samples of 103 brands of bottled water and found that approximately 25 percent of the bottles were tap water. Yep, tap water. Right out of the sink faucet. If the label says "from a municipal source" or "from a community water system," it's good old tap water. And you just paid 6 bucks for that gallon of water. Tap water from the kitchen faucet costs around $6.00 per 1,000 gallons of water. If you drink only bottled water, you'll spend about $1,400 annually to get your recommended daily amount of water, as opposed to 49 cents for one year's supply of just-as-healthy-tap water. Use the calculator at www.newdream.org to calculate your savings based on your actual bottled water consumption—most likely you'll save somewhere in the vicinity of $1,000 per year. Gulp.

But I'm not finished yet. The NRDC found that over 13 percent of the brands tested had more bacteria than allowed under government guidelines. Bottled water is less regulated than tap water. In fact, the plants that produce bottled water are tested only once per month for coliform bacteria (the bugs that reside in the rectum) whereas city tap water is tested over 100 times per month. Does anyone see a problem here? Bottled water made in your very own state doesn't have to be tested at all for coliform bacteria; however, if the bottled water crosses the state line it must be tested for the bugs. Does that make any sense to anyone?

About 20 percent of the waters contained industrial chemicals with scary names like toluene and xylene, as well as chemical used in manufacturing plastics such as phthalate, adipate, and styrene. These so-called "plasticizers" act as hormone disrupters in the human body. A hormone disruptor mimics the hormone estrogen and therefore can change the hormonal milieu in the human body. Some researchers consider these "plasticizers" found in various products to be one of the reasons for the rise in hormone-dependent cancers including breast and prostate cancer.

Well, okay, so what if it has a few bacteria and a slew of chemicals contained within that bottle? It tastes sooooooo much better than the blah-stuff that comes out of the tap, right? Think again. In blind taste studies bottled water did not come out way ahead of the tap water. In fact, in those blind taste studies 45% of the tasters preferred city water as compared to 12% who chose Evian, 19% who chose O-2, and 24% who chose Poland Spring. This study was performed on the *Good Morning America* show in May 2001. A similar study in England found that 60% of the tasters could not differentiate between the local tap water and the bottled water.

One of the funnier studies was from a trendy, celebrity-watching, fashion-forward chic restaurant in southern California. The water was served by a "water sommelier" who asked diners whether they wanted the free city tap water or bottled water. The diners had three choices of bottled water—each of which cost $7 per bottle. Their choices included the French water L'eau Du Robinet (which in French actually means "faucet water"), Aqua de Culo (which is Spanish for "ass water"), and Amazone ("filtered through the Brazilian rain forest's natural filtration system," which, of course, means "ground water"). The majority of diners chose one of the fancy bottled waters—all of which were poured out of the same faucet as the city tap water. And they paid seven dollars a bottle for their hi-falutin' taste preferences. (*Scientific American*, July 2003; Michael Shermer, www.skeptic.com)

Water, fear of, also known as hydrophobia. Hydrophobia literally means the intense fear of water. Probably the most well-known hydrophobic condition is rabies. The patient with late-stage rabies has difficulty with swallowing and panics when presented with liquids to drink.

Water content and food. All foods contain water, even those that seem to be as dry as a bone. For example, corn flakes—would you think that a bowl of cornflakes would contain any water at all unless the milk was poured over it? Well, think again. For every 100 grams of corn flakes, you have 4 grams of water. Even peanuts contain water—1 gram of water per 100 grams of peanuts. Cucumbers are obvious with 95 grams of water per 100 grams of cucumber. Potatoes have 80 grams of water per 100 grams of potatoes and a banana is not far behind the potato with 75 grams of water per 100 grams of banana.

Water and fluid replacement. Just exactly what do we need to replace every day? The average daily urine output for adults is about 1.5 liters (6.3 cups). You lose close to an additional liter (about 4 cups) though breathing, sweating, and bowel movements. Food usually accounts for 20 percent of your total fluid intake, so if you consume 2 liters of water or other beverages per day (a little more than 8 cups) along with your normal diet, you will typically replace your lost fluid.

Reminds me of my safari in Africa. Somebody forgot the corkscrew and for several days we had to live on nothing but food and water. —W.C. Fields

---

Water and weight loss. Finally, an explanation as to why drinking copious amounts of water while dieting contributes to weight loss. When fluid intake is restricted, the resting metabolic rate drops 2–3%. The resting metabolic rate is the rate at which a person at rest burns calories. Since the resting rate accounts for most of the calories burned during the day—even if you get lots of exercise—even a small decline can make it hard to lose weight. Therefore, drinking five to eight glasses of water a day boosts the resting metabolic rate and assists with weight loss.

Water and weight loss, part 2. One of the most effective ways to lose weight is to drink water before meals. Nutritionists from Virginia Tech found that subjects who drank 16 ounces of water (2 glasses) before each of their three daily meals lost 50% more weight than the control subjects.

The study volunteers, 48 overweight and obese men and women, were put on a low-calorie diet for 12 weeks. Half were given no instructions about what to drink; the other half were instructed to drink two glasses of water shortly before their meals. The first group lost 11 pounds on average, but the water group lost more—15.5 pounds on average. Interestingly, the diet also seemed to stick. A year after the study, the water drinkers had continued the regimen on their own and lost additional weight. Who knows why it works? Water is filling, water has no calories, and water may take the place of other high-calorie drinks that might be consumed. (Davy B. Virginia Tech University, Department of Nutrition)

Water safety around the world. More people die each year from drinking unsafe water than from all forms of violence, including war. 884 million people—one in eight living people today—do not have access to safe drinking water. The percentage of the population with access to safe water in each of the following countries is: Ethiopia—18%, Sudan—45%, Pakistan—56%, Mexico—72%, USA—99%. (Source: Water Quality and Health Council: Chlorine Chemistry Council.)

ASPARAGUS TIP

It takes an astounding quantity of water to grow some to grow some of the most common crops. For example, it takes 20,000 liters of water to grow 2.2 pounds or 1 kg of coffee; 11,000 liters of water to produce the feed for one cow to provide one quarter-pounder; 7,000 liters for one cotton T-shirt; 5,000 liters for 2.2 pounds of cheese; 5,000 liters for 2.2 pounds of rice; 3,000 liters for 2.2 pounds of sugar; 2 liters for a cow to produce 1 liter of milk, and 1000 liters for 2.2 pounds of wheat. Here's another way to look at the above data: Every teaspoonful of sugar in your coffee requires 50 cups of water to grow it. Growing the coffee itself requires 1120 cups of water. You could fill 25 bathtubs with water that grows the 250 grams of cotton needed to make a single T-shirt. And to put it one last way, the typical burger guzzling, coffee-drinking, T-shirt-clad Texan consumes as much as a hundred times his own weight in water every day. (Pearce, F. When the Rivers Run Dry. Beacon Press, March 2006)

Americans use 5.7 billion gallons of water per day—just to flush the toilet. We flush more water down the toilet than the 95 million Brits and Canadians use for all of their needs. (Fishman C. The Big Thirst. Free Press, 2011)

Watercress is pleasant enough in a salad or sandwich, but when placed alongside a hamburger it is merely an annoyance. —Fran Leibowitz

---

WATERMELON

Watermelon. Watermelons were originally domesticated in central and southern Africa over 6,000 years ago. Watermelon is not only considered a food plant, but also a source of water in arid regions where water is scarce.

In fact, watermelon has been referred to as a "botanical or living canteen." Egyptians first cultivated watermelon 5,000 years ago. It was so revered in Egypt it was buried in the tombs of Egyptian kings.

Watermelon arrived in the New World with European colonists and African slaves in the early 1600s in Massachusetts. Watermelon seeds were widely dispersed by African slaves in eastern North America; however, the southeastern states were found to have the best climate and soil conditions to grow this delicious melon.

Thomas Jefferson grew watermelons at Monticello, Henry David Thoreau grew watermelons in Concord, Massachusetts, and Mark Twain couldn't say enough about the delights of watermelon: "It is chief of this world's luxuries, king by the grace of God over all the fruits of the earth. When one has tasted it, he knows what the angels eat." Indeed, what would a summer be without watermelon-eating contests, watermelon-size contests, and watermelon seed-spitting contests?

So, what's so special about watermelon? It has a water content of 92 percent, it's packed with antioxidants including vitamin C (12.5 mg or 21% of the daily value), beta-carotene (467 micrograms), and lycopene (9 to 13 milligrams in a cup and a half). Watermelon has the highest concentration of any other fresh fruit or vegetable, and delivers more nutrients per calorie than many fruits. Speaking of calories it only has 46 calories per cup. It also contains 876 IUs of vitamin A (18% of the daily value). Looking for a potassium-containing melon? Watermelon contains 173 mg per cup. And, last but not least, watermelon is totally 100% fat-free.

So, what can watermelon do for you? Regular consumption of watermelon increases the blood concentrations of lycopene (40% more than raw tomatoes) and beta carotene, which have been shown to protect against heart disease and possibly certain cancers including prostate, bladder and cervical. Regular consumption of watermelon also increases levels of arginine, a potent vasodilator. Arginine has been shown to reduce blood pressure, blood sugar, and the vascular complications of sickle cell disease. (Effectiveness of Arginine as a Treatment for Sickle Cell Anemia. Clinical Trials.gov) (Edwards AJ, Vinyard BT, et al. Consumption of watermelon juice increases plasma concentrations of lycopene and β-carotene in humans. *Journal of Nutrition* 2003;133(4):1043–1050)

Watermelon storage and the retention of nutrients. Store a whole watermelon at room temperature if you want maximal retention of its nutrients. Once cut, store in the refrigerator.

Wax. Lemons and limes are often waxed to protect them from moisture loss en route to the store. Before you cut off a piece of the skin for your vodka and tonic, or before you grate the peel to make a tasty zest for a recipe, scrub the peel with a vegetable brush to remove the wax. If you forget to do this, don't worry. A little wax will not compromise your digestive system.

Wedding cake. A physician was addressing a large audience in Tampa, Florida. He was ranting that the "material that we put into our stomachs is enough to have killed most of us sitting here years ago. Red meat is awful, soft drinks corrode your stomach lining, Chinese food is loaded with MSG, high fat diets can be disastrous, and none of us realize that long-term harm caused by germs in our drinking water. But there is ONE thing that is most dangerous of all—and we all have, or will, eat it. Would anyone care to guess what food causes the most grief and suffering for years after eating it?"

After several seconds of quiet, a small 75-year-old Jewish man in the front row raised his hand and said… "Vedding cake?"

WEIGHT GAIN

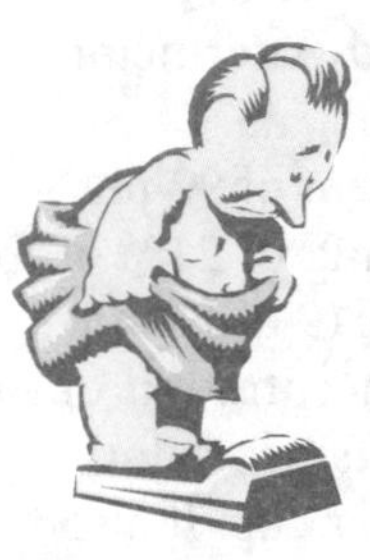

Weight gain and drugs. In 2004, 32.6 million Americans purchased outpatient prescriptions for antidepressants, stimulants, antipsychotics and tranquilizers, up from 21 million in 1997. Overall, around 50 million Americans—one in 6 of the population—currently take at least one psychotropic drug. From a look at the numbers, it seems that they could potentially be causing a significant and growing portion of American's obesity problem. After 10 years on Lithium, for example, two-thirds of patients gained approximately 10 kg or 22 pounds.

The atypical antipsychotic drug, olanzapine (Zyprexa) is also associated with weight gain. One-third of the patients who have taken the drug for a year gain at least 10 kilograms (22 pounds) and half of these patients gain at least 30 kg. Drugs that make you gain weight include selected anti-depressants amitriptyline (Elavil), mirtazepine (Remeron), fluoxetine (Prozac), parxetine (Paxil), and the mood stabilizers including lithium, and valproate (Depakote), and certain antipsychotics.

Other well-known drugs that pack on the pounds include drugs for benign prostatic hyperplasia such as doxazosin (Cardura XL) and terazosin (Hytrin), drugs for diabetes including the sulfonylureas (glyburide and glipizide) and rosiglitazone (Actos), beta-blockers including propranolol/Inderal, metoprolol/Lopressor/Toprol, atenolol/Tenormin, and anticonvulsants including valproic acid/Depakote, carbamazepine/Tegretol, and gabapentin/Neurontin. (*Environmental Nutrition,* September 2008)

Weight gain and dinosaurs. And you think you feel fat after a weekend of splurging. The largest dinosaurs could pack on the pounds at a rate faster than you could ever imagine. The apatosaurus, formerly known as the brontosaurus, puts on more than 30 pounds per day during the adolescent growth spurt. The argentinosaurus, the heaviest dinosaur that has ever roamed the earth, would have gained more than 100 pounds a day during its most rapid growth spurts. And you're still lamenting about your extra five pounds over the Christmas holidays. (*Nature,* July 26, 2001)

Patient's past medical history has been remarkably insignificant, with only a 40-pound weight gain in the past 3 days.
—Physician notes taken from a patient's hospital chart.

Weight gain and heart disease risk in women. A study in the February 8, 1995, Journal of the American Medical Association suggests that women who gain even a modest amount of weight with aging face an increased risk of heart disease, compared to those who manage to keep their weight on an even keel. The findings were surprising:

- Women who gain 11 to 17 pounds over their weight at age 18 run an increased risk of heart disease, as compared to peers who had gained fewer than 11 pounds.
- Women who gain 17 to 24 pounds showed a 64% greater risk.
- Women who gain 44 pounds or more face the most serious threat: a 250% greater risk of cardiovascular disease.

More recent studies continue to confirm the relationship between weight gain and heart disease risk. In a 2006 study in Circulation, even a modest weight gain of 8 pounds during adulthood was associated with a 27% increased risk of heart disease compared with women with a stable weight after adjusting for physical activity and other cardiovascular risk factors. (Li TY et al. Obesity as compared with physical activity in predicting risk of coronary artery disease in women. *Circulation.* 2006;113:499–506)

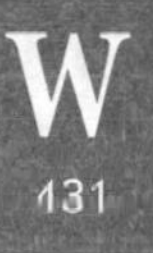

Weight gain and foods that pack on the pounds. There appears to be a shift in the conventional wisdom that a "caloric is a calorie is a calorie," and that if you take in only a certain amount of calories you can either lose weight or you can maintain your weight. Well, whoever said that conventional wisdom is always right?

A new study in the June 23, 2011 *New England Journal of Medicine* found specific foods tend to pack on the pounds more than others. Much to my horror, potatoes are the leader of the pack. A single-serving bag of potato chips added to one's daily intake tacked on 1.69 pounds over a four year period. Boiled, mashed or baked potatoes added about a half a pound, but French fries were the clear winner packing on 3.5 pounds over a four year period. Right behind the potato was a sugar-containing soft drink. One a day for four years added another pound.

OK, then, which foods lowered weight? Adding a daily serving of yogurt knocked off nearly a pound over four years, while adding a serving of nuts or fruit was associated with a loss of about a loss of about a half a pound each. An extra serving of whole grains, vegetables or diet soft drinks reduced weight slightly.

Weight gain and hypothyroidism. The issue of weight gain and hypothyroidism has been exaggerated. Although many women would like to blame their weight gain on thyroid problems, hypothyroidism typically isn't the culprit. An underactive thyroid is more often associated with smaller, unexplained weight gains of 5, 10, or 15 pounds. Rarely, if ever, does the weight gain exceed 20 pounds. So, if you've gained that 44 pounds since high school, only 20 at the most can be blamed on your thyroid if you're diagnosed with hypothyroidism.

Weight gain and television viewing. The average American watches more than 4 hours of TV each day or approximately 28 hours of TV per week. This would equal 2 months of nonstop TV-watching per year. In a 65-year life, the average American will have spent 9 years glued to the television. YIKES. Researchers at the University of Minnesota School of Public Health followed the habits of more than 1,000 men and women who were trying not to gain weight. They monitored eating habits, exercising habits, and television viewing time. By the end of the year, those who spent the most time in front of the TV gained the most weight. Among high-income women, each extra hour of TV viewed per day led to an extra one-half pound of weight gained over the year. Multiply that times 30 years and you have gained 15 pounds just watching TV. Well, at least we can blame part of our weight gain on the television. (*American Journal of Public Health,* February 1998; TV-Free America, 1322 18th St., Washington DC; http://www.csun.edu/science/health/docs/tv&health.html)

TV trivia:

- Percentage of households in the U.S. that possess at least one television—99.
- Number of TV sets per average U.S. household—2.24
- Percentage of U.S. households with three or more TV sets—66.
- Number of hours per day that TV is on in an average U.S. home—6 hours, 47 minutes
- Percentage of Americans who regularly watch TV while eating dinner—66
- Number of hours of TV watched annually by Americans—250 billion
- Percentage of Americans that say they watch too much TV—49
- Number of minutes per week that parents spend in meaningful conversation with their children—3.5
- Number of minutes per week that the average American child watches TV—1,680
- Hours per year the average American youth spends in school—900
- Hours per year the average American youth watches TV—1500

Your body is excess baggage you must carry through life. The more excess baggage, the shorter the trip. —Arnold H. Glasgow

---

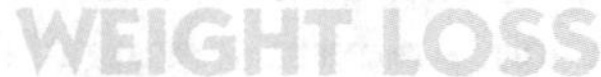

WEIGHT LOSS

Weight loss and exercising. There are a zillion benefits to exercise, but recent studies have suggested that the food part of the equation is much more important than the activity part. Weight loss is 85% reduction in food intake and only about 15% exercise. (*Nutrition Action Healthletter,* May 2010)

Weight loss and "fidgeting factor." Investigators at the Mayo Clinic have finally confirmed what many of us have already suspected: Those of us who "fidget" are much less likely to gain weight by overeating.

Non-obese patients in the study were all placed on a 1,000-calorie diet, in addition to their weight-maintenance requirements. Their total energy expenditure was measured through an elaborate technique that took into account things such as basal metabolism rates, postprandial thermogenesis, and volitional exercise. After all of those variables were added, subtracted, multiplied, and divided, the remaining energy expenditure was classified as non exercise-activity thermogenesis, also known as NEAT—the expenditures due to fidgeting, maintenance of posture, and other physical activities of daily life. Two-thirds of the subjects' increases in total energy expenditure proved to be in this category. Moreover, changes in NEAT accounted for tenfold difference in fat storage, and directly predicted resistance to weight gain associated with overfeeding.

As an addendum to that study…same Mayo Clinic researchers put special sensors into the underwear of 20 volunteers and monitored their every movement. Bottom line—the ten lean participants were more active even after they were "required" to gain weight for the study. Move, move, move. (Levine JA, Eberhard NL, Jensen MD. Role of nonexercise activity thermogenesis in resistance to fat gain in humans. *Science* 1999; 283; 212; Johannson DL, Ravussin E. Spontaneous physical activity: relationship between fidgeting and body weight control. *Current Opinion in Endocrinology, Diabetes, Obesity.* October 2008; 15(5):409–415)

If you want to lose 170 pounds right away,
get rid of your husband. —George Burns

Weight loss—gender differences. Take a man and a woman who are both sedentary, 35 years of age, 225 pounds and 5'7." If these two did everything exactly alike, the man would lose more weight than the women and he would win a weight loss contest hands down. If the man and woman just sat in a room for a day, he would have a 300-calorie advantage. Why? Men have more muscle mass and muscle uses more energy than fat, therefore the man burns more energy just to live. Women have more fat tissue compared to skeletal muscle tissue. The predominance of estrogen and progesterone predispose her to water retention and subcutaneous fat accumulation. Why? Teleologically this provides nutrition for a developing fetus if food and water are scarce—in other words, this fat and water retaining "gift" is for the survival of the species during times of draught and starvation. The abundance of testosterone in the male reduces subcutaneous fat and builds more muscle mass. (Baugh M. Sports Nutrition: The Awful Truth, 2005)

Weight loss. Slow down there, sister. The faster you eat, the fatter you get. People who eat their meals in five minutes flat are three times more likely to get fat. A Japanese study found that the speed at which we eat may be even more important that what we eat. Why? Gobbling down meals bypasses the "I'm full" signal, also known as the satiety signal, so fast eaters wind up consuming many more calories than those who take it slowly. It takes 20 minutes for the hypothalamus to register the "I'm full" signal. Who's to blame for this speed-eating? Modern society will take the brunt of the blame. Fewer families eat together, more people are eating while watching TV or being distracted in some other way, and people eat "fast food" as fast as they can pull out of the fast-food drive-through lane. All of the above promote hasty eating and hefty waistlines. (Denney-Wilson E, Campbell K, *British Medical Journal* October/November 2008)

Do not, I repeat, *do not* eat at buffet restaurants or at the breakfast buffet table.

Weight loss. Smaller plates, smaller cups, smaller boobs, smaller butts. University of Illinois at Champaign-Urbana researchers invited fellow faculty, students, and staff to a party at which they would serve themselves at an "all-you-can-eat" ice cream buffet. Those who were given larger bowls and a soup spoon consistently served themselves more ice cream than those with smaller bowls and smaller spoons. Those with the larger spoons served themselves 14.5% more, whereas those with the larger bowls served themselves a whopping 31% more.

Weight loss and sleep duration. In a randomized crossover study, 10 overweight middle-aged adults whose caloric intake was restricted to 90% of their resting metabolic rate were assigned to 5.5 or 8.5 hours of sleep daily for 14 days; three months later they were assigned to the other sleep schedule for another 14 days. Fat loss, fat-free body mass, and several endocrine hormones were monitored.

At the end of the study the mean weight loss with each treatment was about 3 kilograms. However, people who slept for 8.5 hours lost 56% of weight as fat, whereas people who slept for 5.5 hours lost 25% of weight as fat. In addition, sleep-deprived participants had lower resting metabolic rates and 24-hour plasma epinephrine levels, and they reported greater hunger. (Nedeltcheva AV et al. Insufficient sleep undermines dietary efforts to reduce adiposity. *Ann Intern Med* 2010 Oct 5; 153:435)

In a second study, mean adjusted weight gains after 12 years of following 60,000 non-obese women found that after age adjustment, women who reported ≤ 5 hours of sleep nightly weight an average of 2.47 kg (6 pounds) more than those who reported sleeping for the median duration of 7 hours. Mean adjusted weight gains after 10 years for women who slept ≤ 5, 6, or 7 hours were 5.63 kg, 5.16 kg, and 4.91 kg, respectively. (Patel SR et al. Association between reduced sleep and weight gain in women. *Am J Epidemiol* 2006 Nov 15; 164:947–54)

Bottom line? Grab that pillow and hit the sack. Adequate sleep *is* important in efforts to lose body fat.

Weight loss. Weight loss, despite normal or even greatly increased food intake occurs in three conditions:

- Grave's disease—hyperthyroidism
- Uncontrolled diabetes mellitus in which calories are lost through glycosuria
- Intestinal malabsorption

Weight loss and specific foods to kick-start energy expenditure. Now that we have seen what foods top the list for packin' on the pounds, here is a list of foods that might help to take it off. There is evidence that the five following foods may just be the ticket to boosting metabolism. And, here they are:

1. Green tea
2. Almonds
3. Garbanzo beans (chickpeas)
4. Tofu
5. Brown rice

So, what is it about each of the above foods that give metabolism a boost.

1. The polyphenols in green tea appear to block an enzyme that breaks down norepinephrine, the primary neurotransmitter of the sympathetic nervous system. The higher the levels of norepinephrine, the greater your metabolism and the faster the calories are burned.

2. Almond oil contains phenylethylamine (PEA), a naturally occurring chemical that works similar to amphetamines in revving up metabolism. In addition, PEA improves mood and energy levels, both of which are important in controlling eating by providing the motivation needed to become more physically active.

3. Garbanzo beans contain L-phenylalanine, the essential amino acid that functions as a natural antidepressant, improves memory and mood, and boosts metabolism. L-phenylalanine also helps provide a feeling of satiety, reducing the need to eat more food and still feel satisfied. Other foods that contain L-phenylalanine include soy beans, fish, poultry, almonds, pecans, pumpkin and sesame seeds, lima beans, and lentils.

4. Tofu (one of the top most disliked foods in America) increases the levels of L-tyrosine found in the blood. Tyrosine assists in the production of thyroid hormones that boost metabolism and regulate weight more efficiently. Foods that contain tyrosine include soy beans, egg whites, salmon, turkey breast, canned tuna, Alaskan King Crab, cheese, spinach, watercress, and seaweed. Cottage cheese also packs a powerful tyrosine punch.

5. Brown rice (and other whole grains) is high in chromium, a mineral that is essential for metabolizing protein, carbohydrates, and fat. It also increases tissue sensitivity to insulin, preventing hyperinsulinemia and the as-

sociated weight gain that accompanies excessive insulin production. Chromium has also been shown to increase lean body mass and decrease the percentage of body fat—both factors in weight loss. (Dullo AB et al. Efficacy of a green tea extract rich in catechin polyphenols and caffeine in increasing 24-h energy expenditure and fat oxidation in humans. *Am J of Clin Nutr* 1999; 70(6):1040–1045; *The Lark Letter*, April 2004)

Weight loss and keeping it off—not easy. Research by Rudolph Leibel and colleagues at Columbia University have found that shows when people are overweight and lose weight, their biology changes in a way that makes it hard to keep the weight off. Take two women who weigh 150 pounds. One has always weight 150 pounds and the other was 170 and reduced down to 150. Metabolically, they look very different. To maintain her 150-pound weight, the woman who has dropped from 170 is going to have to exist on 15 percent fewer calories than the woman who was always at 150 pounds.

Weight loss—the 10% rule. For the average American, leaving just 10% behind at each meal every single day—about 83,950 calories per year, or the amount in 300 candy bars—is enough to lead to a 10 pound weight loss over a year's time.

Weight Control Registry. The National Weight Control Registry (1-800-606-6927) was founded in 1994. It is the largest ongoing study of people (about 6,000) who have lost at least 30 pounds and who have kept it off for at least one year. However, the average participant in the study has lost at least 70 pounds and has kept it off for at least 6 years. What's the secret? What do these people DO that works? Seven things helped keep the weight off:

1. Low-calorie diet—generally low in fat and high in carbohydrates
2. Consistent diet from day-to-day
3. Eating breakfast helps to curb hunger throughout the rest of the day
4. Very physically active—walking, swimming, biking, aerobic class
5. Weigh themselves frequently—three quarters weigh themselves at least daily or once a week
6. Watch only a limited amount of TV (about 10 hours a week—a third of the average American
7. They don't let a small weight gain get any bigger—with even a small increase they will modify their diet or pick up the pace with physical activity

Weight Watchers. Weight Watchers emphasizes calorie-controlled, high-fiber eating and healthful lifestyle habits. The 1-2-3 success program assigns members a daily food point allotment averaging 1,250–1,500 calories per day for women. Weekly group meetings with mandatory weigh-ins are part of the package (1-800-651-6000 or www.weight-watchers.com). The new points-plus program was launched in 2011 with a newer version in 2012. (Truby H and Bonham M. What makes a weight loss program successful? *BMJ* 2011 Nov 3: 343d6629. Jolly K et al. Comparison of range of commercial or primary care led weight reduction program with minimal intervention control for weight loss in obesity: Lighten Up randomized controlled trial. *BMJ* 2011 Nov 3:323:d6500)

You know you've reached middle age when your weight-lifting consists merely of standing up. —Bob Hope

---

Wheat. Back to celiac disease in Chapter C—avoid any form of wheat, including bulgur, farina, kamut, spelt, and triticale.

Wheat bran. In the early 1960s and 1970s, the fiber-rich bran from wheat was fed to cattle. We ate the wheat products without the fiber and the cows ate the fiber-rich bran. What happened? We were constipated and the cows were regular. What's wrong with this picture?

Whiskey

Always carry a flagon of whiskey in case of a snake bite and furthermore always carry a small snake. —W.C. Fields

---

Whole wheat vs. whole grain—the whole truth. How do you know that the bread or cereal you buy is whole "whatever"? Whole grain refers to a category of foods that contain the entire grain kernel—the bran, the germ, and endosperm—and all of the nutritional goodies therein, like fiber and antioxidants. A whole grain can be a whole food such as brown rice, popcorn, or oatmeal, or an ingredient such as whole-wheat flour or rye flour. So, the real confusion comes when reading a label. So, *read the label.* Ingredients are listed by order of volume, so that first ingredient should be whole wheat or another whole grain. Beware of words like bromated, bleached, and wheat; only "whole wheat" or "100% whole wheat" as the first ingredient is the "real" thing. Most bread made with whole wheat or oats contains two to three grams of fiber per slice.

Another clue: If the front of the package says "100% whole grain," then all of the grains listed in the ingredients ***must*** be whole. If the front of the package just says "whole grain," then at least 51% of the grains on the ingredient list must come from the whole-grain category. "Whole wheat" simply means that the wheat component is whole—it doesn't give you a clue to the other refined or processed grains.

So, choose foods that name one of the following whole-grain ingredients first on the label's list: "brown rice," "buckwheat," "bulgur," "millet," "oatmeal," "quinoa," "rolled oats," "whole-grain barley," "whole-grain corn," "whole-grain sorghum," "whole-grain triticale," "whole oats," "whole rye," "whole wheat," "wild rice."

Foods labeled with the words "multi-grain," "cracked wheat," "seven-grain," or "bran" are usually not whole-grain products.

Wine is living proof that God loves us and likes to see us happy.
—Benjamin Franklin (1738)

Vintners in the Napa Valle area, which primarily produces Pinot Blanc, Pinot Noir, and Pinot Grigio wines, have developed a new hybrid grape that acts as an anti-diuretic. It is expected to reduce the number of trips older people have to make to the bathroom during the night. The wine will be marketed as Pinot More.

WINE

White wine and risk reduction of food borne illness. Can downing a glass of chardonnay reduce the risk of bacterial food poisoning? Well now, this would be a boon to those who are pushing alcohol for everything from a hammertoe to heart disease. A food scientist from Oregon State University seized upon earlier research that showed drinking wine may help people avoid food poisoning. Our friend the food scientist, Mark Daeschel, developed a stomach model by filling a plastic bag with gastric juices and food. To this mix he added strains of *E. coli* and *Salmonella*, as well as 50 grams of Oregon's finest Chardonnay (a white wine) and 50 grams of Oregon's finest Pinot Noir (a red wine). Voilà! He found that Chardonnay neutralized all of the bacteria in just about 60 minutes, whereas the lowly red wine took over 90 minutes. He also tried the same amount of beer and unfermented grape juice and did not find the same bug-killing properties. He attributed the neutralizing effects to the white wine's "high malic and tartaric acids and high alcohol content." He is also working on a white wine spray that can be used to disinfect countertops…a little spritz for the counter, a little spritz for the person doin' the spritzin'. Works for me. (Los Angeles Times, 10/24/2002)

Oenophile (EE–nuh–fyl)–someone who enjoys wine, especially a connoisseur. From the Greek oinos (wine) and phile (love). The earliest documented use of the word was in 1930.

Wine and World War II. The French helped save the Brits by providing an important piece of information supplied by a vintner in the south of France. The vintner informed the British that Hitler had placed a huge order for wine "with special corking for a hot climate." The British figured out where that hot climate was and they were prepared for the Nazi invasion of Northern Africa. (Katja Thimm, Der Spiegel)

All I need is an onion, a little bit of bread, and a bottle of red...
—Alice Prin, cabaret singer (1901–1953)

Wishbone. We have all grabbed an end of the slippery little wishbone and made a wish before pulling it apart. But what does a chicken use its wishbone for? It must have a function in the bird, or it wouldn't be there, right? Right. Each end of the wishbone is attached to one of the bird's two scapulae, or shoulder bones. Rapid compression of the wishbone during flight squeezes air back and forth between the two lungs and between various sacs that serve to cool and lighten the bird's body. By squeezing and expanding these air sacs, the wishbone increases the amount of oxygen available to the lungs, a big bonus during the high-energy, high-oxygen, demanding exertions of flight. Seems to be kind of a waste in chickens, doesn't it? How many chickens do you see gliding through the air flapping their wings? But all birds have wishbones; we're just more familiar with the wishbone from poultry.

Consider the wishbone of the hummingbird. The ten-gram hummingbird uses ten times more oxygen per gram of body weight than the most energetic human. To do this, the hummingbird's heart beats about 1,440 times per minute, compared to the heart of the exercising human that beats anywhere from 110–220 beats per minute. This requires a lot of flapping of those hummingbird wings and lots of wishbone compressions!

Wild rice. Actually, wild rice is a misnomer. It is not a type of rice; it is a grass seed native to North America. It is grown in California and Minnesota and shipped around the U.S. to a supermarket near you. It has 70 calories per half cup, compared to plain ol' white rice that has 110 calories per half cup. It also has some B vitamins. (University of California, *Berkeley Wellness Letter,* Vol. 17, No. 1, October 2000)

Wine. Red wine (purple grape juice) or white wine—what's the difference besides the obvious? The tannins found in red wine are responsible for the inhibition of platelet aggregation, offering protection from strokes and heart attacks (acute coronary syndromes) by reducing clot formation in the arteries. In addition, red wine contains polyphenols. Polyphenols prevent the LDL-cholesterol from oxidizing and forming fatty plaques in the artery walls. In a study of the antioxidant properties of red wine, the antioxidant activity increased significantly within two hours of consumption. Sounds like a perfectly healthy excuse for sipping a glass or two in the evening. (Quantum Sufficit, *American Family Physician* 1995;51(6):1372.)

The following is a reason to *never* quit drinking red wine…

French researchers have pointed out a possible rebound effect for individuals who stop drinking red wine. This rebound effect increases platelet stickiness and in turn increases the risk of clot formation and the possibility of a stroke or acute coronary syndrome—at least in rats. After depriving rats of alcohol for 18 hours, platelet-clotting responses rose by 124% in those given straight 6% ethanol and 46% in those drinking white wine. However, clotting responses decreased by 59% in those given red wine. It appears as if the naturally-occurring compound, tannin, is responsible for preventing this rebound effect. (Streppel MT, et al. Long-term wine consumption is related to cardiovascular mortality and life expectancy independently of moderate alcohol intake: the Zutphen Study. *Journal of Epidemiology and Comm Health.* 2009;63:534–540)

If drinking is beneficial, these findings suggest that those who drink wine in moderate amounts may accrue more benefits than do drinkers of other alcoholic beverages. (Gronbaek M et al. Type of alcohol consumed and mortality from all causes, coronary heart disease, and cancer. *Annals of Internal Medicine* 19 September 2000;133:411–19)

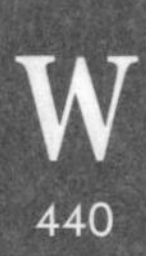

Wine and omega-3 fatty acids. The Lyon Diet Heart Study showed that moderate wine consumption in patients with coronary heart disease was associated with higher levels of omega-3 fatty acids. Why and how were not discussed but since we all know the benefits of omega-3 fatty acids this is certainly an intriguing finding for all of the oenophiles reading this book. (deLorgeril M, et al. Interactions of wine drinking with omega-3 fatty acids in coronary heart disease patients: a fish-like effect of moderate wine drinking. *Am Hear J.* 2008;155:175–181; di Giuseppe R, et al. European Collaborative Group of the IMMIDIET Project. Alcohol consumption and n-3 polyunsaturated fatty acids in healthy men and women from 3 European populations. *Am J Clin Nutr* 2009 89:354—362)

Question: Do you know what that indentation at the bottom of a wine bottle is called?

Answer: a kick or a punt.

Wisconsin. The Centers for Disease Control has given the state of Wisconsin the distinction as being numero uno for adult binge-drinking. Twenty-three percent of the adults in Wisconsin consume five or more drinks in one sitting.

Witch's Brew. Three plants, Atropa belladonna (nightshade), Hyoscyamus Niger (henbane), and Mandragora officinarum (mandrake), have a rich and vivid history as plants used for poisoning purposes, soothsaying, magic, and witchcraft. In ancient Greece, it was believed that inhaling a smoldering henbane plant made one prophetic. (Henbane, by the way, is the plant from which Scopolamine is made, and Scopolamine, as we know it in clinical medicine, induces "twilight" sleep.) In ancient Rome wine was mixed with the deadly nightshade plant to experience hallucinations.

The writings of the Middle Ages are replete with stories of witchcraft and devil worship. None other than Anres Laguna, the physician to Pope Julius III in 1545, wrote one such description of a "green unguent" (ointment) known as Witch's Brew: "…a jar half-filled with a certain green unguent…with which they were anointing themselves…was composed of herbs...which are hemlock, nightshade, henbane, and mandrake: of which unguent…I managed to obtain a good canister full…which I used to anoint from head-to-toe the wife of the hangman (as a remedy for her insomnia). On being anointed, she suddenly slept such a profound sleep, with her eyes open like a rabbit (she also fittingly looked like a boiled hare), that I could not imagine how to wake her…"

As the story continued in Dr. Laguna's writings, she was finally aroused 36 hours after her "anointment" with the green stuff. When she was awakened, she appeared to be quite grouchy about being disturbed from her deep sleep. She snapped at Dr. Laguna: "Why do you wake me at such an inopportune time? I was surrounded by all of the pleasures and delights of the world." Upon further questioning, she described the pleasures and delights as vivid episodes of flying and orgasmic adventures. She experienced evenings of debauchery at various banquets, music halls, and dances, where she "coupled with young men" which she "desired the most."

At some point in the Middle Ages it was discovered that if the constituents of Witch's Brew were combined with fats or oils they would penetrate the skin and could be easily absorbed through the sweat glands in the axillary areas (armpits) or body orifices (vagina and rectum being the two that come to mind). You might ask at this point why the oral route was not considered? Because the potion was too deadly if taken by mouth. Application of the ointment via the armpits or "private parts" allowed the psychoactive drugs to reach the bloodstream and brain without passing through the GI tract and risking poisoning from the products of liver metabolism.

Numerous writings from the Middle Ages contain statements about the mode of application of the "Witch's salves" or "Witch's ointments." For example, in the writings of Lady Alice Kyteler in 1324, the inquisitor states: "… in rifling the closet of the ladie, they found a pipe of ointment, wherewith she greased a staffe (i.e., broomstick), upon which she ambled and galloped through thick and thin." Whoopee! In another writing from the fifteenth century records of Jordanes de Bergamo: "… But the vulgar believe, and the witches confess, that on certain days and nights they anoint a staff and ride on it to the appointed place or anoint themselves under the arms and in other hairy places..."

And now, you know the rest of the story. This, my faithful readers, is why so many of the pictures during the period of the Middle Ages depict the witches riding broomsticks through the sky! Gives new meaning to the witch riding the broomstick at Halloween, doesn't it?

Women's website for Heart Health. How about a heart-healthy website just for women? This web site is sponsored by the American Medical Women's Association and the National Association of Margarine Manufacturers. Now that's a match, considering margarine's rather poor image as a heart-healthy food...oops, I forgot, soft margarines have been vindicated. Anyway, check out www.healthyfridge.org for tips on what to eat, when to eat it, how to eat it, cook it, prepare it, and the latest research on food and women.

Worcestershire sauce. One of the major claims of Worcestershire sauce is that is it one of the hardest words to say and/or to spell. Its other major claim to fame is that there would be no Bloody Mary in the world without it. But it was discovered somewhat by accident by two "chemists" who opened a shop in Worcester, England. Their names were John Lea and William Perrins and they named their shop after themselves—Lea & Perrins.

The recipe for Worcestershire sauce was actually a recipe they were asked to make by a customer. The customer had visited Bengal and had returned with the unusual recipe. Lea and Perrins mixed it up, and after tasting it they decided it was not fit for human consumption. For whatever reason they did not discard the sauce. They stored the jars of the "mixture" in the cellar and forgot about them. Years later, as they were cleaning out the cellar, they rediscovered the jars of the Bengal recipe. They tasted it again and a star was born! It was delicious the second time around. The liquid had aged and matured. They marketed the concoction as Lea & Perrins Worcestershire Sauce, and it quickly became popular around the world.

Wrigley, William, Jr. It all started in 1891 when Jr. moved to Chicago to open a new market for selling William Sr.'s soap. Along with the soap he would give a little gift of baking powder. The baking powder became more popular than the soap. So, he changed his focus in 1892 and sold baking powder. He also changed his little gift and gave chewing gum. The story repeats itself. The chewing gum became more popular than the baking powder. He changed his focus again and in 1893 he started selling Wrigley's Juicy Fruit and Spearmint gums. And the rest is history.

Never eat more than you can lift.

—Miss Piggy

X-Rated

XXX Sugar. No, this isn't about a triple X-rated adult sugar. Powdered or confectioner's sugar is granulated sugar that has been crushed into a fine powder with a small amount of cornstarch added to prevent clumping. The XXXs are the designation as to the fineness of the powder and go all the way up to XXXXXXXXXXXX (or 12 X)! You'll usually find XXX or XXXX in the baking section of your grocery store.

Xenical (Orlistat, 120 mg as a prescription) (Alli—over-the-counter orlistat, 60 mg). Xenical is a diet drug that interferes with the breakdown, digestion, and absorption of dietary fat in the gut. It is for individuals who have a hard time cutting back on fat intake and who have a body mass index (BMI) greater than 30, or greater than 27 with concomitant medical conditions hypertension, diabetes, or elevated cholesterol.

Orlistat is notorious for its gastrointestinal side effects which can include "anal leakage" with oily, loose stools. Fortunately for family and friends, these decrease with time. So hang in there with the anal leakage.

Xenical inhibits fat absorption by 30%. It does not reduce appetite nor does it speed up metabolism. It's not a great weight-loss drug, so the search is still on for the optimal drug to help shed those pounds.

On May 26, 2010, the FDA notified healthcare professionals and patients about a revised label reflecting new safety information about rare cases of severe liver injury that have been reported with the use of Xenical. The warning also applies to the over-the-counter form of Xenical, Alli.

Xylitol (zi-la-tol). Xylitol is a popular sugar substitute, also known as a "sugar alcohol," used in sugarless chewing gum and candy. Manufacturers use it because it adds bulk and sweetness to foods, with only about half of the calories of sugar. And foods with sugar alcohols can be labeled "sugar free" which is always a big seller. Xylitol in sugarless gum and candy also has an extra zip—it stimulates saliva flow, suppressing cavity formation and flushing away food particles and dead cells that lead to halitosis. It's found in a variety of other products as well, including baked goods, chewable vitamins, throat lozenges, and over-the-counter medications. Xylitol is derived from birch bark and is considered to be totally safe for human consumption… BUT, it is LETHAL for dogs. (See Chapter D for Doggie Don'ts)

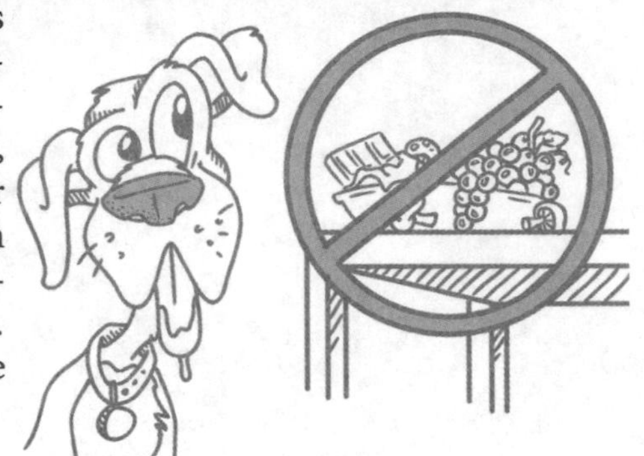

CHAPTER Y

Cogito ergo spud. (I think, therefore I yam).

—graffito

YAMS

Yams. Is a yam a sweet potato? No. There are more than 600 species of wild yams known to yam aficionados; however, only 12 are safe to consume. The yam we're most familiar with in the U.S. is the *Diascorea villosa*—otherwise known as the Mexican wild yam. The root of this tuberous plant is a dietary staple in Mexico and has also been used in many herbal products.

Yam scam. Here's the scoop about "The Wild Yam Scam." Topical "natural" wild yam extract creams have been sold for years for the treatment of menstrual and menopausal symptoms. Unfortunately, nary a single standardized, evidence-based study has demonstrated any effectiveness whatsoever. WHY?

Yams do *not* contain any *active* hormones, including the hormones progesterone, estrogen, or dehydroepiandrosterone (DHEA). So, slathering a barrel of cream from the extract from wild yams, whether they are from Mexico or Montana, will *not* help hot flashes, sleep disturbances, period irregularities, or any other symptoms of menopause, perimenopause, or menstruation. Allow me to explain.

Yams contain a steroid called diosgenin that can be converted to the hormone progesterone, but this conversion can only take place in a laboratory test tube (in vitro). It cannot and will not convert to an active form in the human body (in vivo). The so-called "natural" progesterone creams are not natural at all. These creams contain an added form of micronized progesterone made in the laboratory by a pharmaceutical company. A compounding pharmacy has the capability of doing this, but this brings us to the second caveat.

Yam cream that has the added micronized progesterone and is rubbed on the skin cannot be absorbed in reliable therapeutic doses. So even though this form of progesterone is absorbed through the skin, studies have shown time and again, that it is very difficult to achieve therapeutic blood levels with this route of administration.

So, what is a hot-flashing, sleep-deprived, postmenopausal woman to do? You can take "natural" progesterone as a pill, Prometrium*, or you can insert a vaginal progesterone gel, Crinone/Prochieve or insert a vaginal suppository, Endometrin. All of the aforementioned forms are prescription drugs. Steer clear of the over-the-counter creams, lotions, and potions. As mentioned earlier, few of them, if any of them, contain active ingredients. And, for heaven's sake, don't consume massive quantities of wild yams. You'll get a sure-fired case of orange-tinted skin, but not a single reduction in the number or symptoms of those hot flashes.

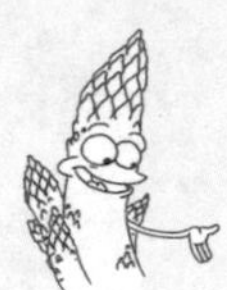

ASPARAGUS TIP

Prometrium has a peanut base—beware if you have peanut allergies.

(Sego S. Wild Yam. *The Clinical Advisor.* 2012 (February):100–102; Wu WH, Liu LY, Chung CJ, et al. Estrogenic effect of yam ingestion in healthy postmenopausal women. *J Am Coll Nutr.* 2005;24:235–243)

Yogurt. Where does yogurt come from? It starts out as milk, is fermented by bacteria, and is usually thickened with nonfat milk solids. The bacteria, *lactobacillus bulgaricus* and *streptococcus thermophilus,* are referred to as "starter" cultures. They convert lactose, the main carbohydrate in milk, into lactic acid, which curdles milk proteins into the consistency of yogurt.

And, here's the good news for individuals who are lactose intolerant. You can certainly tolerate yogurt, because the "live and active" cultures do the work of digesting lactose for you.

You just can't beat a cup of plain yogurt, low-fat yogurt, or fat-free yogurt when it comes to calcium (400–450 mg) and calories (100). That's more calcium than a cup of 1% or fat-free milk. And, like milk, a cup of plain yogurt contains protein, vitamin B12, riboflavin (vitamin B2), potassium, magnesium, and zinc. Unlike milk, most yogurt is not fortified with vitamin D; however, many forms of yogurt today do have vitamin D added.

Most of the health benefits of yogurt are linked to the bacterial cultures. The problem is the survival of these "starter" cultures in the cold cruel world of the gastric environment of the stomach. A gastric pH of 2 is not conducive to a long healthy life if you are a *Lactobacillus bulgaricus* or a *Streptococcus thermophilus.* Some manufacturers have begun to add "probiotics" to yogurt.

Probiotics are "live and active" cultures that survive the hostile environment of the stomach pH. (see chapter P for a discussion on Probiotics)

Yohimbine. A warning about recommending the "herbal Viagra." Yohimbine, from the bark of a West African tree, has long been described as a "male potency enhancer." The distributors of yohimbine have also described it as herbal Viagra; however, *buyer beware.* It has not been effective as a sexual enhancer in men with normal sexual function; however, it may have some effect in men with psychological erectile dysfunction. Yohimbine has also been suggested as an antidote to the sexual side effects of the serotonin reuptake inhibitors (SRIs) such as paroxetine (Paxil), fluoxetine (Prozac), citalopram (Celexa), and sertraline (Zoloft).

Studies in rats were quite promising, and in this case it's too bad that human results don't mimic the results of rat studies. Male rats given yohimbine were able to copulate 45 times in 15 minutes with their female partners. The female partners were not amused.

Unfortunately yohimbine has a few side effects that can send you straight to the emergency room, bypassing the bedroom. These include increased blood pressure, numerous drug and food interactions (MAO inhibitors, chocolate, aged cheeses, beer, wine, nuts, aged red meats), nervousness, anxiety, tachycardia, hypertensive crisis, and hallucinations.

YO-YO DIETING

Yo-yo dieting. This method of dieting is used by hundreds of thousands of women around the country. Up 10 pounds, down 15 pounds. Up 12 pounds, down 8 pounds—the yo-yo effect. For years experts thought the yo-yo diet was bad for you-you, and that future attempts at losing weight would be much more difficult due to permanent changes in metabolic rates. Fortunately, that's not the case. A major review of three decades of studies concluded that metabolism does not change with this type of diet and it's no easier, nor is it any harder, to lose weight the next time around.

Yo-yo dieting in men and the risk of gallstones. Hey guys, are you constantly taking weight off and putting it on again? The yo-yo cycle of dieting? Well, researchers have analyzed data from 51,529 men enrolled in the Health Professionals Follow-Up Study and they found that men who repeatedly go through weight loss-weight gain cycles increase their risk of gallstone disease by about 50% compared with men who maintain a stable weight. Men whose weight varied by less than 10 pounds increased their risk by about 10% while those who regularly lost and then gained 50 pounds or more had a 51% increase in the risk of gallstone disease. (*Archives of Internal Medicine,* 2006)

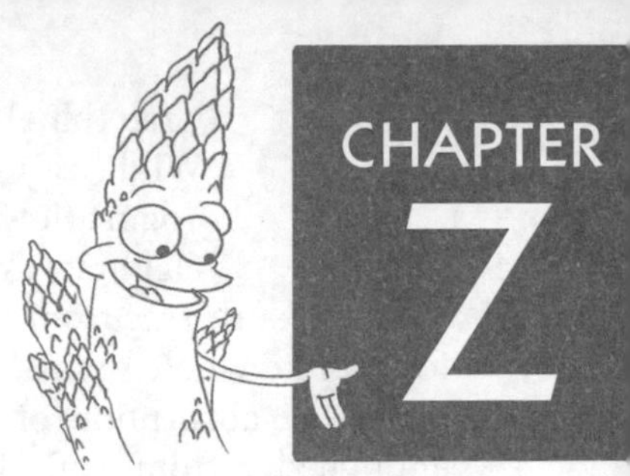

CHAPTER Z

I refuse to spend my life worrying about what I eat. There is no pleasure worth forgoing just for an extra three years in the geriatric ward..

—John Mortimer

Zest. Zest is a food ingredient prepared by scraping or cutting from the outer, colorful skin of citrus fruits such as lemon, orange, citron, and lime. Zest is used to add flavor or "zest" to a dish. A good example is the lemon zest added to a lemon meringue pie. Another common example is the zest of a lime, cut into a long spiral, or "twist," that is added to various cocktails such as martinis and vodka tonics. Zest is also a brand name of a bar of soap… don't mistakenly scrape or cut this for a food-enhancing effect.

ZINC

Zinc. Zinc is the second most abundantly distributed trace element in the body after iron. Zinc plays an important role in cell division, cell growth, wound healing, the breakdown of carbohydrates, and maintenance of a healthy immune system, specifically T-cell maturation. Zinc, along with antioxidants, has been shown to delay the progression of age-related macular degeneration. The recommended daily allowance (RDA) of zinc for women is 9 mg per day and 11 mg per day for men. There's no harm in taking a multivitamin with 15 mg for zinc and 2 mg of copper, but don't regularly take supplement with more than 30 mg of zinc. That much, combined with what people normally get from foods, may put you over the Tolerable Upper Intake Level of 40 mg per day. (*Dietary Guidelines for Americans,* 2010)

The best sources of zinc include:

Oysters 3 oz. .... 28.3 mg
TOTAL raisin bran 1 cup .... 15.0 mg
Ground beef (5% fat) 1 patty .... 5.3 mg

Crab (blue) 3 oz. .... 3.6 mg
Wild rice 1 cup.. 2.2 mg
Yogurt (lowfat, plain) 8 oz.................... 2.0 mg
Oat bran 1 cup .... 1.2 mg

We absorb zinc from animal foods better than plant foods because plant foods, like whole grains, contain substances known as phytates which can block the absorption of certain nutrients like zinc. If you're not getting enough zinc from your diet consider taking a multivitamin which will provide enough zinc to meet the daily needs.

Zinc and the common cold. Can zinc supplements actually prevent the common cold? According to a study by Kurugol the answer is yes, the mean number of colds in children can be reduced by taking prophylactic oral zinc sulphate 15 mg daily. The mean number of colds in the zinc group was 1.2 versus 1.7 in the control group during the 7-month study period. The dose was increased to 30 mg of zinc at the onset of a cold and until symptoms resolved. (Kurugol, et al. The prophylactic and therapeutic effectiveness of zinc sulphate on common cold in children. *ActaPaediatrica.* 2007;95(10:1175–1181)

A meta-analysis found that the beneficial effect of zinc for the common cold is small at best. One of the studies found a positive effect of zinc nasal gel on cold symptoms and duration but three other studies found no benefit from zinc lozenges and zinc nasal spray.

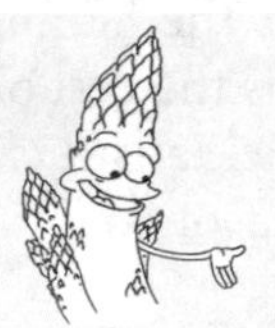

ASPARAGUS TIP

One very important finding: Intranasal zinc preparations have been associated with partial or complete loss of smell. This loss is permanent. YIKES.

(Caruso TJ et al. Treatment of naturally acquired common colds with zinc: A structured review. *Clin Infect Dis* 2007 Sep 1;45:569)

Zinc and infections in the elderly. Zinc supplementation in the elderly has been show to significantly reduce the number of infections and to reduce inflammatory mediators and oxidative stress. The amount of zinc used in the study was 45 mg per day of elemental zinc gluconate, and the length of the study was one year. (Prasad AS, et al. Zinc supplementation decreases incidence of infections in the elderly: effect of zinc on generation of cytokines and oxidative stress." *The Am J Clin Nutri* 2007;85(3):837–844)

Zinc and the gastrointestinal tract. Zinc malabsorption can occur with mucosal disease of the small intestine (celiac disease is a good example), as well as a deficiency of a cofactor necessary for its absorption. Dietary zinc may help maintain cell integrity and control inflammation in the gastrointestinal tract. Symptoms include a reduced ability to taste, inflammation of the skin around the mouth, anus, hands and feet. Other symptoms of zinc deficiency include failure to thrive in infants, chronic diarrhea, edema (swelling), decreased appetite, erectile dysfunction, delayed wound healing, and the loss of hair. Treatment with zinc sulfate produces a dramatic clinical recovery. Getting enough zinc in the diet may also reduce the risk of developing gastroenteritis.

Zinc and immune function. Individuals with zinc deficiency have abnormal T-helper cell function. Since the T-helper cell is responsible for cell-mediated immunity and the immune response to viruses, fungi, cancer cells, parasites, and protozoa, replacing zinc to normal levels would theoretically boost the immune response to both these pathogens and to cancer.

Zinc poisoning and denture cream. Thirty five million Americans wear dentures. Zinc has been used as a color blocker and bonding agent in denture creams for years until reports of excess zinc poisoning began to show up in the literature. The clinical manifestations of zinc excess include neuropathy, balance problems, numbness and tingling, weakness, and other neurological manifestations. On February 18, 2010 Glaxo-Smith-and Kline stopped selling a number of Super Poli-Grip and Fixodent denture creams and paid out $120 million dollars in lawsuit damages.

Zinc and sperm counts. Guys, do you need a sperm count boost? You just might want to take folic acid and zinc on a daily basis in order to pump up the sperm. Researchers found that men who took 5 mg of folic acid and 66 mg of zinc per day boosted sperm counts by 74 percent in just 26 weeks. These doses are slightly higher than the recommended daily amounts of each but talk to your fertility specialist to see if it's an acceptable amount for you. (*Fertility and Sterility,* March 2002)

Think of sperm swimming upstream. For all but one of them, it's going to be a very bad day. —Howard Anderson

---

Zinc and macular degeneration. Dietary intake of both vitamin E and zinc has been shown to be inversely related to the development of macular degeneration. (vanLeeuwen et al. Dietary intake of antioxidants and risk of age-related macular degeneration. *JAMA* 2005; 294:3101–3107)

Zinc and vegans/vegetarians. Zinc deficiency is uncommon in the United States because most people consume enough animal products in their diet to provide adequate zinc. Vegans are especially at high risk for deficiency. Taking an extra zinc supplement is not necessary; however, if you are a vegan, peruse the above list of zinc-containing foods and make an effort to consume any of the plant foods that contain zinc on a daily basis. If none of the above appeal to you, zip to the health food store for a multivitamin with zinc.

Zinfandel grape. This red wine grape was first used in California to make "jug" wines. However, in the past two decades, fueled by the popularity of zinfandel wines, it has been developed into one of the best of the red varietal grapes and is the most widely grown grape in the state. The zinfandel grape is of European origin, but has become known as "California's grape" for two reasons: It has been grown in California since the late nineteenth century, and zinfandel wines from that state have been a major contribution to the world of wine. There are both red and white zinfandels, with the white zinfandel considered to be a "blush" wine.

Zucchini. The zucchini is an American squash with an Italian name. Zucchini is the diminutive form of the Italian zucca, meaning "gourd." "Courgette" is the British word for zucchini. Zucchini is also known as summer squash, yellow crookneck squash, and yellow straightneck squash.

One-half cup of cooked zucchini slices, with the skin, has 1 gram of dietary fiber, 220 IU of vitamin A (5.5% of the RDA for a woman, 4.5% of the RDA for a man), and 4 mg vitamin C (6.5% of the RDA for both genders. One-half cup of yellow squash (either crookneck or straightneck) has 260 IU of vitamin A and 5 mg of vitamin C.

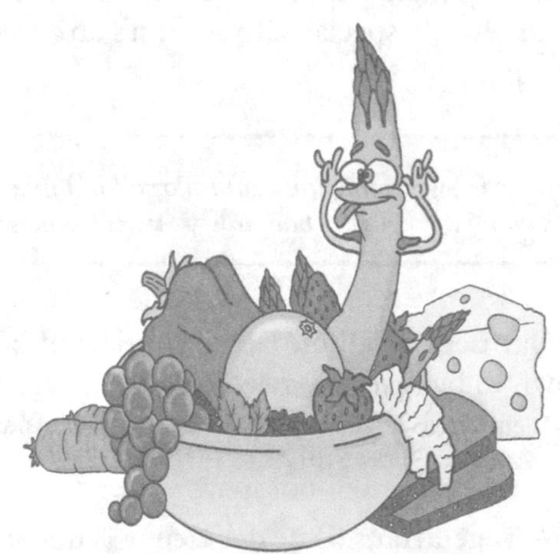

INDEX

E

F

M

N

O

T

X

Y

Z

ORDER FORM

Order an extra copy or two of *Kiss My Asparagus.*

# Ordered	Title	Price	Sub Total
______	*Kiss My Asparagus*	$25*	______
	Shipping $5 1st book $3 each additional book		______
		Total	______

*$30 in Canada

Mailing Information

Name ______________________________

Address ______________________________

City ______________ **State** ________ **Zip** ______________

Phone ______________________________

Send check made payable to BARB BANCROFT to:
CPP Associates Inc
3100 N. Sheridan Road #9C
Chicago IL 60657
Questions? 708-867-8824

We also accept MasterCard and Visa

MC or VISA # ______________________________
(circle one)

Exp. date ______________

Signature ______________________________

Fax orders to: 708 867 8825
Barb's Website: http://barbbancroft.com
eMail: BBancr9271@aol.com

kma0812